Nutrition and Athletic Performance

Nutrition and Athletic Performance

Editor

Stephen Ives

MDPI • Basel • Beijing • Wuhan • Barcelona • Belgrade • Manchester • Tokyo • Cluj • Tianjin

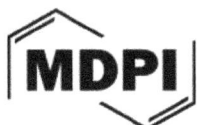

Editor
Stephen Ives
Skidmore College
USA

Editorial Office
MDPI
St. Alban-Anlage 66
4052 Basel, Switzerland

This is a reprint of articles from the Special Issue published online in the open access journal *Nutrients* (ISSN 2072-6643) (available at: https://www.mdpi.com/journal/nutrients/special_issues/Athletic_Performance).

For citation purposes, cite each article independently as indicated on the article page online and as indicated below:

> LastName, A.A.; LastName, B.B.; LastName, C.C. Article Title. *Journal Name* **Year**, *Volume Number*, Page Range.

ISBN 978-3-0365-4835-7 (Hbk)
ISBN 978-3-0365-4836-4 (PDF)

© 2022 by the authors. Articles in this book are Open Access and distributed under the Creative Commons Attribution (CC BY) license, which allows users to download, copy and build upon published articles, as long as the author and publisher are properly credited, which ensures maximum dissemination and a wider impact of our publications.

The book as a whole is distributed by MDPI under the terms and conditions of the Creative Commons license CC BY-NC-ND.

Contents

About the Editor vii

Preface to "Nutrition and Athletic Performance" ix

Diego Fernández-Lázaro, Juan Mielgo-Ayuso, Jesús Seco Calvo, Alfredo Córdova Martínez, Alberto Caballero García and Cesar I. Fernandez-Lazaro
Modulation of Exercise-Induced Muscle Damage, Inflammation, and Oxidative Markers by Curcumin Supplementation in a Physically Active Population: A Systematic Review
Reprinted from: *Nutrients* **2020**, *12*, 501, doi:10.3390/nu12020501 1

Mojtaba Kaviani, Philip D. Chilibeck, Spencer Gall, Jennifer Jochim and Gordon A. Zello
The Effects of Low- and High-Glycemic Index Sport Nutrition Bars on Metabolism and Performance in Recreational Soccer Players
Reprinted from: *Nutrients* **2020**, *12*, 982, doi:10.3390/nu12040982 21

Kengo Ishihara, Natsuki Uchiyama, Shino Kizaki, Emi Mori, Tsutomu Nonaka and Hiroshi Oneda
Application of Continuous Glucose Monitoring for Assessment of Individual Carbohydrate Requirement during Ultramarathon Race
Reprinted from: *Nutrients* **2020**, *12*, 1121, doi:10.3390/nu12041121 35

Jorge Pérez-Gómez, Santos Villafaina, José Carmelo Adsuar, Eugenio Merellano-Navarro and Daniel Collado-Mateo
Effects of Ashwagandha (*Withania somnifera*) on VO_{2max}: A Systematic Review and Meta-Analysis
Reprinted from: *Nutrients* **2020**, *12*, 1119, doi:10.3390/nu12041119 47

Csilla Ari, Cem Murdun, Craig Goldhagen, Andrew P. Koutnik, Sahil R. Bharwani, David M. Diamond, Mark Kindy, Dominic P. D'Agostino and Zsolt Kovacs
Exogenous Ketone Supplements Improved Motor Performance in Preclinical Rodent Models
Reprinted from: *Nutrients* **2020**, *12*, 2459, doi:10.3390/nu12082459 59

Álvaro Huerta Ojeda, Camila Tapia Cerda, María Fernanda Poblete Salvatierra, Guillermo Barahona-Fuentes and Carlos Jorquera Aguilera
Effects of Beta-Alanine Supplementation on Physical Performance in Aerobic–Anaerobic Transition Zones: A Systematic Review and Meta-Analysis
Reprinted from: *Nutrients* **2020**, *12*, 2490, doi:10.3390/nu12092490 77

Carlos Rodrigo Soares Freitas Sampaio, Felipe J. Aidar, Alexandre R. P. Ferreira, Jymmys Lopes dos Santos, Anderson Carlos Marçal, Dihogo Gama de Matos, Raphael Fabrício de Souza, Osvaldo Costa Moreira, Ialuska Guerra, José Fernandes Filho, Lucas Soares Marcucci-Barbosa, Albená Nunes-Silva, Paulo Francisco de Almeida-Neto, Breno Guilherme Araújo Tinoco Cabral and Victor Machado Reis
Can Creatine Supplementation Interfere with Muscle Strength and Fatigue in Brazilian National Level Paralympic Powerlifting?
Reprinted from: *Nutrients* **2020**, *12*, 2492, doi:10.3390/nu12092492 97

Tomáš Hlinský, Michal Kumstát and Petr Vajda
Effects of Dietary Nitrates on Time Trial Performance in Athletes with Different Training Status: Systematic Review
Reprinted from: *Nutrients* **2020**, *12*, 2734, doi:10.3390/nu12092734 107

Pavel Kysel, Denisa Haluzíková, Radka Petráková Doležalová, Ivana Laňková, Zdeňka Lacinová, Barbora Judita Kasperová, Jaroslava Trnovská, Viktorie Hrádková, Miloš Mráz, Zdeněk Vilikus and Martin Haluzík
The Influence of Cyclical Ketogenic Reduction Diet vs. Nutritionally Balanced Reduction Diet on Body Composition, Strength, and Endurance Performance in Healthy Young Males: A Randomized Controlled Trial
Reprinted from: *Nutrients* **2020**, *12*, 2832, doi:10.3390/nu12092832 125

Néstor Vicente-Salar, Guillermo Santos-Sánchez and Enrique Roche
Nutritional Ergogenic Aids in Racquet Sports: A Systematic Review
Reprinted from: *Nutrients* **2020**, *12*, 2842, doi:10.3390/nu12092842 137

Monique D. Dudar, Emilie D. Bode, Karly R. Fishkin, Rochelle A. Brown, Madeleine M. Carre, Noa R. Mills, Michael J. Ormsbee and Stephen J. Ives
Pre-Sleep Low Glycemic Index Modified Starch Does Not Improve Next-Morning Fuel Selection or Running Performance in Male and Female Endurance Athletes
Reprinted from: *Nutrients* **2020**, *12*, 2888, doi:10.3390/nu12092888 157

Maija Marttinen, Reeta Ala-Jaakkola, Arja Laitila and Markus J. Lehtinen
Gut Microbiota, Probiotics and Physical Performance in Athletes and Physically Active Individuals
Reprinted from: *Nutrients* **2020**, *12*, 2936, doi:10.3390/nu12102936 173

Yasuko Yoshida, Keisei Kosaki, Takehito Sugasawa, Masahiro Matsui, Masaki Yoshioka, Kai Aoki, Tomoaki Kuji, Risuke Mizuno, Makoto Kuro-o, Kunihiro Yamagata, Seiji Maeda and Kazuhiro Takekoshi
High Salt Diet Impacts the Risk of Sarcopenia Associated with Reduction of Skeletal Muscle Performance in the Japanese Population
Reprinted from: *Nutrients* **2020**, *12*, 3474, doi:10.3390/nu12113474 205

About the Editor

Stephen Ives

Dr. Stephen Ives, Associate Professor and Associate Chair, Health and Human Physiological Sciences, Skidmore College. I approach the understanding of health and human physiology with an integrative physiological perspective, and thus I am interested in how lifestyle factors such as nutrition influence our health but also our physical capacity for exercise, with a desire to understand these phenomena in a systemic way.

Preface to "Nutrition and Athletic Performance"

The current collection of articles selected for this Special Issue, and now monograph, aimed to increase our understanding of the role of nutrition in athletic performance. The aim was to gather new evidence, or novel syntheses of existing evidence, in various models that address how diet, dietary supplementation, or manipulating the temporal nature of diet/supplementation may alter or influence human performance positively or negatively across broad populations. Indeed, I believe we were successful, as the current collection of papers includes such timely topics as the ketogenic diet or ketone supplementation, the gut microbiome, understanding the role of the glycemic index and timing, as well as supplementation with nitrates, curcumin, beta alanine, and creatine. Some of these papers address the current state of affairs regarding existing practices, which is frequently a forgotten or overlooked aspect that is often crucial before considering dietary manipulation. Importantly, this collection of studies was inclusive of age, sex/gender, ability status, and diversity of sport or activity. I would like to personally thank the authors for contributing to this Special Issue, which will now be memorialized as a monograph, but also the reviewers who provided critical feedback in improving the manuscripts presented herein, but also in reviewing articles that were not deemed acceptable in the journal and Special Issue. I hope that this collection helps the researchers, practitioners, and students who will become the next generation that will continue such academic pursuits.

Stephen Ives
Editor

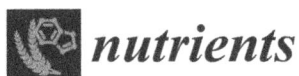

Review

Modulation of Exercise-Induced Muscle Damage, Inflammation, and Oxidative Markers by Curcumin Supplementation in a Physically Active Population: A Systematic Review

Diego Fernández-Lázaro [1,*], Juan Mielgo-Ayuso [2], Jesús Seco Calvo [3], Alfredo Córdova Martínez [2], Alberto Caballero García [4] and Cesar I. Fernandez-Lazaro [1,5]

1. Department of Cellular Biology, Histology and Pharmacology, Faculty of Health Sciences, University of Valladolid, Campus of Soria, 42003 Soria, Spain; fernandezlazaro@usal.es
2. Department of Biochemistry and Physiology, Faculty of Health Sciences, University of Valladolid, Campus of Soria, 42003 Soria, Spain; juanfrancisco.mielgo@uva.es (J.M.-A.); a.cordova@bio.uva.es (A.C.M.)
3. Institute of Biomedicine (IBIOMED), Physiotherapy Department, University of Leon, Campus of Vegazana, 24071 Leon, Spain; dr.seco.jesus@gmail.com
4. Department of Anatomy and Radiology, Faculty of Health Sciences, University of Valladolid, Campus of Soria, 42003 Soria, Spain; albcab@ah.uva.es
5. Department of Preventive Medicine and Public Health, School of Medicine, University of Navarra, IdiSNA, 31008 Pamplona, Spain
* Correspondence: diego.fernandez.lazaro@uva.es; Tel.: +34-975-129-185

Received: 22 January 2020; Accepted: 12 February 2020; Published: 15 February 2020

Abstract: Physical activity, particularly high-intensity eccentric muscle contractions, produces exercise-induced muscle damage (EIMD). The breakdown of muscle fibers and the consequent inflammatory responses derived from EIMD affect exercise performance. Curcumin, a natural polyphenol extracted from turmeric, has been shown to have mainly antioxidant and also anti-inflammatory properties. This effect of curcumin could improve EIMD and exercise performance. The main objective of this systematic review was to critically evaluate the effectiveness of curcumin supplementation on EIMD and inflammatory and oxidative markers in a physically active population. A structured search was carried out following Preferred Reporting Items for Systematic Review and Meta-Analyses (PRISMA) guidelines in the databases SCOPUS, Web of Science (WOS), and Medline (PubMed) from inception to October 2019. The search included original articles with randomized controlled crossover or parallel design in which the intake of curcumin administered before and/or after exercise was compared with an identical placebo situation. No filters were applied to the type of physical exercise performed, the sex or the age of the participants. Of the 301 articles identified in the search, 11 met the established criteria and were included in this systematic review. The methodological quality of the studies was assessed using the McMaster Critical Review Form. The use of curcumin reduces the subjective perception of the intensity of muscle pain; reduces muscle damage through the decrease of creatine kinase (CK); increases muscle performance; has an anti-inflammatory effect by modulating the pro-inflammatory cytokines, such as TNF-α, IL-6, and IL-8; and may have a slight antioxidant effect. In summary, the administration of curcumin at a dose between 150–1500 mg/day before and during exercise, and up until 72 h' post-exercise, improved performance by reducing EIMD and modulating the inflammation caused by physical activity. In addition, humans appear to be able to tolerate high doses of curcumin without significant side-effects.

Keywords: natural polyphenols; curcumin; muscle-damaging exercise; anti-inflammatory; antioxidants; physical activity

1. Introduction

Physical activity, particularly high-intensity eccentric muscle contractions, induces exercise-induced muscle damage (EIMD) [1,2]. EIMD leads to the onset of an inflammatory response that is associated with a decrease in the ability to generate muscle strength, decreased range of motion (ROM), localized swelling, delayed onset muscle soreness (DOMS), and increased muscle proteins in the blood (creatine kinase (CK), lactate dehydrogenase (LDH), and myoglobin (Mb)) [3]. In addition, EIMD triggers inflammatory responses that result in elevations of inflammation markers such as C-reactive protein (CRP) and some inflammatory interleukins (IL-1, IL-6, tumor necrosis factor (TNF-α)) [4]. Similarly, it promotes the production of transcription factors such as nuclear factor kB (NF kB) through the production of reactive oxygen species (ROS) [5].

On the other hand, research indicates that oxidative stress (OS) is evident following EIMD by an increase in ROS [6]. In this sense, endogenous antioxidants may also be up-regulated via exercise, which stimulates an acute OS and inflammatory response [7]. Therefore, inflammatory processes are always linked to OS and must be analyzed and controlled together, because both are directly involved in EIMD [8]. One way to prevent and minimize the effects of OS and the inflammatory process, and attenuate EIMD [9], could be an oral intake of anti-inflammatory or antioxidant supplementation. A natural product that can be used, with potential antioxidant and anti-inflammatory effects, is curcumin (1,7-bis (4-hydroxy-3-methoxyphenyl) 1,6-heptadiene-3,5-dione), which is the main natural bioactive polyphenol of the spice herb turmeric (2%–5% by weight). Curcumin is a highly pleiotropic molecule that interacts with multiple anti-inflammatory and antioxidant pathways [10,11]. The United States Food and Drug Administration (FDA) has listed curcumin as GRAS (generally recognized as safe), and curcumin-containing supplements have been approved for human ingestion [12]. In this way, curcumin used as a pharmaceutical preparation has been shown to be safe, even at high doses. However, it has been shown to cause some gastric irritation in humans, hepatotoxicity in mice, and at high doses, hepatotoxicity in rats. Humans appear to be able to tolerate high doses of curcumin without significant side-effects. This may be because of differences in metabolism of curcumin in humans as compared to susceptible species such as rats. However, when used as a spice, because of its high water content, it could be attacked by aflatoxin-producing fungi, causing kidney, lung, or liver toxicity. It must be taken into account that curcumin as a spice is produced in tropical countries (warm and humid) that favor the growth of fungi [11,12].

Curcumin supplementation could be beneficial for attenuating EIMD given that curcumin has been shown to potentially help alleviate exercise performance decrements following intense and challenging exercise, as a result of membrane protective effects, antioxidants response, and anti-inflammatory action [13,14]. The anti-inflammatory properties attributed to curcumin are due to its ability to inhibit the nuclear factor kappa (NF-κB), which may be a muscle protective and regeneration agent and plays an important role in controlling physiological mechanisms of inflammation and protein breakdown [15]. Curcumin is capable of blocking the activation of TNF-α-dependent NF-κB and the activation pathway induced by ROS [16–18]. Likewise, curcumin could have a low regulatory effect on the expression of the COX-2 enzyme and inhibit pro-inflammatory enzyme 5-LOX (lipoxygenase-5) expression in the leukotriene-producing metabolic pathway [19], as well as the intercellular adhesion molecule 1 (ICAM-1) and vascular cell adhesion molecule 1 (VCAM-1)—a crucial step in the inflammatory response—and decrease inducible nitric oxide synthase (iNOS), which is directly responsible for inflammatory damage by blocking of the cytokines responsible for its activation [19,20]. In this way, curcumin induces the negative regulation of pro-inflammatory interleukins (IL-1, IL-2, IL-6, IL-8, and IL-12), inflammatory cytokines, such as TNF-α and monocyte-1 chemotherapeutic protein (MCP-1), through inhibition of the transcription signaling pathway (JAK/STAT) [11]. In addition, the overexpression of Bcl-2 or Bcl-X L protects cells from apoptosis that counteracts proapoptotic and proinflammatory attacks and restores the anti-inflammatory physiological phenotype [18,21]; curcumin controls the response to thermal shock for attenuated muscle damage [22] and biomarkers of muscle damage, such as CK [11].

In line with this, some studies have shown the effects of curcumin supplementation on OS, inflammation, EIMD, and sport performance with controversial results. These inconsistent results may be due, in part, to differences in doses, timing of supplementation, timing of exercise, exercise model, and experimental design between studies [23]. Previous research has indicated that curcumin may have antioxidant, anti-inflammatory, and analgesic effects on DOMS [24]. Furthermore, similar effects of curcumin have been described by Tanabe et al. [1], who found that ingestion before exercise could attenuate acute inflammation, and after exercise, it could attenuate muscle damage and facilitate faster recovery. Drobnic et al. [5] reported a reduction in muscular trauma with a moderate reduction in pain with curcumin supplementation. In contrast, Sciberras et al. [4] did not reveal any statistical difference between intervention with curcumin and placebo in levels of IL-6 and IL-10. In addition, markers of oxidative stress were only slightly increased after exercise in both groups, which does not allow a comparison of the effects of curcumin versus placebo [5], and there were no differences in terms of changes in maximal voluntary contraction (MVC) and serum CK activity [25]. Finally, not all observed changes in performance and soreness after exercise in humans [10] have been reproduced on the mouse model [26].

However, it is necessary to clarify the useful doses, timing (before or after exercise), duration of treatment, and the effects of curcumin on OS, inflammation, and EIMD. Therefore, the purpose of this study was to critically evaluate the effectiveness of curcumin supplementation on EIMD, inflammatory, and oxidative markers in a physically active population. In addition, the study shows the effective doses, timing, and duration of treatment for optimal application.

2. Material and Methods

2.1. Search Strategy

The present article is a systematic review focusing on the effect of curcumin supplementation on muscle pain, muscle function, muscle enzyme activity, inflammatory markers, and antioxidant effect and was conducted following the Preferred Reporting Elements for Systematic Reviews and Meta-analysis (PRISMA) guidelines [27] and the PICOS question model for the definition of inclusion criteria: P (population); "healthy exercise practitioners", I (intervention); "supplementation with curcumin", C (comparison); "same conditions with placebo or control group", O (outcomes); "muscle pain, inflammation and/or muscle damage serum markers and antioxidant effect", S (study design); "double- or single-blind design and randomized parallel or crossed".

A structured search was carried out in the databases SCOPUS, Medline (PubMed), and Web of Science (WOS), which includes other databases such as BCI, BIOSIS, CCC, DIIDW, INSPEC, KJD, MEDLINE, RSCI, SCIELO, all of which are high-quality databases which guarantee good bibliographic support. The search covered a time span from March 2015—when Nicol et al. [28] suggested the use of oral curcumin is likely to reduce pain associated with delayed onset muscle soreness (DOMS) with some evidence for enhanced recovery of muscle performance—to November 2019. Search terms were a mix of Medical Subject Headings (MeSH) and free words for key concepts related to curcumin, muscle, exercise, inflammation, and recovery, as follows: ("curcumin" OR "curcuminoids" OR "curcuma longa" OR "turmeric") AND ("muscle damage" OR "delay onset muscle soreness" OR "DOMS" OR "inflammation" OR "inflammatory" OR "inflammatory markers" OR "oxidative stress") AND ("exercise" OR "physical activity" OR "sports"). Through this search, relevant articles in the field were obtained applying the snowball strategy. All titles and abstracts from the search were cross-referenced to identify duplicates and any potential missing studies. Titles and abstracts were then screened for a subsequent full-text review. The search for published studies was independently performed by two authors (DFL and CIFL) and disagreements about physical parameters were resolved through discussion.

2.2. Selection of Articles: Inclusion and Exclusion Criteria

For the articles obtained in the search, the following inclusion criteria were applied to select studies: articles (I) depicting a well-designed experiment that included the ingestion of a dose of curcumin, or a curcumin-containing product, before and/or during exercise in humans; (II) with an identical experimental situation with or without the ingestion of a placebo; (III) with a double- or single-blind design and randomized parallel or crossed design; (V) with clear information on the administration of curcumin (dose of curcumin per kg body mass and/or absolute dose of curcumin on body mass, time of curcumin intake before or after exercise, duration of treatment); (VI) in which curcumin was administered in the form of a beverage, gum, or pills; (VII) in which one of the measured variables was changes in muscle pain, muscle function, muscle enzyme activity, inflammatory markers, or antioxidant effect; (VIII) in which the languages were restricted to English, German, French, Italian, Spanish, and Portuguese. The following exclusion criteria were applied: (I) animal studies, (II) uncontrolled trials, (III) studies using non-standardized turmeric extracts or extracts of unknown curcuminoid content, and (IV) studies performed on subjects with a prior condition of musculoskeletal injury or pain. There were no filters applied to the individuals' fitness level, sex, or age to increase the power of the analysis.

The methodological quality of the articles, evaluated using McMaster's Critical Review Form [29], scored between 12 and 15 points, representing a minimum methodological quality of 75% and a maximum of 93.8%. Of the 11 studies, 7 achieved a "Very Good" quality, 2 a "Good" quality, and 2 studies an "excellent" quality. No study was excluded because it did not reach the minimum quality threshold. Table 1 details the results of the criteria evaluated, where the main deficiencies found in methodological quality are associated with items 5 and 12 of the questionnaire, and comprises a detailed justification of the size of the study and a discussion of relevance of the results to clinical practice, respectively. The objective of this evaluation was to determine the existing methodological limitations in each of the studies and to allow the quality of the results to be comparable between the different study designs.

Once the inclusion/exclusion criteria were applied to each study including authors, year of publication, study design, curcumin administration (dose and timing), sample size, and characteristics of the participants (fitness level and sex), and final outcomes of the interventions were extracted independently by two authors (DFL and CIFL) using a spreadsheet (Microsoft Inc, Seattle, WA, USA). Subsequently, disagreements were resolved through discussion until a consensus was reached.

Table 1. Methodological quality of the studies included in the systematic review.

		References	Drobnic et al., 2014 [5]	Sciberras et al., 2015 [4]	Nicol et al., 2015 [28]	Tanabe et al., 2015 [2]	McFarlin et al., 2016 [30]	Nakhostin-Roohi et al., 2016 [24]	Delecroix et al., 2017 [31]	Tanabe et al., 2018 [1]	Tanabe et al., 2019 [25]	Jäger et al., 2019 [10]	Basham et al., 2019 [32]	T_I
ITEMS		1	1	1	1	1	1	1	1	1	1	1	1	10
		2	1	1	1	1	1	1	1	1	1	1	1	10
		3	1	1	1	1	1	1	1	1	1	1	1	10
		4	1	1	1	1	1	1	0	1	1	1	1	10
		5	0	1	0	1	0	0	0	1	1	1	1	4
		6	0	1	0	1	1	1	1	1	1	1	1	7
		7	1	1	1	1	1	1	1	1	1	1	1	10
		8	1	1	1	1	1	1	1	1	1	1	1	10
		9	1	1	0	1	1	1	0	1	1	1	1	10
		10	1	1	1	1	1	1	1	1	1	1	1	7
		11	1	0	1	1	1	0	1	1	1	1	1	10
		12	1	0	0	0	1	1	0	0	0	0	0	3
		13	0	1	1	1	1	1	1	1	1	1	1	6
		14	1	1	1	1	1	1	1	1	1	1	1	10
		15	1	1	1	1	1	1	0	1	0	1	0	7
		16	1	1	1	0	0	0	1	1	1	1	1	6
		T_S	13	14	12	14	14	13	12	15	14	15	14	
		%	81.3	87.5	75	87.5	87.5	81.3	75	93.8	87.5	93.8	87.5	
		MQ	VG	VG	G	VG	VG	VG	G	E	VG	E	VG	

(T_S) Total items fulfilled by study. (1) Criterion met; (0) Criterion not met. (T_I): Total items fulfilled by items. Methodological Quality (MQ): poor (P) ≤8 points; acceptable (A) 9–10 points; good (G) 11–12 points; very good (VG) 13–14 points; excellent (E) ≥15 points.

3. Results

3.1. Selection of Studies

The literature search provided a total of 301 articles related to the select descriptors, but only 11 articles met all the inclusion/exclusion criteria (Figure 1). The number of the articles to which each exclusion criterion was applied were as follows: 94 papers were removed because they were duplicates. After the elimination of duplicate articles, 207 articles were selected for examination by title and abstract, of which 150 were excluded as non-intervention studies and 38 as unrelated to the search topic. The full texts of the remaining 19 publications were evaluated according to the inclusion criteria, from which three studies were eliminated because they were conducted in animal populations, four because they used unhealthy subjects, and one because they did not measure any of the variables included in this study.

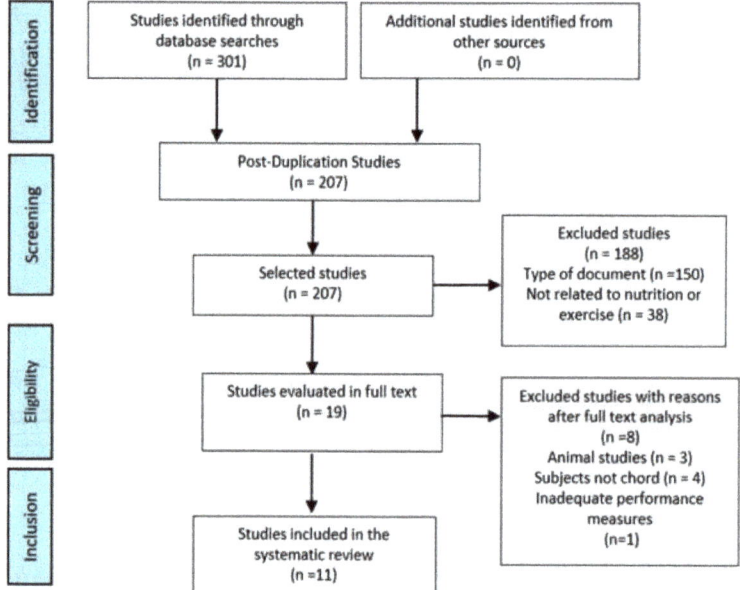

Figure 1. Selection of Studies.

3.2. Characteristics of the Studies

The participants 'samples (n = 237) included individuals of both genders (187 men and 50 women), where 10 were elite athletes, 131 were moderately active people, and 96 were people who were asked not to undergo pre-study training (Table 2). In ten of the eleven articles, some commercial supplement of curcumin in capsules of standardized composition and known bioavailability was used, while Nicol et al. [28] opted for a pharmaceutical preparation of curcumin capsules using a specific composition protocol for research. In addition, Delecroix et al. [31] chose a combination of curcumin plus piperine in the composition. Regarding the daily dose of curcumin, seven studies used doses ranging from 150 to 1500 mg [1,2,4,5,10,24,25,30,32], and two studies tested higher doses of about 5 g [28] and 6 g [31] daily. In nine of the included studies, supplementation was given before and after exercise [1,2,5,10,25,28,30–32], Sciberras et al. [4] used curcumin before exercise, and Nakhostin-Roohi et al. [24] supplemented with curcumin after exercise. Finally, treatment duration ranged from one to fifty-six days, with three studies of four days [1,5,31], two of six days [28,30], two of seven days [1,25], two of one day [2,24], one of twenty-eight days [10], and one of fifty-six days [32], respectively.

Table 2. Characteristics of participants and interventions in the studies included in the review.

Level of Participants	Elite Athletes	1 Study [31]
	Moderately Active	5 Studies [4,5,10,28,32]
	No Regular Training before the Study	5 Studies [1,2,24,25,30]
Type of Administration of Curcumin	Commercially available curcumin supplement	10 studies [1,2,4,5,10,24,25,30–32]
	Curcumin capsule made for the study	1 study [28]
Dosage Used	150 mg/day	1 study [24]
	180 mg/day (2 doses of 90 mg/day)	2 studies [1,25]
	300 mg /day (2 doses of 150 mg/day)	1 study [2]
	400 mg/day	1 study [30]
	400 mg /day (2 doses of 200 mg/day)	1 study [5]
	500 mg / day	1 study [4]
	5 g/day (2 doses of 2.5 g/day)	1 study [28]
	6 g of curcumin + 60 mg of piperine/day (3 doses of 2 g of curcumin + 20 mg of piperine/day)	1 study [31]
	600 mg/day (3 doses of 200 mg of curcumin)	1 study [10]
	1500 mg/day (3 doses of 500 mg of curcumin)	1 study [32]
Moment of Supplementation	Before Exercise	1 study [4]
	Before and After Exercise	9 studies [1,2,5,10,25,28,30–32]
	After Exercise	1 study [24]
Duration of Treatment	1 day	2 studies [2,24]
	4 days	3 studies [4,5,31]
	6 days	2 studies [28,30]
	7 days	2 studies [1,25]
	56 days	1 study [10]
	28 days	1 study [32]

3.3. Outcome Measures

Table 3A–C includes information about the author/s and year of publication; the sample investigated, with details of fitness level, sex, and the number of participants; the study design cites the control group if the study included one; the supplementation protocol that specifies the type of curcumin used, the dose, and the time at which it was administered; the parameters analyzed or main effects on muscle damage; and finally, results or main conclusions.

Table 3. Summary of studies included in this systematic review.

A. Summary of Studies Included in This Systematic Review.

Author/s—Year	Study Design	Population	Intervention	Analyzed Results	Main Conclusions
Drobnic et al., 2014 [5]	Randomized controlled trial single-blind	20 moderately active men (38.1 ± 11.1 years and 32.7 ± 12.3 years)	200 mg curcumin capsules (Phytosome Meriva) twice a day 48 h before exercise and for 24 h after	Evidence of muscle injury by MRI	↓ RT and LT posterior and medial
				CRP, hsCRP, ERS, MCP-1, FRAP, CAT, GPx, CK	↑ CRP, hsCRP, ERS, MCP-1, FRAP, CAT, GPx, CK
				IL-8	↓ IL-8
Sciberras et al., 2015 [4]	Double-blind randomized cross-over. Subjects performed three trials in total (supplement/placebo and control)	11 male recreational athletes (35.5 ± 5.7 years)	500 mg of curcumin in capsules (Meriva Curcumin) 72 h before and immediately before exercise	Intensity of pain	↑ Intensity of pain
				RPE	↑ RPE
				Cortisol, PCR, Hto, Hb,	↑ Cortisol, PCR, Hto, Hb,
				WBC, Neutrophils, IL-6,	WBC, Neutrophils, IL-6,
				IL1-RA, IL-10	IL1-RA, IL-10
				Questionnaire DALDA	↑ "better than usual"
Nicol et al., 2015 [28]	Double-blind crossover randomized controlled trial	17 moderately active men (33.8 ± 5.4 years)	2.5 g of curcumin in capsules, 48 h before the exercise and for 72 h after	Muscle pain—VAS	↓ Muscle pain: squatting jump (1.5–1.1; ± 1.2); Stretch butt (−1.0a–1.9; ± 0.9); Sitting on one leg (−1.4a–1.7; 90% CL ± 1.0)
				Jump height to one leg	↑ Jump 1 leg (15%; 90% CL ± 1 2%)
				CK	↓ CK 24 and 48 h before (−22%; 90% CL ± 22%), (−29%; ± 21%)
				IL-6	↑ IL-6 at 0-h (31%; ± 29%) and 48 h (32%; ± 29%) ↓ 24 h post-exercise (−20%; ± 18%)
				TNF-α	↑ TNF-α
Tanabe et al., 2015 [2]	Single-blind crossover randomized controlled trial	14 young men without regular resistance training (23.5 ± 2.3 years)	150 mg curcumin capsules (Theracurcumin Theravalues) twice a day 1 h before exercise and 12 h later	MVC Torque	↓ MVC Torque
				ROM	↑ ROM
				Upper arm circumference	↑ Upper arm circumference
				Muscle pain—VAS	↑VAS
				CK	↓ CK (maximum activity)
				IL-6	↑ IL-6
				TNF-α	↑ TNF-α

B. Summary of Studies Included in This Systematic Review (Continued)

Author/s—Year	Study Design	Population	Intervention	Analyzed Results	Main Conclusions

Table 3. Cont.

Study	Design	Subjects	Intervention	Measurements	Results
McFarlin et al., 2016 [30]	Randomized controlled trial double blind	28 men and women without regular resistance training (20 ± 1 ages and 19 ± 2 ages)	400mg curcumin capsules (Long-life) 48h before exercise and for 72h after	Subjective quadriceps pain	↑ Subjective quadriceps pain
				ADL	↑ADL
				CK	↓CK
				TNF-α	↓TNF-α
				IL-6	↑IL-6
				IL-8	↓IL-8
				IL-10	↑IL-10
Nakhostin-Roohi et al., 2016 [24]	Controlled test randomized crossed double-blind	10 young men without regular training with weights (25.0 ± 1.6 years)	150 mg of curcumin in capsules (Theravalues) Immediately after exercise	Muscle pain—VAS	↓ VAS 48–72 h
				TAC	↑TAC
				CK	↓CK
				ALT	↓ALT
				AST	↓AST
Delecroix et al., 2017 [31]	A randomized, balanced cross-over	10 rugby players elite level (20.7 ± 1.4 years)	2 g curcumin + 20 mg of piperine in capsules (MGD Nature) 3 times/day 48h before exercise and for 48 h after exercise	6-s power sprint	< Group reduction EXP: (−1.77 ± 7.25%; 1277 ± 153 W). CON Group (−13.6 ± 13.0%; 1130 ± 241 W)
				CMJ	↑ CMJ (ES = −0.56; CI 90% = 0.81–0.32)
				CK	↑ CK 24, 48, 72 h post-exercise
				Muscle pain—Hooper scale	↑ Muscle pain—Hooper scale
				Subjective quadriceps pain	↑ Subjective quadriceps pain
Tanabe et al., 2018 [1]	Double-blind crossover randomized controlled trial	Exp1: 10 men (28.5 ± 3.4 years) Exp2: 10 men (29.0 ± 3.9 years) Both untrained 3–7 days prior to assay	90mg curcumin capsules (Theracurmin Theravalues) 2 times/day Exp1: 7 days before exercise Exp2: 7 days after exercise	MVC Torque	Exp1:↑ Exp2:↑ MVC Torque
				ROM	Exp1:↑ Exp2:↑ ROM
				Muscle pain -VAS	Exp1:↑ Exp2: ↓ VAS
				T₂	Exp1:↑ Exp2: ↑ T₂
				CK	Exp1:↑ Exp2:↓ CK
				TNF-α	Exp1:↑ Exp2: ↑ TNF-α
				IL-8	Exp1: ↓ Exp2: ↑ IL-8
				d-ROMs	Exp1:↑ Exp2: ↑ d-ROMs
				BAP	Exp1:↑ Exp2: ↑ BAP
Tanabe et al., 2019 [25]	Single-Blind Parallel Randomized Trial	24 young men without intense training during the study period PRE (28.8 ± 3.6 years) POST (29.8 ± 3.4 years) CON (28.0 ± 3.2 years)	90 mg curcumin capsules (Theracurcumin Theravalues) twice a day PRE: 7 days before exercise POST: 4 days after exercise CON: 4 days after exercise	MVC Torque	PRE: ↑ POST: ↑ MVC Torque
				ROM	PRE: ↑ POST: ↑ ROM
				Muscle pain—VAS	PRE: ↑ POST: ↓ VAS
				CK	PRE: ↑ POST: ↑ CK

Table 3. *Cont.*

C. Summary of Studies Included in This Systematic Review (Continued)

Author/s—Year	Study Design	Population	Intervention	Analyzed Results	Main Conclusions
Jäger et al., 2019 [10]	Randomized controlled trial double-blind	63 men (31) and women (32) (21 ± 2 years) physically active meeting ACSM guidelines	G1: Placebo (PLB) G2: 50 mg curcumin in capsules (CurcuWIN®)G3: 200 mg curcumin in capsules (CurcuWIN®)3 times/day (breakfast/lunch/dinner)	Subjective muscle pain anterior, posterior, and total scale 100 mm Maximum extension torque and isokinetic flexion Extension power and isokinetic flexion Isometric torque Measurements: 1 h, 24 h, 48 h, and 72 h post-exercise	↑ Subjective muscle pain (anterior, posterior) G 1, 2, and 3 † Subjective (total) muscle pain G3 1 h and 24 h post-exercise † Maximum bending torque G2 † Bending power G2
Basham et al., 2019 [32]	Randomized controlled trial double-blind	20 men elite level (21.7 ± 2.9 years) physically active compliance with ACSM guidelines	1.5 g curcumin/69 mg curcuminoids 500 mg capsule (CurcuFresh, NOW FoodsUSA) twice a day (2 breakfast/1 dinner)	Oxidative stress Inflammation Muscle damage Muscle pain	↓ CK ($p < 0.0001$) ↓ VAS ($p = 0.012$) &TAC &MDA &TNF-α

(A) ↑: Statistically significant increase; †: change without statistical significance; ↓: Statistically significant decrease; MRI: magnetic resonance imaging; RT: right thigh; LT: left thigh; CRP: C-reactive protein; hsCRP: high sensitivity CRP; ERS: erythrocyte sedimentation; MCP-1: monocyte 1 chemotherapeutic protein; FRAP: Ferric reduction capacity of plasma; CAT: catalase; GPx: glutathione peroxidase; CK: creatine kinase; IL-8: interleukin 8; RPE: subjective perception of effort; Hto: hematocrit; Hb: hemoglobin; WBC: white blood cell count; IL-6: interleukin 6; IL1-RA: interleukin 1-RA; IL-10: interleukin 10; DALDA: daily analysis of life demands in athletes; VAS: visual analog scale; TNF-α: tumor necrosis factor alpha; CVS: maximum voluntary contraction; ROM: range of motion; TAC: Total Antioxidant Capacity; ALT: alanine aminotransferase; AST: aspartate aminotransferase. (B) ADL: Activities of daily living; CMJ: Contra movement jump; MVC Torque: Maximum voluntary contraction torque; ROM: Range of motion; T2: Transverse relaxation time; d-ROMs: Derivatives of reactive oxygen metabolites; BAP: Biological antioxidant potential; EXP: Experimental; CON: Control. (C) &: Unchanged; PLB: Placebo; G: Group; MDA: Malondialdehyde; ACSM: The American College of Sports Medicine.

4. Discussion

The main objective of this systematic review was to critically evaluate the effectiveness of curcumin supplementation on EIMD (muscle pain, muscle performance, and muscle enzyme activity) and inflammatory and oxidative markers in a physically active population. The main results indicated that supplementation with 150 and 1500 mg/day of oral curcumin, both before and up until 72 h after exercise, has been shown to be effective on exercise performance, modulated in part by the reduction of EIMD and inflammation caused by physical activity. However, it was difficult to determine the true efficacy of the antioxidant capacity of curcumin. Due to the differently measured outcomes in the studies, the following outcomes were divided into different groups to provide a clearer analysis. The results could be influenced by type of exercise, amount of each supplement, and duration of the intervention. Participant characteristics, such as age, gender, ethnicity, body composition, training level, differences in training, nutrition, and health status, may also have influenced the results.

4.1. Curcumin Supplementation

The dose of curcumin administered in interventions ranged from 150 to 6000 mg/day, and therefore, the effects of curcumin in a physically active population should be attributed to this dose range. However, the European Food Safety Authority (EFSA) determined the permitted daily intake to be 3 mg/kg body weight [33]. Thus, two investigations justified a dose of 180 mg/day of curcumin following the EFSA recommendation [1,25]. However, other studies [28,30,32] did not base the choice of dose on the same criteria.

Mc Farlin et al. [30] designed a pilot experiment in which they compared the effect of three doses of curcumin (200, 400, and 1000 mg) on inflammatory serum cytokines in order to avoid the use of animal models. These authors concluded that the optimal dose would be 400 mg/day. Furthermore, Nicol et al. [28] selected a dose of 5000 mg/day of natural curcumin based on a study in mice, which resulted in a dose of less than 5% bioavailable curcumin (<200 mg/day of bioactive curcumin). Finally, Basham et al. [32] selected a dose of 1500 mg (69 mg of curcuminoids). This study implemented a newly enhanced absorption and pharmacokinetics of fresh turmeric derived from curcuminoids in comparison with the standard curcumin from dried rhizomers. Dosing was determined via the manufacturer's recommendations [34]. However, most studies investigating curcumin supplementation have utilized dosages ranging from as little as 50 mg/day [35] to 2.5 g/day [28], demonstrating efficacy and safety in humans. Further, internal quality control testing was performed by the manufacturer, ensuring safety and authenticity of the supplement.

Thus, while research using curcumin supplements with improved bioavailability (Meriva Curcumin [4,5]; Theracurcumin Theravalues [1,24,25,36]; Longvida [30]; CurcuWIN [10]; CurcuFresh [32] determined the dose at values between 150 and 1500 mg/day, studies using curcumin naturally [28,31] needed higher doses (5000 to 6000 mg/day) to achieve similar bioavailability.

The Korean Food and Drug Safety Administration has declared turmeric safe and tolerable in humans, and long-term studies with curcumin have revealed no toxic or adverse effects. However, in a supradosing range, with higher doses than the studies described in this manuscript of between 8 and 12 g, some subjects experienced mild nausea or diarrhea [37]. One consideration that should be taken into account in supplementation with curcumin in athletes, who are themselves susceptible to iron deficiencies with or without anemia, is the interaction between high doses of curcumin and the alteration of iron metabolism by the chelation of iron and elevation of hepcidin, which could be another potential cause of decreased iron levels [38]. For this reason, piperine increases in importance because it allows a high bioavailability of curcumin with lower doses [39]. In this sense, Delecroix et al. [31] used curcumin (6 g) plus piperine (20 mg) per day. However, it is not possible to determine the degree of absorption of the different formulations of curcumin because the studies do not reveal the plasma concentrations.

We believe that curcumin can be safely used as a modulating therapy for markers of inflammation and exercise-induced muscle damage. However, in spite of the safety of the curcumin dose, it is necessary to develop more precise criteria according to the type of curcumin administered, the duration of treatment, and the type of sport performed, in order to establish an optimal dose and an effective intake time that are capable of attenuating the effects of exercise on inflammatory responses and muscle damage.

4.2. Exercise-Induced Muscle Damage (EIMD)

EIMD could affect different muscle dimensions such as muscle pain, muscle performance, and muscle enzyme activity.

4.2.1. Effect on Muscle Pain

Muscle pain can be induced by EIMD or an unaccustomed activity [40] and results in discomfort at the site of the injury and loss, among others, of muscle function and strength; hence, it limits physical function for several days after exercise [41]. The potential effect of curcumin supplementation in reducing muscle pain could be due to the effect it has on suppressing the induction of expression of the isoform COX-2 [25], thus avoiding the production of mediating substances, such as prostaglandin E2 (PGE2), histamine, bradykinin, and serotonin derived from COX-2 that activate nerve endings [19]. The action of curcumin decreasing these mediators, especially PGE2, would provide the attenuation of the phenomenon of long-lasting hyperalgesia that occurs in afferent sensory fibers of type C [42].

In this sense, ten studies [1,2,5,10,24,25,28,30–32] evaluate the ability of curcumin to attenuate muscle pain; eight of which do so through the Visual Analog Scale (VAS) [1,2,4,10,24,25,28,32]. Concretely, Nicol et al. [28], described that the intake of 2.5 g of curcumin supplementation in capsules taken 48 h before and 72 h after eccentric exercise caused significant reductions in pain. Aligned with this, in two studies by Tanabe et al. [1,25], a significant reduction in muscle pain was demonstrated by the effect of administering 180 mg of curcumin supplement (90 mg twice daily) in Theracumin-Theravalues capsules, only when administered four [25] and seven [1] days after eccentric contraction exercise. In addition, the curcumin supplementation (1.5 g) resulted in significantly decreased muscle soreness overall (VAS scale 2.88) when compared to the placebo (VAS scale 3.36) ($p < 0.0120$) [32]. The supplementation continued for three days during the follow-up testing sessions; thus, 28 total days of supplementation were implemented. Finally, Nakhostin-Roohi et al. [24] showed that one dose of 150 mg of curcumin supplementation in capsules (Theravalues) taken immediately after exercise significantly reduced muscle pain at 48 and 72 h after eccentric exercise.

However, Jäger et al. [10] showed non-significant improvements in exercise-induced total thigh soreness and indicated that the 200 mg curcumin groups reported 26%, 20%, and 8% less soreness immediately, 24 h, and 48 h after exercise, respectively, as compared the soreness levels that were reported in the PLA and 50 mg curcumin groups; these differences failed to reach statistical significance. The supplementation of curcumin was for eight weeks prior to downhill running protocol VAS. In this sense, Tanabe et al. [2] did not find a significant effect in delayed onset muscle soreness (DOMS) using 150 mg of curcumin or placebo orally before and 12 h after each eccentric exercise.

There are many possible supplementation conditions in terms of dose, frequency, and time points. Nosaka et al. [43] reported that essential amino acid supplementation given both 30 min before and immediately after eccentric exercise did not affect any indicators of muscle damage, but when the supplementation was continued for next four days after exercise, it attenuated increase in muscle soreness and range of motion (ROM). Thus, it is possible that curcumin supplementation has an effect on DOMS if the curcumin is given on recovery days, for a period of at least 3 days, as in [28,32], or for a longer period of time [1,25]. However, a single dose of curcumin (150 mg) immediately after exercise significantly reduced muscle pain [24]. This situation may justify the need for a series of studies to investigate whether curcumin supplementation for recovery immediately after exercise will provide greater effects on muscle damage.

On the other hand, three studies [5,30,31] evaluate the ability of curcumin to attenuate muscle pain using other scales. In particular, Drobnic et al. [5] observed a tendency towards less pain, but no significant improvements, in the lower extremities after 200 mg curcumin supplementation taken 48 h before and 24 h after a downhill race. In addition, Mc Farling et al. [30] investigated subjective quadriceps muscle soreness, finding no significant difference in muscle soreness or activities of daily living soreness between supplementation with curcumin (400 mg; 24 h before and for 72 h after) and placebo. Moreover, Delecroix et al. [31] showed no beneficial effect of curcumin (2 g; 48 h before and for 48 h after) in reducing muscle pain, as evaluated by the Hooper scale and subjective quadriceps muscle soreness.

It is possible that differences in pain perception outcomes in studies that could not establish the same effect are probably due to the subjective perception of the patient's pain intensity. For this reason, a combination of physiological and psychological factors could play an important role in individual perception, thus potentially improving recovery from training [44]. Therefore, it cannot be ruled out that perception, psychological factors, and placebo effects may have influenced the reported results. We described that the doses of curcumin that showed benefits for muscle pain attenuation were in a wide range (150 mg–2.5 g); however, what might be effective is administration immediately after exercise and/or within at least 72 h after exercise.

4.2.2. Effect on Muscle Performance

Muscle damage caused by mechanical stress during eccentric exercise and subsequent inflammatory responses lead to a deterioration of muscle performance. Thus, changes in maximum voluntary contraction (MVC) force, range of motion (ROM), and isokinetic dynamometry reflect the dimension and time progression of EIMD, and therefore, these parameters can be used as markers of athletic performance [1,2,31]. MVC, isokinetic dynamometry, and ROM are diminished by the activation of NF-κB under the high mechanical stress caused by the overuse of some joints in sport, which generates fragments of the extracellular matrix of the bone or cartilage. These fragments are recognized by receptors of innate immunity, which recognize pattern recognition receptors, called toll-like receptors. Cell activation mediated by this process ends between the activation of NF-κB, which is a stimulator of the secretion of inflammatory cytokines (IL-1, IL-1b, IL-2, IL-15, IL-21, TNF-α), chemokines (CCL-19, CCR-7), and metalloproteases (MMP-13, ADAMTS-4), all responsible for producing tissue damage [45]. It is probably the action of curcumin that is responsible for minimizing the incapacitating tissue effects, as it is a therapeutic agent that blocks the signaling pathway of NF-κB. In addition, reducing leucocyte adhesion and migration, and as a result, relieving pain and swelling, improves joint mobility and stiffness [16,37]. Three studies conducted by Tanabe et al. [1,2,25] evaluated MVC and ROM. One of them [2] showed that 150 mg of curcumin both before and 12 h after 50 eccentric contractions of the elbow flexors presented a significantly smaller decreasing magnitude on the MVC. However, ROM decreased significantly at all measurement times (24, 48, 72, and 96 h) in the curcumin group, but there were no significant interaction effects for changes between placebo and curcumin. Another study by the same author [1] demonstrated significantly faster recovery of torque MVC and significant improvements in ROM only when 180 mg of curcumin was ingested after exercise [1]. Moreover, Tanabe et al. [25] found that when 180 mg curcumin was ingested during the four days following exercise, ROM improved significantly after three to four post-exercise days, with no relevant changes in MVC for any of the study conditions. Recently, Jäger et al. [10] reported that only 200 mg (CurcuWIN®) was effective in preventing the observed decreases in peak extension torque values seen 1 and 24 h after exercise that damaged muscles.

In this way, these studies suggest that the intake of a dose of curcumin (90–200 mg) after exercise may be effective as a muscle performance enhancer by benefiting the recovery process.

4.2.3. Effect on Muscle Enzyme Activity

Intense exercise increases the circulating levels of markers for muscle damage such as lactate dehydrogenase (LDH), CK, myoglobin (Mb), and transaminases (alanine aminotransferase (ALT) and aspartate aminotransferase (AST)). All these parameters are indicative of increased EIMD and OS, which negatively affect athletes because they reduce exercise performance and can also put their health at risk [46].

The effect of curcumin on CK enzyme activity levels after exercise was studied in eight investigations included in this systematic review [1,2,5,24,25,28,30,31]. Five of them [1,2,24,28,30] presented significantly lower maximum CK activity in the curcumin-supplemented group compared to the placebo groups. Moreover, although there were no significant differences, three studies [5,25,31] observed that CK levels tended to increase less in the curcumin group. Potentially, the decrease in CK after curcumin supplementation could be attributed to an antioxidant role by neutralizing oxygen free radicals (ROS) produced during the electron transport chain of oxidative phosphorylation, necessary for energy requirements in physical exercise [8]. Another possible mechanism of CK's activity reduction may be the inhibition of the production of histamine and prostaglandin by suppressing the positive regulation of COX-2, a pathway involved in vascular permeability [47]. In local areas with inflammation, they reduce the permeability of the membranes, thus reducing the intracellular–intravascular flow of CK. Thus, the limitation of vascular permeability could be the key factor in reducing inflammation and muscle pain [48]. The differences between studies may be due to dose, timing of curcumin supplementation, and intensity of physical activity. In addition, Nakhostin-Roohi et al. [24] showed ALT and AST at significantly reduced levels in curcumin group.

The findings of this study [24] suggest that a 150 mg dose of curcumin, when administered immediately after exercise, may have protective effects on muscle damage by significantly reducing the levels of three markers of circulating muscle damage (CK, AST, and ALT). It is difficult to concretize supplementation with curcumin because there are many possible supplementation conditions in terms of dose, frequency, and time points where curcumin has been shown to be effective in relation to its potential to decrease muscle damage, which is reflected in decreased CK activity in the supplemented groups.

4.3. Effect on Inflammatory Markers

Curcumin is currently recognized for its potential anti-inflammatory effect [13,15]. In this sense, inflammation is a physiological process in response to physical exercise. Pro-inflammatory cytokines and chemokines produced by immune cells during the immune response interact with their receptors by activating signaling pathways of the inflammatory response [20]. The possible positive effect of curcumin supplementation on inflammatory response may be due to the modulating action of curcumin on inflammatory signaling cascades. These signaling pathways include the nuclear factor κB pathway (NF-κB), the signal transducer and transcription activator Janus kinase (JAK/STAT), and mitogen activated protein kinase (MAPKs). Curcumin inhibits the activation of NF-κB, suppresses the activation and phosphorylation of JAK/STAT proteins, and inhibits MAPK signaling through its interaction with three major members of this pathway, including JNK, p38, and ERK. Bisdemethoxycurcumin suppresses infiltration, activation, and maturation of leukocytes, and also the production of proinflammatory mediators TNF-α, IL-8, and IL-6 at the site of inflammation. Another effect the potential of curcumin is to act as an immunomodulator by intervening in the suppression of immune responses acquired in T cells, inhibiting the activation, differentiation, and production of cytokines [20].

In the studies analyzed in this systematic review, the pro-inflammatory cytokines TNF-α [1,2,28,30,32], interleukin 6 (IL-6) [2,4,28,30], and IL-8 [1,5,30] were evaluated as markers of inflammation. In relation to TNF-α, Nicol et al. [28] and Tanabe et al. [1,2] did not observe any effect of curcumin supplementation on this inflammation marker. However, McFarlin et al. [30] and Basham et al. [32] reported sustained suppression of TNF-α for up to one day after exercise in the curcumin supplemented group compared to the placebo group. Moreover, TNF-α was significantly lower with curcumin at two days and four days and trended towards being lower with curcumin at three days compared to placebo [30]. It is likely that the effectiveness of curcumin on the plasma decrease of TNF-α is dependent on a minimum dose of 400 mg administered before exercise and for 72 h after exercise (at minimum), which may explain the differences with respect to the studies by

Tanabe et al. [1,2]. In addition, commercial formulas of curcumin [30,32] implemented an enhanced absorption and pharmacokinetics as compared to standard preparations of curcumin [28].

On the other hand, curcumin supplementation showed a downward but non-significant trend on IL-6 cytokines derived from exercise practice [2,4,30]. Moreover, Drobnic et al. [5] and Mc Farlin et al. [30] showed that 400 mg of curcumin supplementation (48 h before and 24–72 h after exercise) significantly reduced IL-8 levels. However, Tanabe et al. [1] observed non-significant decreases in IL-8 12 h after exercise, when subjects were supplemented with 180 mg of curcumin for seven days before the eccentric exercise test. The differences in dosage and timing could be the cause of differences in IL-8 regulation. According to these results, it is possible that a minimum of 400 mg of curcumin administered before and for at least 24 h after exercise may be necessary.

In this way, the promoters of IL-6 and IL-8 cytokines possess binding sites for NF-κB, C/EBPβ, and c-Jun [49]. We believe the role of NF-κB inhibition is a therapeutic objective of curcumin in inflammation because of the importance of NF-κB for the regulation of the constitution and expression of IL-6 and IL-8 [49,50]. McFarling et al. [30] concretely observed that significant inhibition of NF-κB could be related to a significant decrease in IL-8 and a downward trend in IL-6. Thus, supplementation with 400 mg of curcumin, two days before and three days after exercise, appears to be effective in attenuating exercise-induced inflammation because of its direct action on NF-κB, which influences the cytokines IL-8 and IL-6.

Other cytokines, such as IL-10 [4,30], with anti-inflammatory properties capable of inhibiting the synthesis of pro-inflammatory cytokines and IL1RA [4], which is a key mediator in the inflammatory response, were evaluated. Lower levels of non-significant IL-10 and IL1RA were reported in the curcumin-administered groups as compared to the placebo group.

4.4. Effect on Oxidative Markers

This mechanical stress derived from exercise triggers an inflammatory response and the production of ROS. ROS are able to maintain inflammation and in general a high degree of oxidative stress by stimulating the activation pathways of transcription factors such as nuclear factor-κB (NF-κB), a pro-inflammatory master switch that controls the production of inflammatory energy, and are involved in cell damage [32]. This sustained inflammatory response and the high degree of oxidative stress lead to the accumulation of neutrophils and increased "inflammatory growth medium" production of oxidative enzymes, cytokines, and chemokines [15]. In every organism, there is a protection system formed by antioxidant compounds and enzymes that participate in the transformations of these species. One of them is the enzyme glutathione peroxidase (GPx). This enzyme uses glutathione to reduce peroxides, thereby protecting membranes and other cellular structures from the action of lipid peroxides and free radicals [51]. In addition, catalase (CAT) is one of the enzymes involved in the destruction of hydrogen peroxide generated during cell metabolism [52]. The overproduction of ROS eventually surpasses the body's antioxidant capacity [15].

Against this background, curcumin could be useful because it has been described as suppressing the activation of NF-κB and the promotion of antioxidant response by the transcription activation of Nrf2, which could neutralize these harmful effects related to ROS [18]. Drobnic et al. [5] observed non-significant increases in GPx and CAT after supplementation with curcumin (200 mg) before and after exercise. Other antioxidant markers, such as reactive metabolites of oxygen serum (d-ROMs) and potential biological antioxidant (BAP) concentrations, were not different between curcumin and placebo trials after supplementation with curcumin (90 mg) before and after exercise [1]. In agreement with this, Basham et al. [32] found that exercise was not different between curcumin and placebo trials in total antioxidant capacity (TAC), and that malondialdehyde is formed by the lipid peroxidation of unsaturated fatty acids and is a marker of oxidative degradation of the cell membrane. It is difficult to determine the efficacy of the antioxidant capacity of curcumin, considering the above results. However, in this study, TAC remained significantly higher in the curcumin group after exercise compared with the levels in the placebo group ($p < 0.05$) [24]. The findings of this study suggest that a 150 mg dose of curcumin may have antioxidant effects. The differences between the studies could be due to the timing of ingestion of curcumin, manifesting only a significant effect when ingested immediately after exercise, as suggested by Nakhostin-Roohi et al. [24].

5. Limitations, Strengths, and Future Lines of Research

The main limitations of the present systematic review are related to the low number of studies investigated on this subject and to the fact that most of them had a relatively small number of participants. Because of this, it is essential to take into consideration that the studies analyzed were conducted in populations with different levels of physical activity and using different research protocols, which increases the heterogeneity between studies. In addition, dosage, duration of treatment, and formulation of curcumin were not uniform across investigations, which could affect some of the results, particularly because of the limitation associated with the bioavailability of the supplement. Likewise, in some of the selected studies, specific diet controls were carried out prior to the study, telling the participants not to eat foods containing curcumin (e.g., curry) or to follow any nutritional guidelines to avoid the main polyphenols in the diet. However, in other studies, only the consumption of anti-inflammatory drugs was limited, whilst it is still possible that some habitual foods produce anti-inflammatory effects. Finally, it should be noted that the studies analyzed only evaluated inflammatory markers from blood samples, but none in muscle tissue.

The development of curcuminoids in nanoformulations to improve the pharmacokinetics, bioavailability, and biological activity of curcuminoids is currently under investigation [53]. Further research is needed to determine whether these new formulations might be more effective in treating inflammation and the time course of exercise-induced muscle damage. Another way to improve bioavailability would be through piperine, as demonstrated by Delecroix et al. [31], who included 6 g of curcumin +60 mg of piperine/day. Piperine is a thermonutrient that exerts its thermogenic action on the epithelial cells of the small intestine, increasing the rate of nutrient absorption and therefore increasing its bioavailability [54].

Although the studies used in this review were not conducted exclusively in a competitive sports population, they provide an adequate justification to support broader research that could eventually confer its acceptance as a standard in the recovery of muscle function and inflammatory parameters in the framework of physical activity. Furthermore, a strength of this systematic review is quality control through PRISMA and Mc Master.

6. Practical Applications

In general, curcumin supplementation could be used during periods of high demand, tournaments, or competitive events to speed up the recovery of muscle function and counteract the size and progress of symptoms associated with exercise-induced muscle pain [14]. In addition, curcumin has been used in various protocols before and/or after exercise, to decrease inflammation and muscle damage through its ability to modulate the inflammatory response and its antioxidant effect. However, implementing curcumin as an ergogenic aid should be considered in light of the sporting objective, since the persistent use of anti-inflammatory substances that benefit recovery could affect training adaptations [55]. However, maximizing resilience at the expense of training adaptations may be desirable in athletes in competitive seasons.

Since the athlete's recovery in a period of high training or competition loads is limited to a specific moment, the decision on the supplementation strategy to be implemented should be made considering the physiological effects of the substance. Along these lines, it could be considered that supplementation with curcumin in combination with one or more substances that act on different physiological mechanisms could result in a synergistic effect on the parameters of inflammation and muscle damage in the recovery process.

Finally, curcumin should always be used as a pharmaceutical preparation and not as a spice to avoid the toxic effects of fungical aphlotoxins. In addition, caution is needed with athletes who are sensitive to gastric irritation.

7. Conclusions

In summary, the use of curcumin reduces the subjective perception of the intensity of muscle pain. Likewise, curcumin is able to decrease muscle damage through the reduction of muscle CK activity and to increase muscle performance. Moreover, supplementation with curcumin exerts a post-exercise anti-inflammatory effect by modulating the pro-inflammatory cytokines TNF-α, IL-6, and IL-8, and curcumin may have a slight antioxidant effect. The minimum optimal dose to achieve a positive impact would be recommended doses between 150 and 1500 mg/day, when administered before and immediately after exercise, and for 72 h after. Finally, curcumin should only be recommended to athletes who are willing to use ergogenic aids to increase performance, and it should be recommended only on an individual basis to modulate some of the muscle damage and inflammation caused by physical activity. Oral curcumin supplementation has been shown to be effective pre and/or post physical activity.

Author Contributions: D.F.-L.: conceived and designed the investigation, analyzed and interpreted the data, drafted the paper, and approved the final version submitted for publication C.I.F.-L. and J.M.-A.: analyzed and interpreted the data, critically reviewed the paper and approved the final version submitted for publication. J.S.C. and A.C.M. and A.C.G.: critically reviewed the paper and approved the final version submitted for publication. All authors have read and agreed to the published version of the manuscript.

Funding: The authors declare no funding sources.

Acknowledgments: The authors are grateful to the Foundation Institute of Health Sciences Studies of Castilla-León (ICSCYL) for its collaboration in infrastructures, bibliographic bases and computer support.

Conflicts of Interest: The authors declare no conflict of interest.

References

1. Tanabe, Y.; Chino, K.; Ohnishi, T.; Ozawa, H.; Sagayama, H.; Maeda, S.; Takahashi, H. Effects of oral curcumin ingested before or after eccentric exercise on markers of muscle damage and inflammation. *Scand. J. Med. Sci. Sport* **2018**, *29*, 524–534. [CrossRef]
2. Tanabe, Y.; Maeda, S.; Akazawa, N.; Zempo-Miyaki, A.; Choi, Y.; Ra, S.G.; Nosaka, K. Attenuation of indirect markers of eccentric exercise-induced muscle damage by curcumin. *Eur. J. Appl. Physiol.* **2015**, *115*, 1949–1957. [CrossRef] [PubMed]
3. Fatouros, I.G.; Jamurtas, A.Z. Insights into the molecular etiology of exercise-induced inflammation: Opportunities for optimizing performance. *J. Inflamm. Res.* **2016**, *9*, 175–186. [CrossRef] [PubMed]
4. Sciberras, J.N.; Galloway, S.D.; Fenech, A.; Grech, G.; Farrugia, C.; Duca, D.; Mifsud, J. The effect of turmeric (Curcumin) supplementation on cytokine and inflammatory marker responses following 2 hours of endurance cycling. *J. Int. Soc. Sports Nutr.* **2015**, *12*, 5. [CrossRef] [PubMed]
5. Drobnic, F.; Riera, J.; Appendino, G.; Togni, S.; Franceschi, F.; Valle, X.; Tur, J. Reduction of delayed onset muscle soreness by a novel curcumin delivery system (Meriva®): A randomised, placebo-controlled trial. *J. Int. Soc. Sports Nutr.* **2014**, *11*, 31. [CrossRef]
6. Schieber, M.; Chandel, N.S. ROS function in redox signaling and oxidative stress. *Curr. Biol.* **2014**, *24*, R453–R462. [CrossRef]
7. He, F.; Li, J.; Liu, Z.; Chuang, C.-C.; Yang, W.; Zuo, L. Redox mechanism of reactive oxygen species in exercise. *Front. Physiol.* **2016**, *7*, 486. [CrossRef]
8. Córdova Martínez, A. *Sports Physiology*, 1st ed.; Synthesis: Madrid, Spain, 2013; pp. 65–74.
9. Braakhuis, A.J.; Hopkins, W.G. Impact of dietary antioxidants on sport performance: A review. *Sports Med.* **2015**, *45*, 939–955. [CrossRef]
10. Jäger, R.; Purpura, M.; Kerksick, C.M. Eight Weeks of a High Dose of Curcumin Supplementation May Attenuate Performance Decrements Following Muscle-Damaging Exercise. *Nutrients* **2019**, *11*, 1692.

11. Kocaadam, B.; Şanlier, N. Curcumin, an active component of turmeric (Curcuma longa), and its effects on health. *Crit. Rev. Food Sci. Nutr.* **2017**, *57*, 2889–2895. [CrossRef]
12. Administration USFaD. *Generally Recognized as Safe (GRAS) FDA*; FDA: Silver Spring, MD, USA, 2016.
13. Gaffey, A.; Slater, H.; Porritt, K.; Campbell, J.M. The effects of curcuminoids on musculoskeletal pain: A systematic review. *JBI Database Syst. Rev. Implement Rep.* **2017**, *15*, 486–516. [CrossRef]
14. Harty, P.S.; Cottet, M.L.; Malloy, J.K.; Kerksick, C.M. Nutritional and Supplementation Strategies to Prevent and Attenuate Exercise-Induced Muscle Damage: A Brief Review. *Sports Med. Open* **2019**, *5*, 1. [CrossRef] [PubMed]
15. Hewlings, S.; Kalman, D. Curcumin: A review of its' effects on human health. *Foods* **2017**, *6*, 92. [CrossRef] [PubMed]
16. Alamdari, N.; O'Neal, P.; Hasselgren, P.-O. Curcumin and muscle wasting—A new role for an old drug? *Nutrition* **2009**, *25*, 125–129. [CrossRef] [PubMed]
17. Derosa, G.; Maffioli, P.; Simental-Mendia, L.E.; Bo, S.; Sahebkar, A. Effect of curcumin on circulating interleukin-6 concentrations: A systematic review and meta-analysis of randomized controlled trials. *Pharmacol. Res.* **2016**, *111*, 394–404. [CrossRef] [PubMed]
18. Noorafshan, A.; Ashkani-Esfahani, S. A review of therapeutic effects of curcumin. *Curr. Pharm. Des.* **2013**, *19*, 2032–2046. [PubMed]
19. Hatcher, H.; Planalp, R.; Cho, J.; Torti, F.; Torti, S. Curcumin: From ancient medicine to current clinical trials. *Cell Mol. Life Sci.* **2008**, *65*, 1631–1652. [CrossRef]
20. Kahkhaie, K.R.; Mirhosseini, A.; Aliabadi, A.; Mohammadi, A.; Haftcheshmeh, S.M.; Sathyapalan, T.; Sahebkar, A. Curcumin: A modulator of inflammatory signaling pathways in the immune system. *Inflammopharmacology* **2019**, *27*, 885–900. [CrossRef]
21. Sahebkar, A.; Cicero, A.F.; Simental-Mendia, L.E.; Aggarwal, B.B.; Gupta, S.C. Curcumin downregulates human tumor necrosis factor-α levels: A systematic review and meta-analysis ofrandomized controlled trials. *Pharmacol. Res.* **2016**, *107*, 234–242. [CrossRef]
22. Dunsmore, K.E.; Chen, P.G.; Wong, H.R. Curcumin, a medicinal herbal compound capable of inducing the heat shock response. *Cri. Care Med.* **2001**, *29*, 2199–2204. [CrossRef]
23. Thitimuta, S.; Pithayanukul, P.; Nithitanakool, S.; Bavovada, R.; Leanpolchareanchai, J.; Saparpakorn, P. Camellia sinensis l. Extract and its potential beneficial effects in antioxidant, anti-inflammatory, anti-hepatotoxic, and anti-tyrosinase activities. *Molecules* **2017**, *22*, 401. [CrossRef] [PubMed]
24. Nakhostin-Roohi, B.; Nasirvand Moradlou, A.; Mahmoodi Hamidabad, S.; Ghanivand, B. The effect of curcumin supplementation on selected markers of delayed onset muscle soreness (DOMS). *Ann. Appl. Sport Sci.* **2016**, *4*, 25–31. [CrossRef]
25. Tanabe, Y.; Chino, K.; Sagayama, H.; Lee, H.J.; Ozawa, H.; Maeda, S.; Takahashi, H. Effective Timing of Curcumin Ingestion to Attenuate Eccentric Exercise-Induced Muscle Soreness in Men. *J. Nutr. Sci. Vitaminol.* **2019**, *65*, 82–89. [CrossRef] [PubMed]
26. Kopec, T.J. Performance Recovery Following Exercise Induced Muscle Damage (EIMD) through an Exhaustive Bout of Exercise. Ph.D. Thesis, University of Alabama, Tuscaloosa, AL, USA, 2016.
27. Hutton, B.; Catalá-López, F.; Moher, D. La extensión de la declaración PRISMA para revisiones sistemáticas que incorporan metaanálisis en red: PRISMA-NMA. *Med. Clin.* **2016**, *147*, 262–266. [CrossRef] [PubMed]
28. Nicol, L.M.; Rowlands, D.S.; Fazakerly, R.; Kellett, J. Curcumin supplementation likely attenuates delayed onset muscle soreness (DOMS). *Eur. J. Appl. Physiol.* **2015**, *115*, 1769–1777. [CrossRef] [PubMed]
29. Law, M.; Stewart, D.; Pollock, N.; Letts, L.; Bosch, J.; Westmorland, M. *Guidelines for Critical Review Form—Quantitative Studies 1998*; McMaster University: Hamilton, ON, Canada, 2008.
30. McFarlin, B.K.; Venable, A.S.; Henning, A.L.; Sampson, J.N.B.; Pennel, K.; Vingren, J.L.; Hill, D.W. Reduced inflammatory and muscle damage biomarkers following oral supplementation with bioavailable curcumin. *BBA Clin.* **2016**, *5*, 72–78. [CrossRef] [PubMed]
31. Delecroix, B.; Abaïdia, A.E.; Leduc, C.; Dawson, B.; Dupont, G. Curcumin and piperine supplementation and recovery following exercise induced muscle damage: A randomized controlled trial. *J. Sport Sci. Med.* **2017**, *16*, 147–153.
32. Basham, S.A.; Waldman, H.S.; Krings, B.M.; Lamberth, J.; Smith, J.W.; McAllister, M.J. Effect of Curcumin Supplementation on Exercise-Induced Oxidative Stress, Inflammation, Muscle Damage, and Muscle Soreness. *J. Diet Suppl.* **2019**, *1*, 1–14. [CrossRef]

33. Authority EFS. Refined exposure assessment for curcumin (E 100). *EFSA J.* **2014**, *12*, 3876. [CrossRef]
34. Krishnakumar, I.; Kumar, D.; Ninan, E.; Kuttan, R.; Maliakel, B. Enhanced absorption and pharmacokinetics of fresh turmeric (Curcuma longa L) derived curcuminoids in comparison with the standard curcumin from dried rhizomes. *J. Funct. Foods* **2015**, *17*, 55–65. [CrossRef]
35. Oliver, J.M.; Stoner, L.; Rowlands, D.S.; Caldwell, A.R.; Sanders, E.; Kreutzer, A.; Jäger, R. Novel form of curcumin improves endothelial function in young, healthy individuals: A double-blind placebo controlled study. *J. Nutr. Metab.* **2016**, *1*, E1089653. [CrossRef] [PubMed]
36. Tabrizi, R.; Vakili, S.; Akbari, M.; Mirhosseini, N.; Lankarani, K.B.; Rahimi, M.; Asemi, Z. The effects of curcumin-containing supplements on biomarkers of inflammation and oxidative stress: A systematic review and meta-analysis of randomized controlled trials. *Phytother. Res.* **2019**, *33*, 253–262. [CrossRef] [PubMed]
37. Daily, J.W.; Yang, M.; Park, S. Efficacy of turmeric extracts and curcumin for alleviating the symptoms of joint arthritis: A systematic review and meta-analysis of randomized clinical trials. *J. Med. Food* **2016**, *19*, 717–729. [CrossRef] [PubMed]
38. Shen, L.; Liu, C.-C.; An, C.-Y.; Ji, H.-F. How does curcumin work with poor bioavailability? Clues from experimental and theoretical studies. *Sci. Rep.* **2018**, *6*, 20872. [CrossRef] [PubMed]
39. Lee, S.H.; Kim, H.Y.; Back, S.Y.; Han, H.-K. Piperine-mediated drug interactions and formulation strategy for piperine: Recent advances and future perspectives. *Expert Opin. Drug Metab. Toxicol.* **2018**, *14*, 43–57. [CrossRef]
40. Proske, U.; Morgan, D.L. Muscle damage from eccentric exercise: Mechanism, mechanical signs, adaptation and clinical applications. *J. Physiol.* **2001**, *537*, 333–345. [CrossRef]
41. Järvinen, T.A.; Järvinen, M.; Kalimo, H. Regeneration of injured skeletal muscle after the injury. *Muscles Ligaments Tendons* **2013**, *3*, 337–345. [CrossRef]
42. Kirkpatrick, D.R.; McEntire, D.M.; Smith, T.A.; Dueck, N.P.; Kerfeld, M.J.; Hambsch, Z.J.; Agrawal, D.K. Transmission pathways and mediators as the basis for clinical pharmacology of pain. *Expert Rev. Clin. Pharmacol.* **2016**, *9*, 1363–1387. [CrossRef]
43. Nosaka, K. Effects of amino acid supplementation on muscle soreness and damage. *Int. J. Sport Nutr. Exerc. Metab.* **2006**, *16*, 620–635. [CrossRef]
44. Cook, C.J.; Beaven, C.M. Individual perception of recovery is related to subsequent sprint performance. *Br. J. Sports Med.* **2013**, *47*, 705–709. [CrossRef]
45. Wainstein, G.E. Patogénesis de la artrosis. *Rev. Med. Clin. Las. Condes.* **2014**, *25*, 723–727.
46. Córdova, A.; Mielgo-Ayuso, J.; Fernandez-Lazaro, C.I.; Caballero-García, A.; Roche, E.; Fernández-Lázaro, D. Effect of Iron Supplementation on the Modulation of Iron Metabolism, Muscle Damage Biomarkers and Cortisol in Professional Cyclists. *Nutrients* **2019**, *11*, 500.
47. Moriyuki, K.; Sekiguchi, F.; Matsubara, K.; Nishikawa, H.; Kawabata, A. Curcumin inhibits the proteinase-activated receptor-2–triggered prostaglandin E2 production by suppressing cyclooxygenase-2 upregulation and Akt-dependent activation of nuclear factor-κB in human lung epithelial cells. *J. Pharmacol. Sci.* **2010**, *114*, 225–229. [CrossRef] [PubMed]
48. Engel, F.A.; Holmberg, H.-C.; Sperlich, B. Is there evidence that runners can benefit from wearing compression clothing? *Sports Med.* **2016**, *46*, 1939–1952. [CrossRef]
49. Georganas, C.; Liu, H.; Perlman, H.; Hoffmann, A.; Thimmapaya, B.; Pope, R.M. Regulation of IL-6 and IL-8 expression in rheumatoid arthritis synovial fibroblasts: The dominant role for NF-κB but not C/EBPβ or c-Jun. *J. Immunol.* **2000**, *165*, 7199–7206. [CrossRef]
50. Dongari-Bagtzoglou, A.I.; Ebersole, J.L. Increased presence of interleukin-6 (IL-6) and IL-8 secreting fibroblast subpopulations in adult periodontitis. *J. Periodontol.* **1998**, *69*, 899–910. [CrossRef]
51. Ranchordas, M.K.; Rogerson, D.; Soltani, H.; Costello, J.T. Antioxidants for preventing and reducing muscle soreness after exercise. *Cochrane Database Syst. Rev.* **2014**, *12*, CD009789.
52. Miranda, C.; Ela, M.; Hernández Lantigua, I.; Llópiz Janer, N. Enzimas que participan como barreras fisiológicas para eliminar los radicales libres: II. Catalasa. *Rev. Cubana Invest. Biomed.* **1996**, *15*, 5–11.
53. Trivedi, M.K.; Mondal, S.C.; Gangwar, M.; Jana, S. Immunomodulatory potential of nanocurcumin-based formulation. *Inflammopharmacology* **2017**, *25*, 609–619. [CrossRef]

54. Patil, U.K.; Singh, A.; Charkraborty, A.K. Role of piperine as a bioavaility enhacer. *Inter. J. Recent Advan. Pharma. Resear.* **2011**, *4*, 16–23.
55. Owens, D.J.; Twist, C.; Cobley, J.N.; Howatson, G.; Close, G.L. Exercise-induced muscle damage: What is it, what causes it and what are the nutritional solutions? *Eur. J. Sport Sci.* **2019**, *19*, 71–78. [CrossRef] [PubMed]

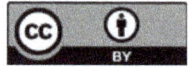

© 2020 by the authors. Licensee MDPI, Basel, Switzerland. This article is an open access article distributed under the terms and conditions of the Creative Commons Attribution (CC BY) license (http://creativecommons.org/licenses/by/4.0/).

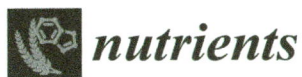

Article

The Effects of Low- and High-Glycemic Index Sport Nutrition Bars on Metabolism and Performance in Recreational Soccer Players

Mojtaba Kaviani [1,2,*], Philip D. Chilibeck [2,*], Spencer Gall [2], Jennifer Jochim [2] and Gordon A. Zello [3]

1. School of Nutrition and Dietetics, Faculty of Pure & Applied Science, Acadia University, Wolfville, Nova Scotia, NS B4P 2R6, Canada
2. College of Kinesiology, University of Saskatchewan, 87 Campus Dr, Saskatoon, SK S7N 5B2, Canada; Spencer.Gall@usask.ca (S.G.); Jennifer.Jochim@usask.ca (J.J.)
3. College of Pharmacy and Nutrition, University of Saskatchewan, 107 Wiggins Rd, Saskatoon, SK S7N 5E5, Canada; gordon.zello@usask.ca
* Correspondence: mojtaba.kaviani@acadiau.ca (M.K.); phil.chilibeck@usask.ca (P.D.C.); Tel.: +1-902-585-1884 (M.K.); +1-306-966-1072 (P.D.C.)

Received: 23 February 2020; Accepted: 31 March 2020; Published: 2 April 2020

Abstract: Consumption of low-glycemic index (GI) carbohydrates (CHO) may be superior to high-GI CHO before exercise by increasing fat oxidation and decreasing carbohydrate oxidation. We compared the effects of pre-exercise feeding of a low-GI lentil-based sports nutrition bar with a high-GI bar on metabolism and performance during a simulated soccer match. Using a randomized, double-blind, counterbalanced, crossover design, participants ($n = 8$) consumed 1.5 g/kg available CHO from a low-GI bar (GI = 45) or high-GI bar (GI = 101) two hours before a 90 min simulated soccer match, and 0.38 g/kg body mass during a 15 min half-time break. The test involved alternating 6 min intervals of paced jogging, running, walking, and sprinting, and 3 min intervals of soccer-specific skills (timed ball dribbling, agility running, heading, kicking accuracy). Carbohydrate oxidation rate was lower during the match after consuming the low-GI compared to high-GI bar (2.17 ± 0.6 vs. 2.72 ± 0.4 g/min; $p < 0.05$). Participants performed better during the low-GI versus high-GI bar condition on the agility test (5.7 ± 0.4 versus 6.1 ± 0.6 s; $p < 0.01$) and heading (i.e., jumping height 24.7 ± 4.3 versus 22.2 ± 4.5 cm; $p < 0.01$) late in the soccer match (72 min). A low-GI lentil-based sports nutrition bar provides a metabolic benefit (lower carbohydrate oxidation rate) and a modest improvement in agility running and jumping height (heading) late in the test.

Keywords: Carbohydrate; high-intensity exercise; fatigue

1. Introduction

Carbohydrate (CHO) is an important source of energy throughout strenuous prolonged exercise. Premature fatigue during prolonged exercise is linked with depletion of carbohydrate stores (i.e., blood glucose and liver and muscle glycogen stores). Thus, carbohydrate consumption before and during exercise improves exercise performance compared with a fasted condition [1,2]. Muscle glycogen concentrations are directly correlated to time to fatigue during moderately strenuous exercise ranging from 60%–80% of maximal oxygen uptake (VO_{2max}) [1]. Thus, endurance and high-intensity intermittent exercise will be adversely affected by reduced glycogen stores. During soccer matches, this would most likely occur in the second half of a game [3–5]. Soccer players with lower levels of muscle glycogen cover less distance and run at lower speeds during the last 15 min of a match [6]. Total number of sprints and markers of acceleration and deceleration capacity are reduced in the last 15 min of the normal duration of a soccer match [7]; therefore, research that targets maintaining these performance outcomes during a soccer match is important.

The glycemic index (GI) differentiates types of carbohydrates based on how fast they cause an increase in blood glucose concentrations [8]. Some studies have indicated consumption of low-GI foods prior to exercise may improve exercise performance compared to high-GI foods [9,10]. Low-GI foods cause a lower insulemic response compared to high-GI foods. Insulin inhibits fat oxidation during exercise [11]; therefore, consumption of low-GI foods might allow increased utilization of fats, lower carbohydrate usage, and preservation of glycogen stores [12–14]. Advantages of carbohydrate ingestion with different GIs prior to prolonged endurance exercises are well documented [15–17]; however, further studies need to address the possible impact of foods with different GIs on high-intensity intermittent exercise, important for many team sports (e.g., soccer, hockey, rugby). It is important to note that, during low to moderate intensity intervals (e.g., rest and recovery times) of high-intensity intermittent exercise, a considerable amount of energy needed for exercising muscles is provided by fat oxidation [18,19]. Our previous studies have shown some metabolic benefits (i.e., lower insulin levels, higher fat oxidation, lower carbohydrate oxidation and reduced lactate levels) when low-GI meals are consumed before interval treadmill exercise programmed to simulate the repeated high-intensity intervals of a typical soccer match, but performance specific to soccer is difficult to evaluate on a treadmill [20–22]. In these previous studies, boiled lentils were compared to high-GI foods (i.e., mashed potatoes with egg whites added to match for protein), but these meals may not be typical before matches for soccer players (or other athletes involved in sports with high-intensity intervals). Endurance athletes often consume sport nutrition bars [23] and surveys of youth soccer players indicate that about 37% consume food, such as sport nutrition bars, up to 1 h before games in an attempt to improve performance [24]; however, the effectiveness of a sport nutrition bar for soccer performance has never been evaluated. From a practical point of view, using sport nutrition bars (high-CHO) can be considered when time is limited before the start of competition. Therefore, the purpose of the current study was to evaluate low- and high-GI sport nutrition bars, consumed before and at half time on metabolism and performance during a soccer-specific field test, which incorporates skills important for soccer performance (i.e., agility running, ball dribbling, kicking accuracy, and ball heading) [25]. We hypothesized that a low-GI sport nutrition bar would be superior to a high-GI sport nutrition bar to improve performance and metabolic responses when consumed before and during a simulated soccer match.

2. Materials and Methods

2.1. Participants

Eight male recreational soccer players participated in this study. Their mean ± standard deviation for age, body mass, and predicted maximal oxygen uptake values were 30 ± 7 years, 76.6 ± 8.6 kg, and 56.5 ± 2.5 mL/kg/min, respectively. The University of Saskatchewan Biomedical Research Ethics board approved the study protocol, and all participants signed a consent form before the study began. The approval number is 12–33. The approval date was February 21, 2012.

2.2. Study Design

Using a randomized, double blind, counter-balanced cross-over design, low-GI and high-GI sport nutrition bars were consumed two hours before and at half time of a simulated soccer match during which soccer-specific skills (agility, ball dribbling, heading, and kicking accuracy) were assessed. Plasma glucose and insulin, non-esterified free fatty acids (NEFA), as well as fat and carbohydrate oxidation were assessed before and during the simulated soccer match.

2.3. Preliminary Test

Participants initially had their maximal aerobic power (VO_{2max}) estimated by a shuttle-run test that involved running 20 m while the speed increased by 0.14 m/s each minute until volitional exhaustion [26]. The purpose of this test was to determine participants' aerobic fitness and to determine maximal running velocity, which was used to set speeds during the exercise tests used to evaluate the different feeding conditions. Participants then performed a familiarization test of the simulated soccer match. This test was identical to the test they performed during the sports bar conditions, but was used as a "practice" run. The purpose of this practice run was to minimize any learning effects from one test to another. The practice trial involved performing 10 six-minute sessions of running between two cones that were 20 m apart, where speed was alternated between sprinting, running, jogging, and walking to simulate the exercise performed during an actual soccer match [21,25]. Speeds of walking, jogging, and running were adjusted according to each participant's predicted maximal aerobic power [26]. The speeds were dictated by "beeps" emitted from a sound system that indicated when the participant was required to reach the next 20 m distance. The speed of walking, jogging, and running were set at 25%, 55%, and 95%, respectively, of the maximal speed reached in the initial maximal shuttle run test [27]. The Bitworks Team Beep Test software (Version 4.1, Bath, UK) was used to write the scripts for each participant. Each 6 min block alternated 60 m of jogging, running, and walking, and 20 m of sprinting. Performance was assessed by tests of either agility running/ball dribbling or kicking/heading of a soccer ball. These pairs of performance tests were alternately performed between the 6 min jogging-running-walking-sprinting sessions with the exception of the first and last 3 min periods of the test during which all four performance tests were completed [25]. The total time of the exercise test (i.e., the 10 six-minute intervals and the testing between intervals) was approximately 90 min which is the same duration as an actual soccer match. The study diagram is shown in Figure 1. This soccer test has been shown to be highly reproducible and is sensitive to improvement with carbohydrate feeding [25]. Separate performance scores were derived for agility, dribbling, kicking accuracy, and heading (Figure 2). Time to complete the agility and ball dribbling courses were recorded for assessment of performance of these tests. The highest vertical jump was recorded for heading performance. A vertical jump measuring device (Vertec, Power Systems (PS), LLC, Knoxville, TN, USA) was used; participants were instructed to use their heads rather than their hands to reach the vanes. Kicking accuracy was scored according to targets set up on a wall net.

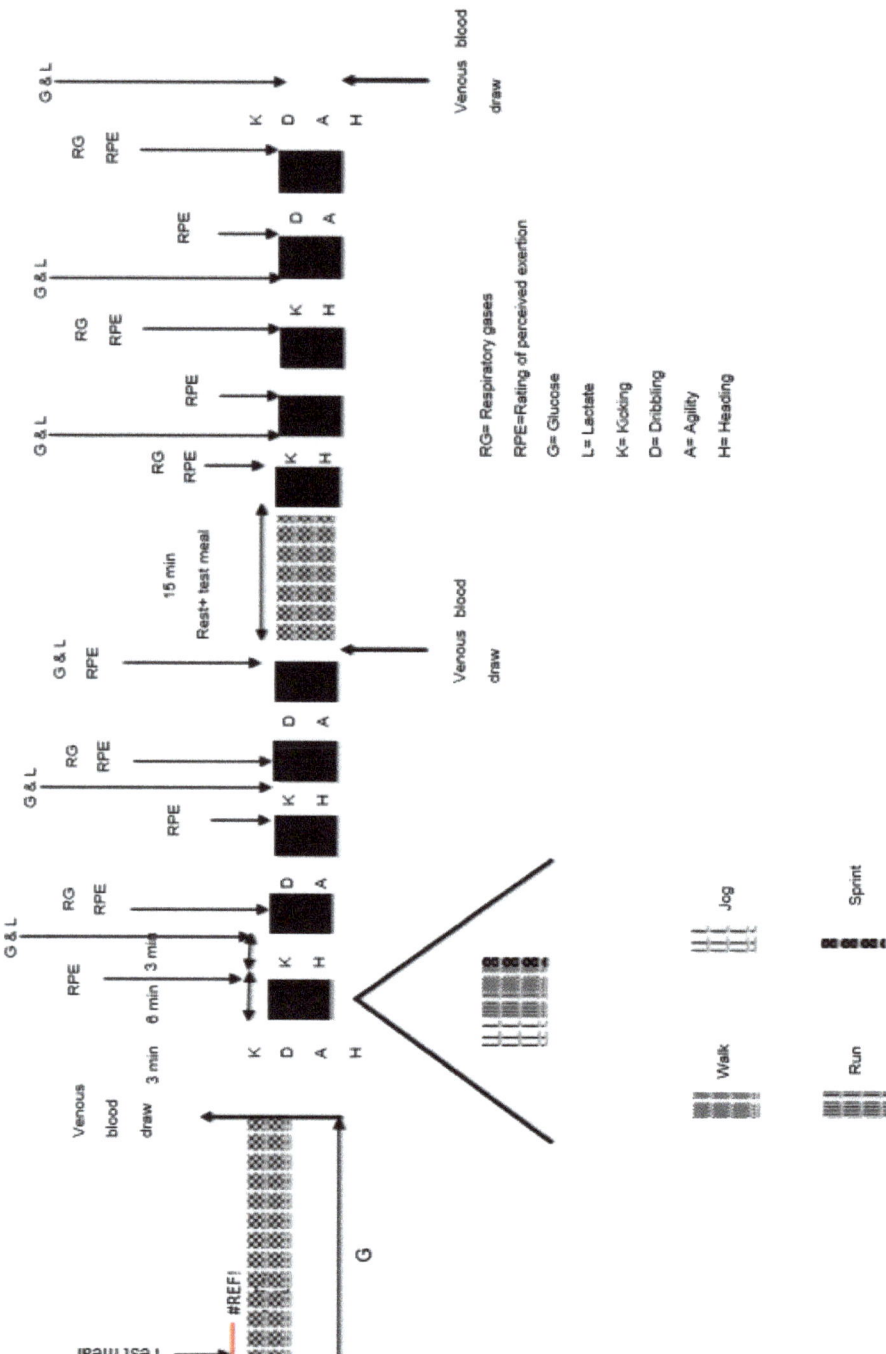

Figure 1. Schematic of the simulated soccer match. "#REF" denotes fingertip blood collection time points for glucose.

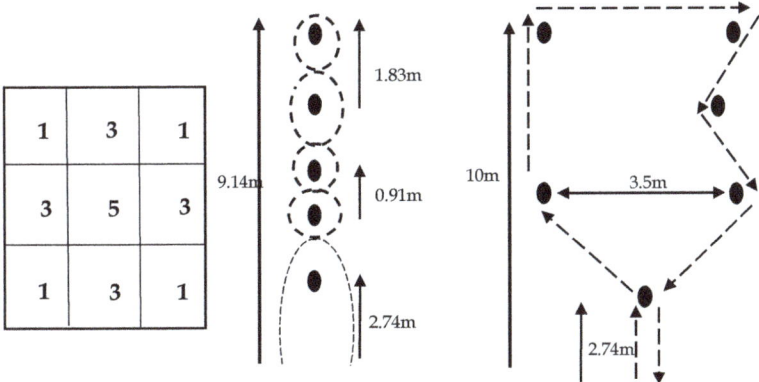

Figure 2. Schematic of the scoring grids for kicking accuracy (**left**), ball-dribbling (**middle**), and agility (**right**) protocols. Arrows represent the distance between the cones. Adopted from Currell et al., [25].

2.4. Experimental Test

Participants reported to the lab on two different occasions after a 12 h fast for a low-GI lentil-based bar (Genki Foods Inc., Winnepegosis, MB, Canada) test and a high-GI bar (Clif Bar Inc. Berelely, CA, USA) test. Each condition was separated by at least one week. The GI of the lentil bar was 45 [28] and the GI of the Clif bar was 101 [29]. The crunchy peanut butter flavor Clif bar was used because it most closely matched the Genki Bar for macronutrients and calories. The characteristics of the nutrition bars for a 70 kg participant are shown in Table 1. The testing was double blind, that is, neither the participant nor the researchers knew what type of nutrition bar was consumed. The blinding was achieved by having a separate research assistant prepare the food and having the participant consume the food in an isolated room two hours before the exercise session. Wrappers were removed from the bars and an appropriate amount of bar was placed in plastic bags. The high- and low-glycemic index sport nutrition bars were similar in appearance (i.e., same color and consistency).

Table 1. Characteristics of the sport nutrition bars for a 70 kg participant.

Description	Low-GI	High-GI
Energy (kcal)	758	761
Fat (g)	19	20
Total Carbohydrate (g)	127	116
Available carbohydrate (g), i.e., Total carbohydrate minus fiber	105	105
Protein (g)	39	31
Glycemic index	45	101

GI, glycemic index.

On each testing day participants were given enough sports bars to consume 1.5 g/kg body mass available CHO, an amount of carbohydrate that was expected to improve performance when given two hours before high-intensity intermittent exercise [20]. This amount is also within the range of recommended CHO intake prior to endurance exercise performance [8]. Participants also consumed 0.38 g/kg available CHO from the bars at half time of the simulated soccer match. Participants had 20 min to consume the bars before the match and 15 min during half time. Furthermore, the exact amount of water consumption was documented in the first trial and then it was replicated in the second trial to minimize the impact of hydration status. The feeding and the simulated soccer match were separated by two hours. Blood glucose was assessed by fingertip sampling before the food consumption and at 5, 15, 30, 60, 90, and 120 min after consumption. Blood samples from an antecubital vein were taken immediately before, at half time, and after finishing the simulated soccer match for assessment of insulin and non-esterified free fatty acid (NEFA) levels. Fingertip blood samples were collected to assess glucose by using a glucose meter (AccuCheck Compact Plus Sarstedt, Nümbrect, Germany). Venous blood samples were maintained in 10 mL tubes (BD Vacutainer SST) for 30 min to clot. The serum was then separated by centrifugation for 15 min at 3500 rpm and stored at −80 °C. Insulin concentrations were determined using an enzyme-linked immunosorbent assay (ELISA) according to the manufacturer's directions (STELLUX®Chemi Human Insulin, Alpco Diagnostics, Salem, MA, USA). The serum NEFA assay was performed using a protocol with an oleic acid standard solution as per the manufacturer's directions (NEFAHR (2), Wako Diagnostics Inc., Richmond, VA, USA). The intra-assay coefficient of variations (CVs) for the insulin, and NEFA assays were <10%. Fingertip blood samples were taken after every second 6 min exercise interval during the simulated soccer match to measure glucose and lactate levels. Blood lactate measurement was assessed using BM-Lactate test strips and the Accutrend®Lactate analyzer (Roche Group; Mannheim, Germany). The K4 b2®(Cosmed USA, Chicago, IL, USA), a portable gas exchange system was used to measure oxygen consumption (VO_2), and carbon dioxide output (VCO_2). Respiratory gases were collected during every second 6 min exercise interval to estimate carbohydrate and fat oxidation. Carbohydrate and fat oxidation rates were estimated from VO_2 and VCO_2 by using stoichiometric equations [30]. Rating of perceived exertion, using the modified 10-point Borg scale, was collected after each 6 min interval [31].

2.5. Dietary and Physical Activity Monitoring

Participants recorded their dietary intake and physical activity for the 24 h before the feeding conditions. These were photocopied and given back to the participants so they could duplicate their diets and physical activity levels during subsequent feeding conditions. This ensured that participants arrived for each exercise feeding condition with similar diets and exercise the previous 24 h.

2.6. Statistical Analysis

All variables were analyzed with a two-factor repeated measures analysis of variance (ANOVA) with factors for food condition (low-GI lentil bar vs. high-GI Clif Bar) and time during the exercise test. When there was a time main effect or an interaction between condition and time, a Least Significant Difference (LSD) post-hoc test was used to determine differences between pairs of means. All variables were also assessed for order effects with a two-factor ANOVA with factors for order (first condition vs. second condition) and time during the exercise test. Significance was accepted at a p-value less than 0.05. All results are reported as means and standard deviations.

3. Results

3.1. Blinding, Order Effects, and Adverse Events

When queried as to which bar condition participants thought they had consumed, two participants guessed correctly, while all others responded that they were unsure; this indicated the success of the blinding. There were no order effects or order*time interactions for any of the outcome variables ($p > 0.05$). There were no adverse events associated with the study. None of the participants complained of gastrointestinal discomfort after consumption of the bars.

3.2. Glucose and Insulin Responses

There was a condition*time interaction for glucose and insulin. The high-GI condition resulted in higher glucose concentrations than the low-GI condition at 105, 90, and 60 min before the simulated soccer match ($p < 0.05$; Figure 3A). The insulin response was higher in the high-GI condition compared to the low-GI condition at two hours after bar consumption ($p < 0.05$; Figure 3B).

3.3. Serum NEFA and Substrate Oxidation

NEFA concentration was not different prior to the exercise test in low-GI vs. high-GI conditions (Figure 4). NEFA concentrations significantly increased in the low-GI and high-GI conditions at 45 min and 90 min of exercise (time main effect, $p < 0.05$; Figure 4). No significant difference was seen between the conditions. During the low-GI condition, carbohydrate oxidation was significantly lower compared to the high-GI condition ($p < 0.05$; Figure 5A). There was no difference between conditions for fat oxidation ($p = 0.14$; Figure 5B). There was a time main effect ($p < 0.05$) for fat oxidation with higher rates at 45–51 min versus 63–69 min and 81–87 min ($p < 0.05$). No significant difference was observed for lactate concentrations between the two conditions (Figure 6). There was a time main effect ($p < 0.01$) for lactate, with values increasing at all time-points, except at 54 min (i.e., after half time) compared to baseline ($p < 0.05$). The lactate at 54 min was lower than at 45 min and 90 min ($p < 0.05$).

3.4. Skill Performance and Rating of Perceived Exertion

There were condition*time interactions for the agility and heading tests ($p < 0.05$). A significant improvement on the agility test and vertical jump height during simulated heading late in the soccer match (72 min) was observed after consuming the low-GI versus high-GI bar (Table 2; $p < 0.01$). No differences were apparent between bar conditions for skills performance of ball dribbling or kicking accuracy (Table 2). There was a time main effect for rating of perceived exertion (RPE; increasing throughout the simulated soccer match; $p < 0.05$); however, no significant difference was observed between the two conditions (mean RPE throughout the 90 min soccer match: low-GI = 5.2 ± 1.5 versus high-GI = 5.4 ± 1.3; $p > 0.05$).

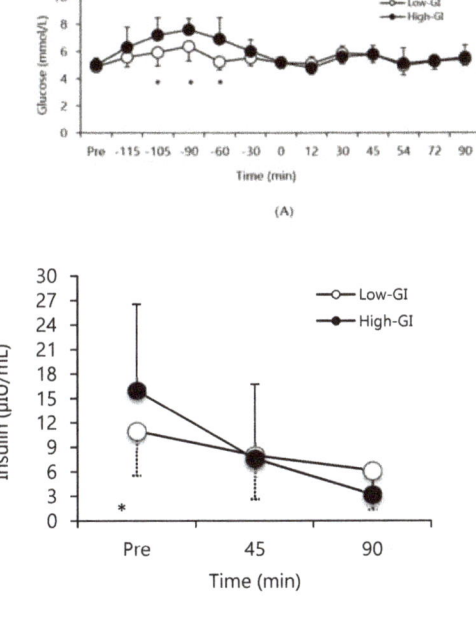

Figure 3. (**A**) Plasma glucose concentrations before and during the simulated soccer match, (**B**) Insulin concentration before, at half time, and at the end of the simulated soccer match (* $p < 0.05$ low-GI vs. high-GI sport nutrition bar). "Pre" denotes fingertip blood sample collection prior to consumption of the sport nutrition bars.

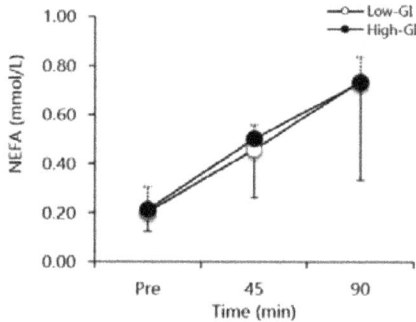

Figure 4. Non-esterified fatty acid concentrations before, at half time, and at the end of the simulated soccer match for low- and high-GI conditions. Values are means ± standard deviation (SD). Time main effect ($p < 0.05$) with 90 min > 45 min > pre ($p < 0.05$). "Pre" denotes venous blood draw prior to the simulated soccer match.

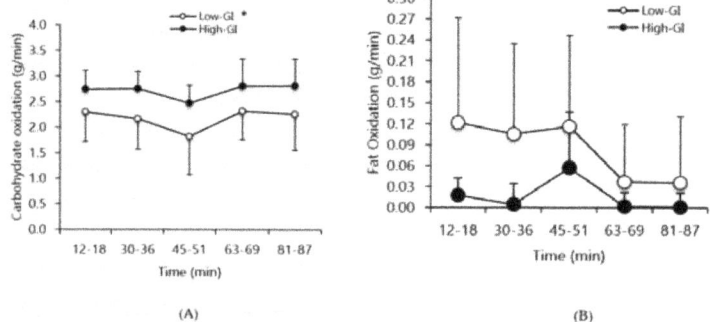

Figure 5. (**A**) Rate of carbohydrate oxidation, (**B**) and fat oxidation during the simulated soccer match in the low glycemic index and high glycemic index conditions. Values are means and SD. * Main effect for condition for carbohydrate oxidation, with the low-GI condition lower than the high-GI condition; $p < 0.05$. There was a time main effect ($p < 0.05$) for fat oxidation (45–51 min > 63–69 min, 81–87 min; $p < 0.05$).

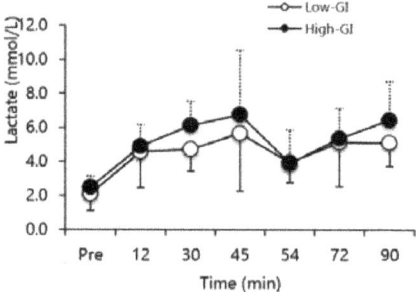

Figure 6. Lactate concentrations before and during the simulated soccer match between low- and high-glycemic index conditions. Values are means ± SD. Time main effect ($p < 0.05$) with all values except 54 min >pre, and 45 min, 90 min >54 min ($p < 0.05$).

Table 2. Performance variables during the simulated soccer match.

Condition	Low-GI						High-GI					
Time (Min)	12	30	45	54	72	90	12	30	45	54	72	90
Ball Dribbling (s)	14.0 ± 2.6	12.8 ± 2.3	11.8 ± 2.0	12.2 ± 2.2	12.6 ± 1.9	12.3 ± 2.1	13.8 ± 2.6	13.1 ± 2.3	12.1 ± 2.2	12.6 ± 1.9	12.1 ± 2.4	12.7 ± 2.7
Heading (cm)	20.5 ± 6.5	24.4 ± 4.1	24.1 ± 4.4	23.3 ± 3.5	24.7 ± 4.3 *	23.3 ± 0.9	20.3 ± 7.9	23.8 ± 4.8	23.5 ± 5.2	22.5 ± 5.2	22.2 ± 4.9	22.5 ± 5.1
Kicking (arbitrary units)	10.0 ± 5.7	11.8 ± 3.0	11.1 ± 5.5	13.1 ± 7.1	12.4 ± 4.0	9.1 ± 4.3	10.8 ± 6.5	10.1 ± 5.4	9.3 ± 5.9	9.0 ± 2.3	12.1 ± 4.5	12.8 ± 6.2
Agility (s)	6.1 ± 0.4	6.0 ± 0.6	6.0 ± 0.6	5.9 ± 0.5	5.7 ± 0.4 *	6.0 ± 0.6	6.1 ± 0.4	6.1 ± 0.6	5.9 ± 0.6	6.1 ± 0.5	6.1 ± 0.6	5.8 ± 0.6

Values are means and standard deviation (SD). * Significantly different in the low-GI versus high-GI condition ($p < 0.01$).

4. Discussion

The main finding of this study was that a low-GI sport nutrition bar consumed two hours before and at half time during a simulated soccer match elicited lower carbohydrate oxidation throughout the match and improvements in agility performance and heading (i.e., vertical jump height) late in the match compared to a high-GI sport nutrition bar. In line with this potential for CHO supplementation to improve performance, in a systematic review, Russell and Kingsley stated that six out of eight included studies found that CHO ingestion in the form of 6%–8% solution of glucose, sucrose, or maltodextrin (which would have a high-GI; i.e., GI > 70 [8]) was linked with an improvement of at least one aspect of soccer skill performance [32]. However, to the best of our knowledge this is the first study to address the influence of low- and high-GI sport nutrition bars consumed shortly prior to prolonged, high-intensity, intermittent exercise, which is typical for many team sports. Although we found improvements in some performance measures with the low-GI sport nutrition bar condition at the 72 min time point, this did not persist to the 90 min time point of the simulated soccer match (Table 2). This may be due to lack of adequate statistical power, or perhaps the GI of the bar consumed does not make a difference this late in the match (i.e., glycogen depletion may be at a low enough level in both conditions to impair performance).

Our metabolic findings are in agreement with our previous work with soccer players. In our previous work, we showed that low-GI foods (i.e., lentils; with GI ranging from 29–36; where low-GI is defined as < 55 [8]) consumed before a simulated soccer match on a treadmill reduced carbohydrate oxidation [20], increased fat oxidation [21], and tended to reduce glycogen usage [22] compared to conditions where high-GI foods (i.e., instant mashed potatoes, white bread, and egg whites to match for protein; GI ranging from 75–81; where high-GI is defined as > 70 [8]) were consumed before exercise. In these previous studies we did not see any difference between low-GI and high-GI conditions when performance was evaluated by repeated sprints at the end of the simulated treadmill test. The current study used skill performance that was quite different from these previous studies and more specific to soccer performance. The current study also used a dietary condition (i.e., sports nutrition bars) which is more likely to be used by soccer players before matches when less time is available for food consumption [5].

In line with our previous studies [20,22] glucose concentrations were significantly higher in the high-GI condition in the first 60 min following consumption versus the low-GI condition. Consequently, insulin response in the high-GI condition was higher than the low-GI condition, which might explain the higher carbohydrate oxidation during the test in the high-GI condition. Insulin inhibits fat oxidation, necessitating greater carbohydrate oxidation and potentially greater glycogen usage [11]. Muscle glycogen is a major substrate during prolonged intermittent high-intensity exercise to provide high rate of ATP re-synthesis [3,4,33]. In this study, the carbohydrate oxidation rate was lower in the low-GI condition compared to the high-GI condition averaged across all time points (i.e., there was a "condition" main effect), and the potential for glycogen sparing might have contributed to improved exercise performance (i.e., agility running and heading) late in the simulated soccer match. In line with this, Saltin [6] showed that total walking distance and sprinting speed were reduced in soccer players with lower glycogen content versus those with higher glycogen content late in a soccer match. Bendiksen et al. [34] reported that utilization of muscle glycogen was significantly lower in the last 30 min of a match suggesting an important role of sustained availability of glucose later in the match. It should be noted, however, that we did not directly assess muscle glycogen in the current study; therefore, we cannot make conclusions on whether there was sparing of glycogen during the low-GI condition.

It has been postulated that a reduction in lipolysis rate, and therefore NEFA, will occur following high-GI pre-exercise meals [15,35]; however, we found no significant difference between low-GI and high-GI conditions for appearance of NEFA in the blood. This discrepancy might have been related to the greater intensity of our test protocol versus the other studies. During higher intensity exercise, plasma NEFA concentrations decrease while glucose and glycogen utilization increase in skeletal muscle [36]. A limited rate of fat oxidation is thought to be connected with a lower flux of long chain NEFA across the mitochondrial membrane [37,38]. An alternative explanation to the lack of difference in NEFA concentration between conditions may be that the high-GI condition resulted in lower intramyocellular lipids utilization rather than lower lipolysis from adipose tissue.

The main limitation of our study was the assumption that reduced carbohydrate oxidation would lead to sparing of muscle glycogen. Direct analysis for glycogen levels by muscle biopsy would strengthen future studies comparing high- versus low-GI foods. We attempted to standardize glycogen levels between trials by having participants match their dietary intake and physical activity levels the day before each trial. For better control, it would be preferable to provide standardized meals to participants the day before trials. We would expect an increase in NEFA release from adipose tissue with the lower insulin concentration in the low-GI condition, but this was not observed. A limitation is that we did not assess glycerol, which may give more precise data on lipolysis. Another limitation is that we tested athletes after an overnight fast. The typical practice of a soccer player would most likely be to have a small breakfast and then consume a small amount of carbohydrate before the soccer match. We supplied enough of the bars to provide 1.5 g/kg available carbohydrate before the soccer match, an amount of carbohydrate that is recommended for improvement in endurance performance [8]. This required consumption of approximately five bars by each participant which totaled approximately 760 kcal (Table 1). We felt the addition of a breakfast before the bar consumption would result in excess fullness in participants. Additional limitations include a relatively small participant number, and the fact that our soccer match was simulated, rather than being an actual soccer match. Future studies could focus on the effects of consuming the bars before actual soccer matches.

5. Conclusions and Practical Application

Previous studies carried out in our lab using treadmill protocols to measure soccer performance (i.e., 1 min intervals of high-intensity running at the end of a simulated soccer match) were not very specific to soccer performance. This motivated the use of a field simulated soccer test incorporating soccer skills (i.e., agility, dribbling, kicking, and heading) to optimize the specificity of the test to the sport of soccer. Another novel aspect of the study was the assessment of sport nutrition bars given with adequate amount of recommended available carbohydrates (i.e., 1.5 g/kg) before endurance exercise performance. Previous research has generally shown that consumption of sports nutrition bars has no effect on endurance exercise performance [39–41]; however, these studies evaluated the effect of only a single sports nutrition bar before exercise. This would deliver well below the recommended amount of available carbohydrate for improving exercise performance; therefore, consumption of higher number of sports nutrition bars might seem practical. Sport nutrition bars containing high-CHO can act as an immediate snack, in particular, when soccer players are under time constraints before matches.

In conclusion, a low-GI sport nutrition bar consumed before a simulated soccer match elicited a lower carbohydrate oxidation rate and a modest improvement in performance (i.e., better agility and heading performance late in a simulated soccer match) versus a high-GI sport nutrition bar. Further studies are required to investigate how sport nutrition bars varying in GIs could impact soccer skill performance during prolonged match play (i.e., over/extra time, penalty kicks) when carbohydrate stores will be further depleted.

Author Contributions: The study was designed by P.D.C. and G.A.Z.; data were collected by M.K., J.J., and S.G.; data interpretation, analysis, and manuscript preparation were undertaken by M.K., P.D.C., and G.A.Z. All authors approved the final version of the paper. All authors have read and agreed to the published version of the manuscript.

Funding: This study was funded by Agri-food Canada and the Saskatchewan Pulse growers. The sponsors had no role in the design, execution, interpretation, or writing of the study.

Conflicts of Interest: The authors declare no conflict of interest.

References

1. Hermansen, L.; Hultman, E.; Saltin, B. Muscle glycogen during prolonged severe exercise. *Acta Physiol. Scand.* **1967**, *71*, 129–139. [CrossRef] [PubMed]
2. Jeukendrup, A. A step towards personalized sports nutrition: Carbohydrate intake during exercise. *Sports Med.* **2014**, *44* (Suppl. 1), S25–S33. [CrossRef] [PubMed]
3. Balsom, P.; Gaitanos, G.; Soderlund, K.; Ekblom, B. High intensity exercise and muscle glycogen availability in humans. *Acta Physiol. Scand.* **1999**, *165*, 337–345. [CrossRef] [PubMed]
4. Balsom, P.; Wood, K.; Olsson, P.; Ekblom, B. Carbohydrate intake and multiple sprint sports: With special reference to football (soccer). *Int. J. Sports Med.* **1999**, *20*, 48–52. [CrossRef] [PubMed]
5. Hills, S.P.; Russell, M. Carbohydrates for soccer: A focus on skilled actions and half-time practices. *Nutrients* **2017**, *10*, 22. [CrossRef]
6. Saltin, B. Metabolic fundamentals in exercise. *Med. Sci. Sports Exerc.* **1973**, *5*, 137–146. [CrossRef]
7. Russell, M.; Sparkes, W.; Northeast, J.; Cook, C.J.; Love, T.D.; Bracken, R.M.; Kilduff, L.P. Changes in acceleration and deceleration capacity throughout professional soccer match-play. *J. Strength Cond. Res.* **2016**, *30*, 2839–2844. [CrossRef]
8. Little, J.P.; Chilibeck, P.D.; Bennett, C.; Zello, G.A. Food for endurance: The evidence, with a focus on the glycaemic index. *CAB Rev. Perspect. Agric. Vet. Sci. Nutr. Nat. Resour.* **2009**, *4*, 1–13. [CrossRef]
9. Burdon, C.A.; Spronk, I.; Lun Cheng, H.; O'Connor, H.T. Effect of glycemic index of a pre-exercise meal on endurance exercise performance: A systematic review and meta-analysis. *Sports Med.* **2017**, *47*, 1087–1101. [CrossRef]
10. Heung-Sang Wong, S.; Sun, F.H.; Chen, Y.J.; Li, C.; Zhang, Y.J.; Ya-Jun Huang, W. Effect of pre-exercise carbohydrate diets with high vs low glycemic index on exercise performance: A meta-analysis. *Nutr. Rev.* **2017**, *75*, 327–338. [CrossRef]
11. Sidossis, L.S.; Stuart, C.A.; Shulman, G.I.; Lopaschuk, G.D.; Wolfe, R.R. Glucose plus insulin regulate fat oxidation by controlling the rate of fatty acid entry into the mitochondria. *J. Clin. Investig.* **1996**, *98*, 2244–2250. [CrossRef] [PubMed]
12. Febbraio, M.A.; Keenan, J.; Angus, D.J.; Campbell, S.E.; Garnham, A.P. Pre-exercise carbohydrate ingestion, glucose kinetics, and muscle glycogen use: Effect of glycemic index. *J. Appl. Physiol.* **2000**, *89*, 1845–1851. [CrossRef] [PubMed]
13. Stevenson, E.J.; Williams, C.; Mash, L.E.; Phillips, B.; Nute, M.L. Influence of high-carbohydrate mixed meals with different glycemic indexes on substrate utilization during subsequent exercise in women. *Am. J. Clin. Nutr.* **2006**, *84*, 354–360. [CrossRef] [PubMed]
14. Wu, C.L.; Nicholas, C.; Williams, C.; Took, A.; Hardy, L. The influence of high-carbohydrate meals with different glycaemic indices on substrate utilisation during subsequent exercise. *Br. J. Nutr.* **2003**, *90*, 1049–1056. [CrossRef]
15. Thomas, D.E.; Brotherhood, J.P.; Brand, J.C. Carbohydrate feeding before exercise: Effect of glycemic index. *Int. J. Sports Med.* **1991**, *12*, 180–186. [CrossRef]
16. Wu, C.L.; Williams, C. A low glycemic index meal before exercise improves endurance running capacity in men. *Int. J. Sport Nutr. Exerc. Metab.* **2006**, *16*, 510–527. [CrossRef]
17. Kaviani, M.; Chilibeck, P.D.; Jochim, J.; Gordon, J.; Zello, G.A. The glycemic index of sport nutrition bars affects performance and metabolism during cycling and next-day recovery. *J. Hum. Kinet.* **2019**, *66*, 69–79. [CrossRef]
18. Mohr, M.; Krustrup, P.; Bangsbo, J. Match performance of high-standard soccer players with special reference to development of fatigue. *J. Sports Sci.* **2003**, *21*, 519–528. [CrossRef]
19. Reilly, T. *The Science of Training—Soccer*; Routledge: London, UK, 2007.
20. Bennett, C.B.; Chilibeck, P.D.; Barss, T.; Vatanparast, H.; Vandenberg, A.; Zello, G.A. Metabolism and performance during extended high-intensity intermittent exercise after consumption of low- and high-glycaemic index pre-exercise meals. *Br. J. Nutr.* **2012**, *108*, 81–90. [CrossRef]
21. Little, J.P.; Chilibeck, P.D.; Ciona, D.; Vandenberg, A.; Zello, G.A. The effects of high and low glycemic index foods on high intensity intermittent exercise. *Int. J. Sports Physiol. Perform.* **2009**, *4*, 367–380. [CrossRef]

22. Little, J.P.; Chilibeck, P.D.; Ciona, D.; Forbes, S.; Rees, H.; Vandenberg, A.; Zello, G.A. Effect of Low- and High-Glycemic-Index Meals on Metabolism and Performance During High-Intensity, Intermittent Exercise. *Int. J. Sport Nutr. Exerc. Metab.* **2010**, *20*, 447–456. [CrossRef] [PubMed]
23. Clark, N. Eating before competing. *Physiol. Sports Med.* **1998**, *26*, 73–74. [CrossRef] [PubMed]
24. Manore, M.M.; Patton-Lopez, M.M.; Meng, Y.; Wong, S.S. Sport nutrition knowledge, behaviors and beliefs of high school soccer players. *Nutrients* **2017**, *9*, 350. [CrossRef] [PubMed]
25. Currell, K.; Conway, S.; Jeukendrup, A.E. Carbohydrate ingestion improves performance of a new reliable test of soccer performance. *Int. J. Sport Nutr. Exerc. Metab.* **2009**, *19*, 34–46. [CrossRef] [PubMed]
26. Ramsbottom, R.; Brewer, J.; Williams, C. A progressive shuttle run test to estimate maximal oxygen uptake. *Br. J. Sports Med.* **1988**, *22*, 141–144. [CrossRef] [PubMed]
27. Nicholas, C.W.; Nuttall, F.E.; Williams, C. The Loughborough Intermittent Shuttle Test: A field test that simulates the activity pattern of soccer. *J. Sports Sci.* **2000**, *18*, 97–104. [CrossRef]
28. Chilibeck, P.D.; Rooke, J.; Zello, G.A. Development of a lentil-based sports nutrition bar. *Appl. Physiol. Nutr. Metab.* **2011**, *36*, 308–309.
29. Gretebeck, R.J.; Gretebeck, K.A.; Tittelbach, T.J. Glycemic index of popular sports drinks and energy foods. *J. Am. Diet. Assoc.* **2002**, *102*, 415–417. [CrossRef]
30. Péronnet, F.; Massicotte, D. Table of nonprotein respiratory quotient: An update. *Can. J. Sport Sci.* **1991**, *16*, 23–29.
31. Borg, G.A. Perceived exertion—Note on history and methods. *Med. Sci. Sports Exerc.* **1973**, *5*, 90–93. [CrossRef]
32. Russell, M.; Kingsley, M. The efficacy of acute nutritional interventions on soccer skill performance. *Sports Med.* **2014**, *44*, 957–970. [CrossRef] [PubMed]
33. Nicholas, C.W.; Williams, C.; Boobis, L.H.; Little, N. Effect of ingesting a carbohydrate electrolyte beverage on muscle glycogen utilisation during high intensity, intermittent shuttle running. *Med. Sci. Sports Exerc.* **1999**, *31*, 1280–1286. [CrossRef] [PubMed]
34. Bendiksen, M.; Bischoff, R.; Randers, M.B.; Mohr, M.; Rollo, I.; Suetta, C.; Bangsbo, J.; Krustrup, P. The Copenhagen Soccer Test: Physiological response and fatigue development. *Med. Sci. Sports Exerc.* **2012**, *44*, 1595–1603. [CrossRef] [PubMed]
35. Wee, S.L.; Williams, C.; Tsintzas, K.; Boobis, L. Ingestion of a high-glycemic index meal increases muscle glycogen storage at rest but augments its utilization during subsequent exercise. *J. Appl. Physiol.* **2005**, *99*, 707–714. [CrossRef] [PubMed]
36. Romijn, J.A.; Coyle, E.F.; Sidossis, L.S.; Gastaldelli, A.; Horowitz, J.F.; Endert, E.; Wolfe, R.R. Regulation of Endogenous Fat and Carbohydrate-Metabolism in Relation to Exercise Intensity and Duration. *Am. J. Physiol.* **1993**, *265*, 380–391. [CrossRef]
37. Coyle, E.F.; Jeukendrup, A.E.; Wagenmakers, A.J.M.; Saris, W.H.M. Fatty acid oxidation is directly regulated by carbohydrate metabolism during exercise. *Am. J. Physiol. Endocrinol. Metab.* **1997**, *273*, E268–E275. [CrossRef]
38. Jeukendrup, A.E. Regulation of fat metabolism in skeletal muscle. *Ann. N.Y. Acad. Sci.* **2002**, *967*, 217–235. [CrossRef]
39. Kolkhorst, F.W.; MacTaggart, J.N.; Hansen, M.R. Effect of a sports food bar on fat utilisation and exercise duration. *Can. J. Appl. Physiol.* **1998**, *23*, 271–278. [CrossRef]
40. Oliver, S.K.; Tremblay, M.S. Effects of a sports nutrition bar on endurance running performance. *J. Strength Cond. Res.* **2002**, *16*, 152–156.
41. Rauch, H.G.; Hawley, J.A.; Woodey, M.; Noakes, T.D.; Dennis, S.C. Effects of ingesting a sports bar versus glucose polymer on substrate utilisation and ultra-endurance performance. *Int. J. Sports Med.* **1999**, *20*, 252–257. [CrossRef]

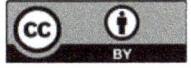

© 2020 by the authors. Licensee MDPI, Basel, Switzerland. This article is an open access article distributed under the terms and conditions of the Creative Commons Attribution (CC BY) license (http://creativecommons.org/licenses/by/4.0/).

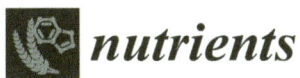

Article

Application of Continuous Glucose Monitoring for Assessment of Individual Carbohydrate Requirement during Ultramarathon Race

Kengo Ishihara [1,2,*], Natsuki Uchiyama [1], Shino Kizaki [1], Emi Mori [1,3], Tsutomu Nonaka [4] and Hiroshi Oneda [5]

1. Department of Food Sciences and Human Nutrition, Faculty of Agriculture, Ryukoku University, Shiga 520-2194, Japan
2. Department of Life Science, Manchester Metropolitan University, Manchester M1 5GD, UK
3. Department of Food and Nutrition, Jin-ai Women's College, Fukui 910-0124, Japan
4. Tail Ender's Trail Running Life, Tokyo 176-0004, Japan
5. Nagatasangyo Co., Ltd, Shiso 671-2544, Japan
* Correspondence: kengo@agr.ryukoku.ac.jp; Tel.: +81-77-599-5601

Received: 6 March 2020; Accepted: 14 April 2020; Published: 17 April 2020

Abstract: Background: The current study intended to evaluate the feasibility of the application of continuous glucose monitoring to guarantee optimal intake of carbohydrate to maintain blood glucose levels during a 160-km ultramarathon race. Methods: Seven ultramarathon runners (four male and three female) took part in the study. The glucose profile was monitored continuously throughout the race, which was divided into 11 segments by timing gates. Running speed in each segment was standardized to the average of the top five finishers for each gender. Food and drink intake during the race were recorded and carbohydrate and energy intake were calculated. Results: Observed glucose levels ranged between 61.9–252.0 mg/dL. Average glucose concentration differed from the start to the end of the race (104 ± 15.0 to 164 ± 30.5 SD mg/dL). The total amount of carbohydrate intake during the race ranged from 0.27 to 1.14 g/kg/h. Glucose concentration positively correlated with running speeds in segments ($P < 0.005$). Energy and carbohydrate intake positively correlated with overall running speed ($P < 0.01$). Conclusion: The present study demonstrates that continuous glucose monitoring could be practical to guarantee optimal carbohydrate intake for each ultramarathon runner.

Keywords: sports nutrition; continuous glucose monitoring; carbohydrate; trail running; Freestyle Libre

1. Introduction

For the first time in human history, in 2019, Eliud Kipchoge ran the marathon distance in under two hours. Recent advances in the area of sports science significantly contributed to his success. In terms of exercise nutrition, it has been recommended to consume 90 g/h of carbohydrates for endurance exercise [1,2]. This amount has been suggested based on the maximum oxidation of carbohydrate as an energy substrate [3,4] and it is noted that the rate-limiting step to oxidizing this amount of carbohydrate is the gastrointestinal absorption process [1].

A longer distance marathon is known as an ultramarathon, and the popularity of these events has increased in recent years [5]. The total energy expenditure of a 160 km ultramarathon reaches about 13,000 kcal [6]. Thus, nutritional strategies have to be considered for ultramarathon runners wanting to improve their race results, but also for those focusing primarily on finishing the event.

GI distress, which is frequently experienced by runners during all types of endurance exercise, makes the current carbohydrate intake recommendation difficult to achieve [7–10]. Several observation studies have shown that carbohydrate intake during ultramarathon races is lower than the current recommendation for carbohydrate intake. In addition to these statements and recommendations, the optimal nutritional strategies for ultramarathons have been proposed based on a baseline metabolic model [11]. It has been reported that only one study [12] achieved the carbohydrate amount suggested in the current recommendation, while others achieved less than the 60 g/h lower level of the recommendation. The lowest observed average was 31 g/h in slower runners [13].

A recently published position statement of the International Society of Sports Nutrition recommended the consumption of 150–400 kcal/h (carbohydrate, 30–50 g/h) [9]. Recent practical recommendations for ultramarathon events offered advice to consume tolerable carbohydrate intake quantities during exercise, which corresponded to 0.8–1.0 g/kg/h of carbohydrate [14]. These values were provided by comparing the race diet between fast and slow runners [13] or by comparing the carbohydrate intake of finishers and non-finishers [12].

Optimal nutrition results in a decreased risk of energy depletion, better performance [10], the prevention of acute cognitive decline, and improved athlete safety on ultramarathon courses with technical terrain or those requiring navigation [9]. However, it may prove difficult for the runner to execute the precise nutrition plan [11] and the carbohydrate requirement for ultramarathon racing varies greatly depending on the individual [9].

The aim of this study was to evaluate the feasibility of continuous glucose monitoring to improve the carbohydrate intake of ultrarunners using a continuous glucose monitoring system [15,16].

2. Materials and Methods

2.1. Study Design

This observational study was designed to determine the minimum carbohydrate requirement to maintain blood glucose level and race speed during ultramarathons. All procedures were approved by the Ryukoku University Human Research Ethics Review Board (No. 2016-08-02). All research procedures complied with the code of ethics of the World Medical Association (Declaration of Helsinki). Written informed consent was obtained from all the participants before the commencement of the study.

2.2. Study Population

Seven runners (4 male and 3 female) without injuries volunteered to participate in the study. All the runners had completed 2 to 3 races certified by the International Trail Running Association and the sum of finisher's points exceeded 12 in the last 3 years, demonstrating their experience in running Ultramarathons. Participant characteristics are presented in Table 1.

Table 1. Clinical characteristics of male and female subjects.

	Male	Female	P
Age (year)	41.5 ± 6.2	42.6 ± 1.2	0.627
Height (cm)	172.9 ± 2.7	158.0 ± 6.5	0.019
Weight (kg)	66.0 ± 9.3	47.9 ± 3.8	0.036
BMI (kg/m^2)	22.2 ± 2.8	18.9 ± 0.7	0.116
Lean body mass (kg)	56.3 ± 5.9	40.7 ± 4.3	0.012
Fat mass (kg)	22.2 ± 2.8	18.9 ± 0.7	0.116

Values are means ± SD (male, $n = 4$; female, $n = 3$).

2.3. Race Course

The present study was conducted during the 2019 Ultra trail Mt. Fuji (https://www.ultratrailmtfuji.com/), held during the last week of April, around Mt. Fuji in Japan (ambient temperature range: 2.3–19.9 °C). The distance of the course covered 165 km and the total elevation was 7942 m. The course included trails, rocks, paths, grasslands, and pavements. The course was divided into 11 segments by 10 timing gates where each runner's passing time was recorded electronically. Distances between each timing gate were 15 ± 5.4 SD km and varied from 7 to 28 km. Running time and speed between each timing gate were obtained from the official race web site. Running time between each timing gate was 1:58 ± 0:48 and 2:18 ± 0:52 h:m for the top 5 male and female finishers, respectively. All the runners had to run with backpacks to carry necessities, including food, and they could replenish food and fluid at each timing gate.

2.4. Running Speed Data Collection and Standardization

Running speed between each timing gate and overall running speed were obtained from the official race web site. The standard running speed of male and female participants (designated as 100%) for each segment were calculated by averaging the top five male and female finishers, respectively. The running speed of subjects in each segment was standardized using the following formula. The standardized running speed exceeds 100% only when running at a pace comparable to the top 1 and 2 places in each gender:

$$\%\text{Running speed} = (\text{The subject's running speed}) / ((\text{Average of top 5 finishers' running speed in each gender})) \times 100, \quad (1)$$

2.5. Glucose Data Collection and Standardization

Blood glucose profile was monitored by a minimally invasive method known as flash glucose monitoring (FGM). Its details have been reported elsewhere [15,17,18]. Briefly, the FGM system (FreeStyle Libre; Abbott Diabetes Care, Alameda, CA) mechanically reads and continuously measures glucose concentration in the interstitial fluid collected from cells immediately below the skin and produces the corresponding ambulatory glucose profile. Subjects were asked to attach the device more than 1 day before the race. The FGM sensor was applied at the back of the upper arm and glucose concentrations were obtained every 15 min [17].

The glucose concentration of each runner during the race was standardized by subtracting the resting fasting glucose concentration of the runner and was expressed as an increase from resting fasting glucose level (Δglucose). The average, highest, lowest, and the difference between the highest and lowest levels of Δglucose in each segment were used as representative values in each segment (Figure 1).

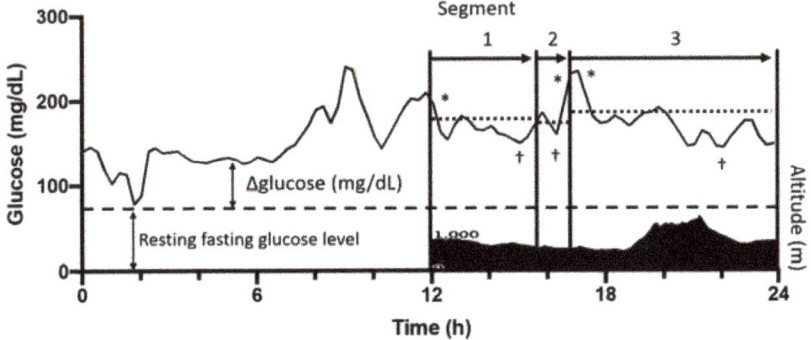

Figure 1. Schematic presentation of the standardization of glucose levels during the race. The overall race course was divided into 11 segments (arrows) by 10 timing gates. The altitude profile of the race course (filled area) and the change of glucose level (solid line) of the first 12 h of the race is shown as a representative result. ΔGlucose level was obtained by subtracting the resting fasting glucose concentration of each runner (dashed line). *, highest value of Δglucose in each segment; †, lowest value of Δglucose in each segment; dotted line, average value of Δglucose in each segment. Running speed (%) was calculated by dividing each runner's running speed by the average running speed of top 5 finishers.

2.6. Diet Supply Data Collection

Runners were asked to record their entire food and drink intake throughout the race. They reported the timing and volume of consumed food products and fluids based on pictures taken throughout the race. Food products and fluids consumed more than 60 min before the race start were not included in the calculation of nutritional intake. The energy and carbohydrate intake during the race were calculated based on the nutrition information provided by manufacturers. If data was not available, intakes were calculated based on the standard tables of food composition in Japan 2015 - (7th revised edition) [19]. The energy and carbohydrate intake were expressed relative to kg of pre-race body weight, per hour of running time. All foods were categorized with reference to previous research [20] as: sports drinks (isotonic and hypertonic formulas), gels, cola, other fluids (all other drinks consumed), sweets, fruits, bars, noodles, bread, rice products and other solids (all other products consumed).

2.7. Statistics

The data reported in the text, tables, and figures are presented as means and standard deviations, unless otherwise specified. Data were processed and analyzed in GraphPad Prism for Mac (version 8.3.1, GraphPad Inc., San Diego, CA, USA). Pearson's correlation coefficients were used to investigate the associations between running speed, glucose level, and carbohydrate intake. One-way ANOVA followed by Tukey's post-hoc test were used to compare the differences between each runner's blood glucose level. Results were considered significant when $P < 0.05$.

3. Results

3.1. General Results

The running speed of the participants ranged from 3.90 to 7.22 km/h with a standardized running speed ranging from 49.0% to 90.1%.

3.2. Relationship between Glucose Level and Running Speed

All participants were within the expected normoglycemic range during exercise (72–252 mg/dL) with the exception of one participant who exhibited a lowest value of 61.9 mg/dL as shown in Table 2. Carbohydrate mainly supplied total energy intake during the race (77.6 ± 8.58SD% of total energy intake).

Table 2. The total energy and nutrient intake, and glucose concentration during the ultramarathon.

	Subject	FS	1	2	3	MS	4	5	6	7
Sex		F	F	F	M	M	M	M	M	M
Running speed	(%)	100	89.5	87.9	72.9	100	90.1	70.0	62.0	49.0
	(min/km)	6.37	5.70	5.60	4.64	8.01	7.22	5.60	4.96	3.90
Energy intake (kcal/kg/h)		-	5.40	4.79	1.91	-	4.37	3.03	1.41	1.46
Carbohydrate intake (g/kg/h)		-	1.14	1.04	0.34	-	0.85	0.64	0.27	0.28
Protein intake (g/kg/h)		-	0.132	0.061	0.042	-	0.143	0.051	0.021	0.021
Fat intake (g/kg/h)		-	0.037	0.040	0.046	-	0.040	0.036	0.030	0.029
Glucose (mg/dL)										
During race	Average	-	131	137	104	-	145	134	121	164
	SD	-	11.9	30.2	15.0	-	20.4	20.2	22.9	30.5
	Highest	-	173	224	151	-	193	198	189	240
	Lowest	-	105	79	62	-	100	94	83	103
Resting fasting		-	53	58	40	-	57	68	83	98

FS and MS, female and male standard running speed, which correspond to the average of the top 5 finishers in each sex. F, female; M, male.

Each runner consumed carbohydrates from liquids, gels, fruits, sweets or solids as shown in Table 3. Six of 7 runners consumed more than 55% of their carbohydrates from liquids and gels (55.3% to 74.8%) except for one runner (28.4%, subject 3). Carbohydrate intake from solids ranged from 21.1% to 42.8% in the six runners and 63.8% in the other runner, who showed the highest fat intake among 7 runners (subject 3).

Table 3. Carbohydrates consumed per product type (g/kg/h).

Subject	1	2	3	4	5	6	7	% of Total
Liquids and gels	0.85	0.71	0.10	0.57	0.35	0.16	0.16	**58.8 ± 15.1**
Sports drink	0.34	0.05	0.04	0.01	0.00	0.05	0.04	11.8 ± 10.8
Cola	0.00	0.08	0.00	0.05	0.03	0.06	0.02	6.9 ± 7.5
Gel	0.51	0.57	0.04	0.51	0.32	0.05	0.06	37.2 ± 19.6
Other liquid	0.00	0.01	0.01	0.01	0.00	0.01	0.03	3.0 ± 4.3
Fruits and sweets	0.05	0.06	0.03	0.01	0.06	0.00	0.00	**4.2 ± 3.7**
Fruit	0.04	0.04	0.02	0.01	0.06	0.00	0.00	3.8 ± 3.5
Sweet	0.01	0.02	0.00	0.00	0.00	0.00	0.00	0.4 ± 0.7
Solids	0.24	0.27	0.21	0.27	0.23	0.10	0.12	**37.0 ± 13.9**
Bar	0.05	0.00	0.00	0.05	0.00	0.00	0.00	1.6 ± 2.7
Noodle	0.02	0.02	0.08	0.00	0.00	0.01	0.00	4.2 ± 8.1
Bread	0.00	0.05	0.05	0.01	0.04	0.04	0.03	7.9 ± 6.5
Rice product	0.00	0.19	0.09	0.18	0.15	0.04	0.08	18.9 ± 9.7
Other solid	0.17	0.01	0.00	0.04	0.03	0.01	0.00	4.4 ± 4.9
Total	1.14	1.04	0.34	0.85	0.64	0.27	0.28	

Subject numbers are identical to Table 2. The subtotal of each category is shown in bold.

The average, highest, lowest, and the difference between the highest and lowest levels of Δglucose in 11 segments were subjected to correlation analysis between running speed and blood glucose level. Figure 2 shows the relationship between glucose level and running speeds in each segment. The lowest ($r^2 = 0.2397$, $P = 0.0028$; $r^2 = 0.1397$, $P = 0.0501$ for male and female, respectively) and average ($r^2 = 0.1650$, $P = 0.0155$; $r^2 = 0.0531$, $P = 0.2381$ for male and female, respectively) levels of Δglucose had a significant positive correlation with running speed, but not for the highest levels of Δglucose ($r^2 = 0.0005$, $P = 0.8952$; $r^2 = 0.0125$, $P = 0.5704$ for male and female, respectively) in male runners. Similar but not significant tendencies were observed in female runners. Interestingly, a significant inverse correlation ($r^2 = 0.1198$, $P = 0.0417$; $r^2 = 0.0107$, $P = 0.6011$ for male and female, respectively) was observed between running speed and the difference between highest and lowest (D) in male runners.

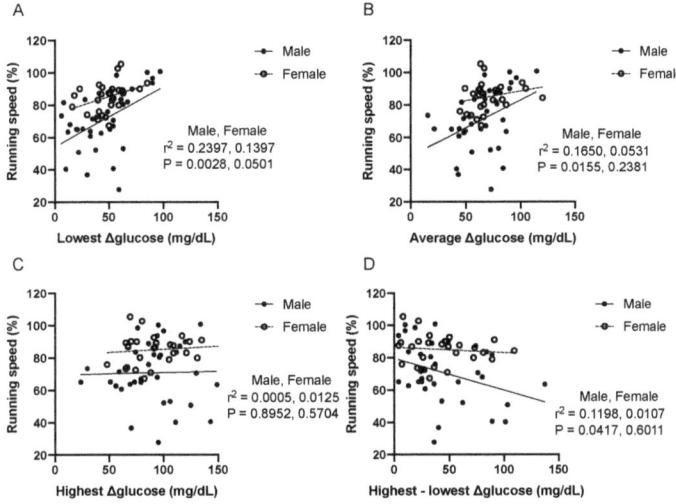

Figure 2. Scatter plots showing relationships between glucose level and running speed. The lowest (**A**), average (**B**), highest (**C**), and difference between highest and lowest (**D**) value of Δglucose levels were calculated as described in Figure 1. Each plot indicates one segment.

3.3. Relationship between Energy and Carbohydrate Intake and Running Speed

Energy intake exhibited a significant positive correlation with running speed ($r^2 = 0.8142$, $P = 0.0054$). Energy intake ranged from 1.41 to 5.40 kcal/kg/h, which is the equivalent of 86.2 to 226.7 kcal/h. A significant correlation was also found between carbohydrate intake and running speed ($r^2 = 0.7955$, $P = 0.0070$). Carbohydrate intake ranged from 0.27 to 1.14 g/h/kg (1.1 to 4.6 kcal/h/kg), which is the equivalent of 16.3 to 52.9 g/h. The energy intake from carbohydrates contributed 63% to 87% of the total energy consumed during the race. No significant correlations were observed between running speed and energy intake from protein and fat (Figure 3).

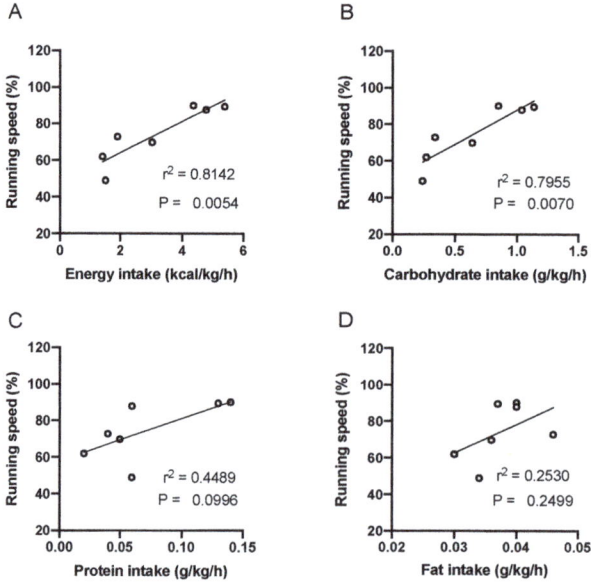

Figure 3. Scatter plots showing relationships between nutrient intake and running speed. The intake of energy (**A**), carbohydrate (**B**), protein (**C**), and fat (**D**) were calculated based on consumed food products and fluids. Each plot indicates one runner.

3.4. Relationship between the Amount of Carbohydrate Intake and Maintenance of Glucose Level during Race

Carbohydrate intake of the seven participants varied within the range of 0.27 to 1.14 g/kg/h and the carbohydrate intake of four subjects (0.27, 0.28, 0.34, and 0.64 g/kg/h) were less than the recently published practical recommendations for ultramarathons. The lowest Δglucose levels of the four subjects were 55.5%, 27.2%, 54.3%, and 66.9% compared to that of the subject who consumed 0.85 g/kg/h, respectively ($P < 0.05$). Likewise, the average level of Δglucose of the four subjects were 48.2%, 68.6%, and 73.6% compared to that of the subject who consumed 0.85 g/kg/h, respectively ($P < 0.05$). Runners who consumed 1.04 or 0.28 g/kg/h of carbohydrate showed higher values in the highest Δ glucose levels and the difference between the highest and lowest blood glucose among seven runners, which seemed to be their specific characteristics ($P < 0.05$, Figure 4).

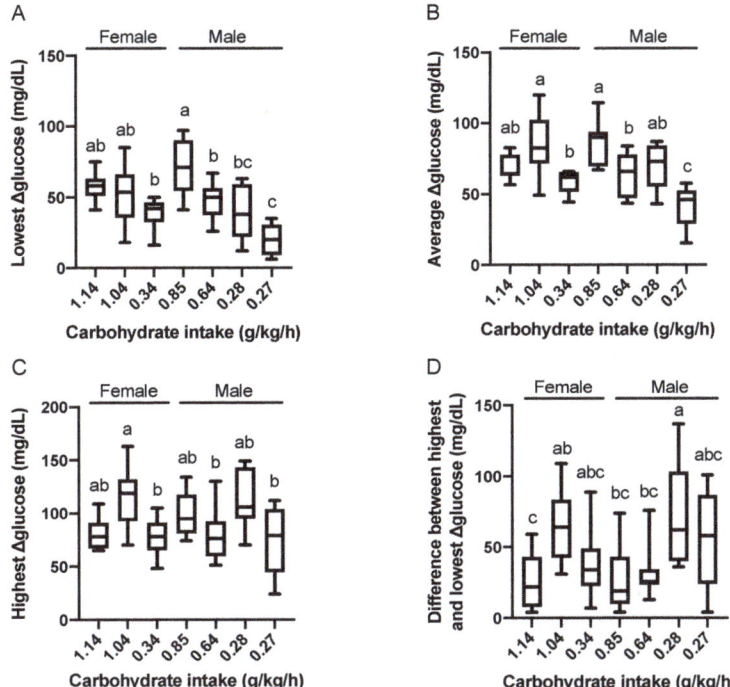

Figure 4. Relationships between carbohydrate intake and the lowest (**A**), average (**B**), highest (**C**), and the difference between the highest and lowest (**D**) value of Δglucose levels. Carbohydrate intake of each runner is expressed in the X-axis. Data are expressed using box-and-whisker plots to indicate the minimum, first quartile, median, third quartile, and maximum. Bar height indicates the average of the dots. Values without common superscript are significantly different, $P < 0.05$

4. Discussion

The aim of this study was to evaluate the feasibility of continuous glucose monitoring to improve the carbohydrate intake [9,13] of ultrarunners using a continuous glucose monitoring system. Overall carbohydrate intake in three of seven subjects were far below the recommended carbohydrate intake (30–50 g/h or 0.8 g/kg/h). A significant positive relationship was observed between higher carbohydrate intake and faster running speed as was expected from the results of previous studies [12,13]. The present study demonstrates that the avoidance of relatively low blood glucose concentrations, achieved through the intake of sufficient carbohydrates, impaired running speed during the ultramarathon. Conversely, there was no association between the highest blood glucose concentrations obtained with running speed, indicating that control of glucose homeostasis, rather than the rapid availability of carbohydrates, is the key determinant of performance. Runners consuming less than 0.8 g/kg/h of carbohydrates tended to have a reduced running speed associated with a result of low blood glucose.

Carbohydrate intake of 30–60 g/h is an established recommendation for endurance sports, with even higher amounts (i.e., up to 90 g/h and a glucose:fructose ratio of 2:1) being advocated for exercise bouts lasting more than 3 h [1,2]. However, there is a disparity between this recommendation and actual intakes in ultramarathon runners. Observation studies have demonstrated that actual carbohydrate intake during ultramarathons is less than 60 g/h in most runners [6,13,21], including slower runners consuming 37 g/h [14], with very few runners taking more than 60g of carbohydrates [22,23]. There are numerous barriers to achieve consumption of 90 g/h of a multiple-transportable carbohydrate blend. First, the absolute exercise intensity of an ultramarathon is not as high as some other endurance activities because of its extremely long duration (6, 13, 24, 48, 72 h, 6 or 10 days) [24]. Secondly, the rate-limiting step for oxidizing 90 g of carbohydrate per hour is intestinal absorption which may be affected by undertaking exercise of this intensity and duration due to changes in splanchnic blood flow. In addition, ultramarathon runners lose appetite as a result of heat, endotoxin, or vertical shaking of their digestive system during rough terrain races [24–26]. Thirdly, a practical limitation is that ultramarathon runners have to carry their food and fluid in their backpacks during long hours of racing, resulting in an increase in exercise intensity due to the additional weight being carried [14]. Fourthly, runners may have physical difficulties in consuming foods when they are keeping balance with both hands when running down steep mountains or climbing steep slopes.

For these reasons, discrepancies easily occur between the recommended amount and the actual amount of carbohydrate intake. However, the optimal amount of carbohydrate varies greatly depending on the individual [9]. Therefore, the application of a continuous glucose monitoring system could be a practical and fast method to estimate optimal carbohydrate intake for each runner.

Given the duration typical of ultramarathons (6 to 48 h), it is not feasible to meet carbohydrate consumption in its entirety during a race. Energy deficiency is common in ultramarathons [8–10,12,13,20,21,27]. Several studies using a doubly labeled water technique or respiratory gas analysis have estimated that energy expenditure during ultramarathons is about 13000 kcal [6,28,29]. The amount of carbohydrates consumed during a 160 km ultramarathon can be speculated from indirect calorimetry. The respiratory exchange ratio was 0.91 during the first 64.5km of the 160km race [29] and was 0.85 immediately after the 330km race [30]. Therefore, carbohydrate oxidation likely provided 50.0%–68.3% of energy expenditure, which is equal to 6500–9100 kcal (1625–2275 g) in the 160 km race.

Gluconeogenesis and hepatic glycogenolysis play an important role to maintain blood glucose levels during prolonged exercise in a fasted or carbohydrate deficient status. Previous studies have reported rates of gluconeogenesis and hepatic glycogenolysis as 0.07 g/kg/h and 0.03 g/kg/h, respectively, in a resting state in low carbohydrate-fed subjects [31]. The sum of these two values (0.1 g/kg/h), endogenous glucose production, would be the minimum amount of carbohydrate required to maintain blood glucose during a resting state. The endogenous glucose production significantly increases to 0.36 g/kg/h during exercise at 55% of peak power output [31] or to 0.48 g/kg/h during exercise at the lactate threshold level in fasted, well trained subjects [32]. Consistently with these findings, three subjects in the present study with a carbohydrate intake of less than 0.48 g/kg/h could not maintain their blood glucose concentrations during the ultramarathon race.

The main limitation of this study is the small number of participants. The present study supports the effectiveness of a recently published position statement of the International Society of Sports Nutrition [10] and practical recommendation for ultramarathon participants to prevent hypoglycemia during exercise. Relationships among carbohydrate intake, the lowest Δglucose, and running speed are relevant in male runners rather than female runners. These observations coincide with the previously reported gender-specific differences in fuel utilization during exercise. Women showed higher lipid oxidation caused by higher plasma adiponectin [33], higher muscle triglyceride utilization [34], low plasma glucose [35], and higher fasting hepatic glucose uptake [36] compared to men. However, more subjects are required to conclude that the observed differences between male and female runners were derived from gender-specific factors.

Hydration and GI distress are negligible factors affecting running speed. Hydration is a factor causing GI distress [37], but these factors could not be standardized in the study. Dehydration issues were not observed, which may be associated a steady rain during the race. These two factors should be quantitatively assessed and statistically analyzed as a factor affecting running speed in larger numbers of participants.

The insufficient standardization of food intake before and during the race is another limitation. The following factors should be appropriately controlled in future research: pre-race meals within 48 h of the start of the race, caffeine intake, gastrointestinal distress, and objective recording of food and drink intake by action cameras as reported [20].

Another limitation of this study is a slower rise and generally lower glucose peak values in the FGM system used in the present study as compared with the blood sampling, and this may underestimate the effect of carbohydrate ingestion on glucose response [18]. Nevertheless, the non-invasive and fast understanding of fluctuations of glucose level according to the specific characteristics of each athlete would be useful to plan and modify a personal nutrient strategy during an ultramarathon race.

The other limitation of the present study was large fluctuations in running speed in the ultramarathon. The running speeds in 11 segments varied in a range of 5.5 to 14.3 km/h and 4.8 to 11.8 km/h even in top five male and female runners, respectively. We speculated that these fluctuations in running speed were mainly associated with two factors: terrain [26] and physiological changes such as muscle fatigue and energy deficiency. Therefore, the running speeds of the subjects were standardized using the top 5 finishers to explore the relationship between blood glucose levels and running speed. The precise and objective power meters for running, which are already applicable in cycling studies [38], or accurate physical workload calculation based on GPS monitoring, would enable more accurate analysis between running performance and blood glucose.

5. Conclusions

In conclusion, the present study demonstrates that continuous glucose monitoring could be practical to guarantee optimal carbohydrate intake for each ultramarathon runner. Decreases in blood glucose during ultramarathons may be attributed to many factors, including sub-optimal carbohydrate intake. Additionally, individual characteristics such as the sex, age, or energy intake of each runner may have had a greater influence on blood glucose fluctuations across the race; thus, utilizing a continuous glucose monitor may help inform better race nutrition strategies.

Author Contributions: Conceptualization, K.I.; methodology, K.I., E.M. and T.N.; software, K.I., N.U. and S.K.; validation, K.I. and T.N.; formal analysis, K.I.; investigation, K.I., N.U., S.K. and T.N.; resources, K.I. and H.O.; data curation, K.I., N.U., S.K. and T.N; writing—original draft preparation, K.I.; writing—review and editing, K.I. and T.N.; visualization, K.I. and T.N.; supervision, K.I.; project administration, K.I.; funding acquisition, K.I. and H.O. All authors have read and agreed to the published version of the manuscript.

Funding: This research was funded by RYUKOKU University and Nagatasangyo.co. (Hyogo, Japan).

Acknowledgments: We express our gratitude and deep appreciation to Gethin H. Evans, PhD in Manchester Metropolitan University for supporting academic writing. We thank Masumi Nakao, Yuko Koshiba, Shin Uehira and Yasuhito Okumura for recruiting participants. We also thank all the participants for their cooperation in the investigation.

Conflicts of Interest: The author declare that his study has been financed by RYUKOKU university and Nagatasangyo.co. (Hyogo, Japan). They did not participate in the experimental design, data collection, data analysis, interpretation of the data, writing of the manuscript, or in the decision to publish the results.

References

1. Jeukendrup, A.E. Carbohydrate intake during exercise and performance. *Nutrition* **2004**, *20*, 669–677. [CrossRef] [PubMed]
2. Burke, L.M.; Hawley, J.A.; Wong, S.H.S.; Jeukendrup, A.E. Carbohydrates for training and competition. *J. Sports Sci.* **2011**, *29*, S17–S27. [CrossRef] [PubMed]
3. Hawley, J.A.; Dennis, S.C.; Noakes, T.D. Oxidation of Carbohydrate Ingested During Prolonged Endurance Exercise. *Sport. Med. An Int. J. Appl. Med. Sci. Sport Exerc.* **1992**, *14*, 27–42. [CrossRef] [PubMed]
4. Wagenmakers, A.J.M.; Brouns, F.; Saris, W.H.M.; Halliday, D. Oxidation rates of orally ingested carbohydrates during prolonged exercise in men. *J. Appl. Physiol.* **1993**, *75*, 2774–2780. [CrossRef]
5. Nikolaidis, P.; Knechtle, B. Age of peak performance in 50-km ultramarathoners – is it older than in marathoners? *Open Access J. Sport. Med.* **2018**, *9*, 37–45. [CrossRef]
6. Arribalzaga, M.; Ruano, M.; Saiz, S. Review of the Food Guidelines in Continuous Ultramarathon. *J. Nutr. Food Sci.* **2017**, *7*, 635.

7. Pfeiffer, B.; Stellingwerff, T.; Hodgson, A.B.; Randell, R.; Pöttgen, K.; Res, P.; Jeukendrup, A.E. Nutritional intake and gastrointestinal problems during competitive endurance events. *Med. Sci. Sports Exerc.* **2012**, *44*, 344–351. [CrossRef]
8. Wardenaar, F.C.; Dijkhuizen, R.; Ceelen, I.J.M.; Jonk, E.; de Vries, J.H.M.; Witkamp, R.F.; Mensink, M. Nutrient Intake by Ultramarathon Runners: Can They Meet Recommendations? *Int. J. Sport Nutr. Exerc. Metab.* **2015**, *25*, 375–386. [CrossRef]
9. Tiller, N.B.; Roberts, J.D.; Beasley, L.; Chapman, S.; Pinto, J.M.; Smith, L.; Wiffin, M.; Russell, M.; Sparks, S.A.; Duckworth, L.; et al. International Society of Sports Nutrition Position Stand: Nutritional considerations for single-stage ultra-marathon training and racing. *J. Int. Soc. Sports Nutr.* **2019**, *16*, 1–23. [CrossRef]
10. Williamson, E. Nutritional implications for ultra-endurance walking and running events. *Extrem. Physiol. Med.* **2016**, *5*, 13. [CrossRef]
11. Pruitt, K.A.; Hill, J.M. Optimal pacing and carbohydrate intake strategies for ultramarathons. *Eur. J. Appl. Physiol.* **2017**, *117*, 2527–2545. [CrossRef]
12. Stuempfle, K.J.; Hoffman, M.D.; Weschler, L.B.; Rogers, I.R.; Hew-Butler, T. Race diet of finishers and non-finishers in a 100 mile (161 km) mountain footrace. *J. Am. Coll. Nutr.* **2011**, *30*, 529–535. [CrossRef] [PubMed]
13. Costa, R.J.S.; Gill, S.K.; Hankey, J.; Wright, A.; Marczak, S. Perturbed energy balance and hydration status in ultra-endurance runners during a 24 h ultra-marathon. *Br. J. Nutr.* **2014**, *112*, 428–437. [CrossRef]
14. Costa, R.J.S.; Knechtle, B.; Tarnopolsky, M.; Hoffman, M.D. Nutrition for Ultramarathon Running: Trail, Track, and Road. *Int. J. Sport Nutr. Exerc. Metab.* **2019**, *29*, 130–140. [CrossRef] [PubMed]
15. Al Hayek, A.A.; Robert, A.A.; Al Dawish, M.A. Evaluation of FreeStyle Libre Flash Glucose Monitoring System on Glycemic Control, Health-Related Quality of Life, and Fear of Hypoglycemia in Patients with Type 1 Diabetes. *Clin. Med. Insights Endocrinol. Diabetes* **2017**, *10*, 1–6. [CrossRef] [PubMed]
16. Sengoku, Y.; Nakamura, K.; Ogata, H.; Nabekura, Y.; Nagasaka, S.; Tokuyama, K. Continuous Glucose Monitoring during a 100-km Race: A Case Study in an Elite Ultramarathon Runner. *Int. J. Sports Physiol. Perform.* **2015**, *10*, 124–127. [CrossRef] [PubMed]
17. Fokkert, M.J.; Van Dijk, P.R.; Edens, M.A.; Abbes, S.; De Jong, D.; Slingerland, R.J.; Bilo, H.J.G. Performance of the freestyle libre flash glucose monitoring system in patients with type 1 and 2 diabetes mellitus. *BMJ Open Diabetes Res. Care* **2017**, *5*, e000320. [CrossRef]
18. Fokkert, M.J.; Damman, A.; Van Dijk, P.R.; Edens, M.A.; Abbes, S.; Braakman, J.; Slingerland, R.J.; Dikkeschei, L.D.; Dille, J.; Bilo, H.J.G. Use of FreeStyle Libre Flash Monitor Register in the Netherlands (FLARE-NL1): Patient Experiences, Satisfaction, and Cost Analysis. *Int. J. Endocrinol.* **2019**, *2019*. [CrossRef]
19. MEXT. *Standard Tables of Food Composition in Japan-2015-(Seventh Revised Version)*; Ministry of Education: Tokyo, Japan, 2015.
20. Arnaoutis, G.; Leveritt, M.; Wardenaar, F.C.; Hoogervorst, D.; Versteegen, J.J.; Van Der Burg, N.; Lambrechtse, K.J.; Bongers, C.C.W.G. Real-Time Observations of Food and Fluid Timing During a 120 km Ultramarathon. *Front. Nutr.* **2018**, *5*, 32.
21. Clark, H.R.; Barker, M.E.; Corfe, B.M. Nutritional strategies of mountain marathon competitors—An observational study. *Int. J. Sport Nutr. Exerc. Metab.* **2005**, *15*, 160–172. [CrossRef]
22. Hoffman, M.D.; Stuempfle, K.J. Hydration strategies, weight change and performance in a 161 km ultramarathon. *Res. Sport. Med.* **2014**, *22*, 213–225. [CrossRef] [PubMed]
23. Zalcman, I.; Guarita, H.V.; Juzwiak, C.R.; Crispim, C.A.; Antunes, H.K.M.; Edwards, B.; Tufik, S.; de Mello, M.T. Nutritional status of adventure racers. *Nutrition* **2007**, *23*, 404–411. [CrossRef]
24. Knechtle, B.; Nikolaidis, P.T. Physiology and pathophysiology in ultra-marathon running. *Front. Physiol.* **2018**, *9*, 634. [CrossRef]
25. Stuempfle, K.J.; Valentino, T.; Hew-Butler, T.; Hecht, F.M.; Hoffman, M.D. Nausea is associated with endotoxemia during a 161-km ultramarathon. *J. Sports Sci.* **2016**, *34*, 1662–1668. [CrossRef] [PubMed]
26. Brown, J.S.; Connolly, D.A. Selected human physiological responses during extreme heat: The Badwater Ultramarathon. *J. strength Cond. Res.* **2015**, *29*, 1729–1736. [CrossRef] [PubMed]
27. Martinez, S.; Aguilo, A.; Rodas, L.; Lozano, L.; Moreno, C.; Tauler, P. Energy, macronutrient and water intake during a mountain ultramarathon event: The influence of distance. *J. Sports Sci.* **2018**, *36*, 333–339. [CrossRef] [PubMed]

28. Hill, R.J.; Davies, P.S. Energy expenditure during 2 wk of an ultra-endurance run around Australia. *Med. Sci. Sports Exerc.* **2001**, *33*, 148–151. [CrossRef]
29. Dumke, C.L.; Shooter, L.; Lind, R.H.; Nieman, D.C. Indirect calorimetry during ultradistance running: A case report. *J. Sports Sci. Med.* **2006**, *5*, 692–698.
30. David Cotter, J.; Gatterer, H.; Vernillo, G.; Savoldelli, A.; Skafidas, S.; Zignoli, A.; La Torre, A.; Pellegrini, B.; Giardini, G.; Trabucchi, P.; et al. An Extreme Mountain Ultra-Marathon Decreases the Cost of Uphill Walking and Running. *Front. Physiol.* **2016**, *7*, 530.
31. Webster, C.C.; Noakes, T.D.; Chacko, S.K.; Swart, J.; Kohn, T.A.; Smith, J.A.H. Gluconeogenesis during endurance exercise in cyclists habituated to a long-term low carbohydrate high-fat diet. *Authors. J. Physiol. C* **2016**, *594*, 4389–4405. [CrossRef]
32. Emhoff, C.A.W.; Messonnier, L.A.; Horning, M.A.; Fattor, J.A.; Carlson, T.J.; Brooks, G.A. Gluconeogenesis and hepatic glycogenolysis during exercise at the lactate threshold. *J. Appl. Physiol.* **2013**, *114*, 297–306. [CrossRef] [PubMed]
33. Geer, E.B.; Shen, W. Gender differences in insulin resistance, body composition, and energy balance. *Gend. Med.* **2009**, *6*, 60–75. [CrossRef] [PubMed]
34. Wismann, J.; Willoughby, D. Gender Differences in Carbohydrate Metabolism and Carbohydrate Loading. *J. Int. Soc. Sports Nutr.* **2006**, *3*, 28–35. [CrossRef] [PubMed]
35. Soeters, M.R.; Sauerwein, H.P.; Groener, J.E.; Aerts, J.M.; Ackermans, M.T.; Glatz, J.F.C.; Fliers, E.; Serlie, M.J. Gender-related differences in the metabolic response to fasting. *J. Clin. Endocrinol. Metab.* **2007**, *92*, 3646–3652. [CrossRef]
36. Keramida, G.; Peters, A.M. Fasting hepatic glucose uptake is higher in men than women. *Physiol. Rep.* **2017**, *5*, e13174. [CrossRef]
37. Rehrer, N.J.; Beckers, E.J.; Brouns, F.; Ten Hoor, F.; Saris, W.H. Effects of dehydration on gastric emptying and gastrointestinal distress while running. *Med. Sci. Sports Exerc.* **1990**, *22*, 790–795. [CrossRef]
38. Paton, C.D.; Hopkins, W.G. Tests of cycling performance. *Sport. Med.* **2001**, *31*, 489–496. [CrossRef]

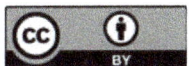 © 2020 by the authors. Licensee MDPI, Basel, Switzerland. This article is an open access article distributed under the terms and conditions of the Creative Commons Attribution (CC BY) license (http://creativecommons.org/licenses/by/4.0/).

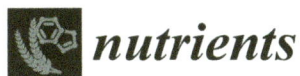

Communication

Effects of Ashwagandha (*Withania somnifera*) on VO$_{2max}$: A Systematic Review and Meta-Analysis

Jorge Pérez-Gómez [1], Santos Villafaina [2,*], José Carmelo Adsuar [1], Eugenio Merellano-Navarro [3] and Daniel Collado-Mateo [4]

1. HEME Research Group, Faculty of Sport Sciences, University of Extremadura, 10003 Caceres, Spain; jorgepg100@gmail.com (J.P.-G.); jadssal@unex.es (J.C.A.)
2. Physical Activity and Quality of Life Research Group (AFYCAV), Faculty of Sport Science, University of Extremadura, 10003 Cáceres, Spain
3. Facultad de Educación, Universidad Autónoma de Chile, Talca 3460000, Chile; emerellano@gmail.com
4. Centre for Sport Studies, Rey Juan Carlos University, Fuenlabrada, 28943 Madrid, Spain; danicolladom@gmail.com
* Correspondence: svillafaina@unex.es; Tel.: +34-927-257-460

Received: 15 March 2020; Accepted: 14 April 2020; Published: 17 April 2020

Abstract: The purpose of this study was to systematically review the scientific literature about the effects of supplementation with Ashwagandha (*Withania somnifera*) on maximum oxygen consumption (VO$_{2max}$), as well as to provide directions for clinical practice. A systematic search was conducted in three electronic databases following the Preferred Reporting Items for Systematic Reviews and Meta-Analyses Guidelines (PRISMA). The inclusion criteria were: (a) VO$_{2max}$ data, with means ± standard deviation before and after the supplement intervention, (b) the study was randomized controlled trial (RCT), (c) the article was written in English. The quality of evidence was evaluated according to the Grading of Recommendations, Assessment, Development and Evaluation (GRADE) approach. A meta-analysis was performed to determine effect sizes. Five studies were selected in the systematic review (162 participants) and four were included in the meta-analysis (142 participants). Results showed a significant enhancement in VO$_{2max}$ in healthy adults and athletes ($p = 0.04$). The mean difference was 3.00 (95% CI from 0.18 to 5.82) with high heterogeneity. In conclusion, Ashwagandha supplementation might improve the VO$_{2max}$ in athlete and non-athlete people. However, further research is need to confirm this hypothesis since the number of studies is limited and the heterogeneity was high.

Keywords: ergogenic aids; maximum oxygen consumption; performance sports; physical fitness

1. Introduction

Maximum oxygen consumption (VO$_{2max}$) is a physiological parameter that defines the aerobic capacity of a person. It is an indicator of the cardiorespiratory fitness that describes health status [1] and sport performance [2]. Focusing on competitive sports, the VO$_{2max}$, together with running economy and the anaerobic threshold, is one of the main factors that determine success in endurance activities [3], and also contributes to increase the team sports performance by increasing work intensity, distance covered, and number of sprints completed [4]. However, from the point of view of the physical training, there are still controversies about the best training intensity to enhance the VO$_{2max}$ [5,6].

Apart from sport performance, VO$_{2max}$ has special interest in the field of health. Low values of VO$_{2max}$ (<17.5 mL·min^{-1}·kg^{-1}) are associated with an increased risk of mortality and loss of independent lifestyle in adults and elderly [7], while high values of cardiorespiratory fitness have been associated with a reduced risk of cardiovascular diseases [8,9]. The VO$_{2max}$ level is also important in children, where a higher aerobic capacity is related to better quality of life [10].

Ashwagandha (*Withania somnifera*) is a plant in the Solanaceae family. The extract of the Ashwagandha root has many biological implications due to its diverse phytochemicals [11], so it has been used, singly or in combination with other natural plants, in many research studies for its properties: anti-diabetic [12], anti-inflammatory [13], anti-microbial [14], anti-tumor [15], anti-stress [16], cardioprotective [17], or neuroprotective [18]. It also displays enhanced endothelial function [11], reduces reactive oxygen species [13], regulates apoptosis [19], and modulates mitochondrial function [11], showing to be effective to treat aging effects [20], anxiety and stress [21], arthritis [22], cognitive functions and memory [23], diabetes [12], epilepsy [24], fatigue [25], neurodegenerative diseases [26], pain [27], thyroid function [28], and skin diseases [29].

In spite of the relevant benefits of supplementation with Ashwagandha, only four meta-analyses have been carried out evaluating its efficacy on anti-inflammatory effects [30], on impotence and infertility treatment [31], on neurobehavioral disorders [32] and anxiety [33]. However, there are no meta-analyses that analyze the effect of Ashwagandha on physical performance. Therefore, the purpose of this study was to systematically review the scientific literature about the effects of supplementation with Ashwagandha on VO_{2max} and to provide practical recommendations. Besides, a meta-analysis was carried out to determine the effect sizes of Ashwagandha on VO_{2max}.

2. Methods

The review was conducted following the statements of the Preferred Reporting Items for Systematic Reviews and Meta-Analyses Guidelines (PRISMA).

2.1. Literature Search

To find the studies reported in the meta-analysis, several electronic databases were screened: PubMed (Medline), Web of Science (which includes other databases such as Current Contents Connect, Derwent Innovations Index, Korean Journal Database, Medline, Russian Science Citation Index, and Scielo Citation Index) and Google Scholar. The search was conducted in September 2019. The search terms were: (a) the type of treatment (Ashwagandha or "*withania somnifera*") and (b) the outcome variable ("oxygen consumption" or "aerobic" or "VO_2"). The search was conducted using the treatment and the outcome variables, separated by the Boolean operator "and".

2.2. Study Selection

The inclusion criteria were: (a) VO_{2max} data, with means ± standard deviation (SD) before and after the supplement intervention; (b) the study was a randomized controlled trial (RCT); (c) the article was written in English. Two independent authors selected the potentially eligible articles from the databases. There were no disagreements.

2.3. Quality of the Evidence and Risk of Bias

The quality of the evidence was categorized using the Grading of Recommendations, Assessment, Development and Evaluation (GRADE) approach. The risk of bias was assessed by the Cochrane Collaboration's tool for assessing risk of bias. This tool classified the selection, performance, detection, attrition, and reporting bias into low, high, or unclear risk of bias.

2.4. Data Collection

Two authors independently extracted data from the studies. The information included: participants, interventions, comparisons, outcomes, and study design (PICOS), following the recommendations from the PRISMA statement. Table 1 shows age, sex, sample size, and condition of the participants. Table 2 presents intervention and the comparison groups, including type of supplementation with the doses, duration of the study, and the daily frequency of the supplementation. Figure 3 displays results for the different outcomes. Study design was not included in any table because all studies were RCT.

Table 1. Characteristics of the sample.

RCT	Weeks	Groups, Sample Size and Sex	Age (Years)	Country	Population
Shenoy 2012	8	AS: 20 (M and F) CG: 20 (M and F)	18–27	India	Elite cyclists
Malik 2013	8	AS: 16 (M) CG: 16 (M)	16–19	India	Hockey players
Choudhary 2015	12	AS: 25 (M and F) CG: 25 (M and F)	20–45	India	Athletes
Tripathi 2016	2	AS: 10 (M) CG: 10 (M)	18–45	India	Healthy adults
Sandhu 2010	8	AS: 10 (M and F) CG: 10 (M and F)	18–25	India	Healthy adults

RCT: randomized controlled trial; AS: Ashwagandha group; M: males; F: females; CG: control group.

Table 2. Characteristics of the interventions.

RCT	Ashwagandha Group Type of Supplementation	Control Group Type of Supplementation	Dose (mg)	Duration of the Study	Daily Frequency	Total Dose (g)
Shenoy 2012	Ashwagandha in gelatin capsules	Capsules containing starch powder	500	8 weeks	twice	56
Malik 2013	Roots of WS	Sugar power was filled in gelatin capsules	500	8 weeks	once	28
Choudhary 2015	One capsule of KSM-66 Ashwagandha	Identical capsules containing sucrose	300	12 weeks	twice	50.4
Tripathi 2016	WS aqueous extract in the capsule form	Maize starch capsule	330	2 weeks	once	4.62
Sandhu 2010	WS filled in gelatin capsules	Capsules filled with flour	500	8 weeks	once	28

RCT: randomized controlled trial; KSM-66: commercial name of an Ashwagandha extract; WS: Withania Somnifera. Total dose was calculated as: total dose (g) = (dose (mg) × daily frequency × study duration (days))/1000.

2.5. Statistical Analysis

The main outcome of this meta-analysis was VO_{2max}. The meta-analysis was conducted using the Revision Manager (RevMan) software (version 5.3) obtained from Cochrane Collaboration web. Post-intervention mean and SD were extracted and used for meta-analyses. All articles reported VO_2 max as mL/kg/min. Mean difference was calculated using a random model. The heterogeneity between the studies was calculated using Tau^2, I^2, and Chi^2 tests. Although there is no consensus about the definition of "mild", "moderate", or "severe" heterogeneity, Higgins and Thompson [34] suggested that values for I^2 higher than 56% would mean large heterogeneity while values lower than 31% would be related to low heterogeneity.

3. Results

3.1. Study Selection

The PRISMA flow diagram is showed in Figure 1. A total of 129 records were identified, 9 of which were removed because they were duplicated. Of the remaining 120 articles, 92 were excluded because they were not related with the topic, 4 studies were not written in English, and 4 were reviews. After reading the remaining 20 articles, another 15 studies did not meet the inclusion criteria and were excluded. Therefore, 5 studies were included in the systematic review. However, the article by Sandhu et al. [35] was excluded from meta-analysis due to the odd results. In this regard, they evaluated healthy young males and females aged between 18 and 25 with body mass index between 18 and 25. Their mean peak VO_{2max} was lower than 14mL/kg/min, which is so much lower than expected for healthy young people and less than half the mean of the rest of the included studies (46.18 mL/kg/min).

We tried to contact with the authors in order to obtain a reason for that, but at the time this article was considered for publication, we did not receive a response. Considering that in the article authors did not explain an incremental test to obtain the VO_{2max}, we believe that they measured the gas exchange at rest, reporting the oxygen consumption (VO_2). Therefore, this article was included in systematic review but not in the meta-analysis.

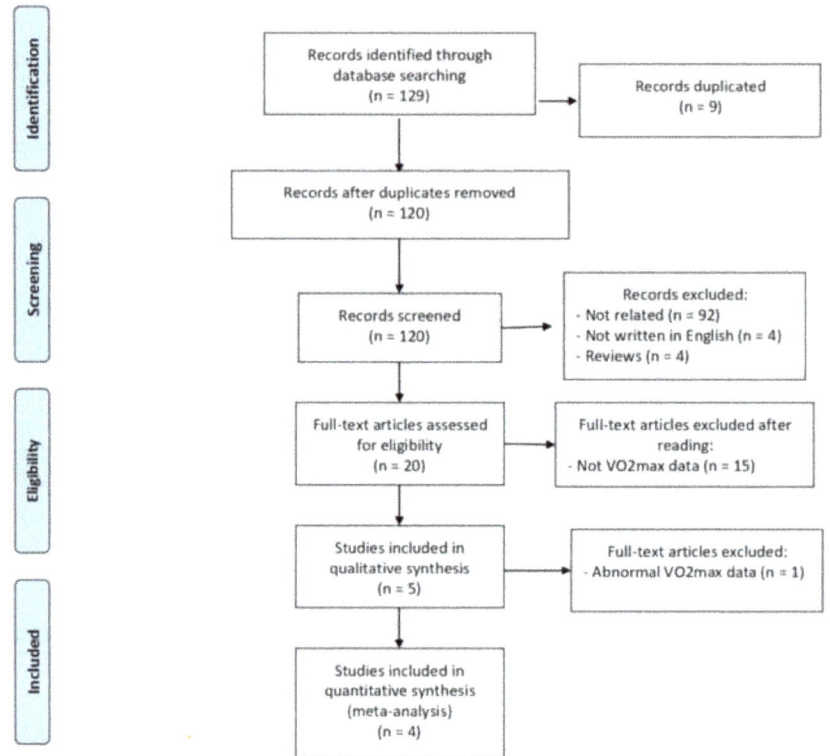

Figure 1. Flow chart delineating the complete systematic review process.

3.2. Quality of Evidence and Risk of Bias

The evidence of the effects on VO_{2max} was initially classified as "high quality" due to all the selected articles were RCT, but the evidence dropped twice because of the small sample size and due to the high degree of heterogeneity. Therefore, the final quality of the evidence was low. The Cochrane Collaboration's tool for assessing risk of bias (Figure 2) showed that the poorer scores were obtained in the performance and detection bias due to unclear reporting.

3.3. Study Characteristics

Study characteristics are summarized in Table 1. The total number of participants included in this systematic review were 162. Of these, 81 belonged to the Ashwagandha group and 81 were the placebo (control) group. The age ranged from 16 to 45 years old. The sample was comprised exclusively of healthy adults and athletes.

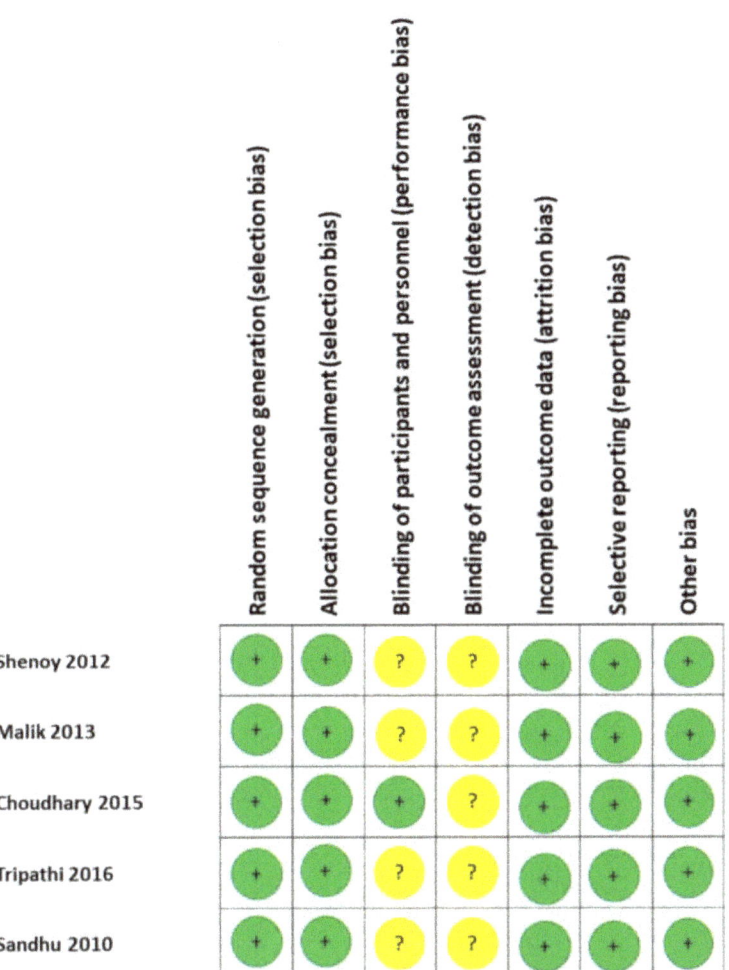

Figure 2. The Cochrane Collaboration's tool for assessing risk of bias.

3.4. Interventions

The characteristics of the Ashwagandha supplementation and placebo group are displayed in Table 2. The doses varied from 300 to 500 mg and the daily frequency intake was once or twice a day. The total duration of the intervention varied from 2 to 12 weeks.

3.5. Outcome Measures

The study of Choudhary et al. [36] found a significant group*treatment interaction in the VO_{2max}. The remaining four articles only found within-group improvement in VO_{2max} after the supplement intervention [35,37–39].

Regarding meta-analysis results, a significant ($p = 0.04$) mean difference was observed. Figure 3 showed a mean difference of 3.00 (95% CI from 0.18 to 5.82). The heterogeneity level was large according to the $I^2 = 84\%$. The quality of the evidence was low according to the GRADE classification.

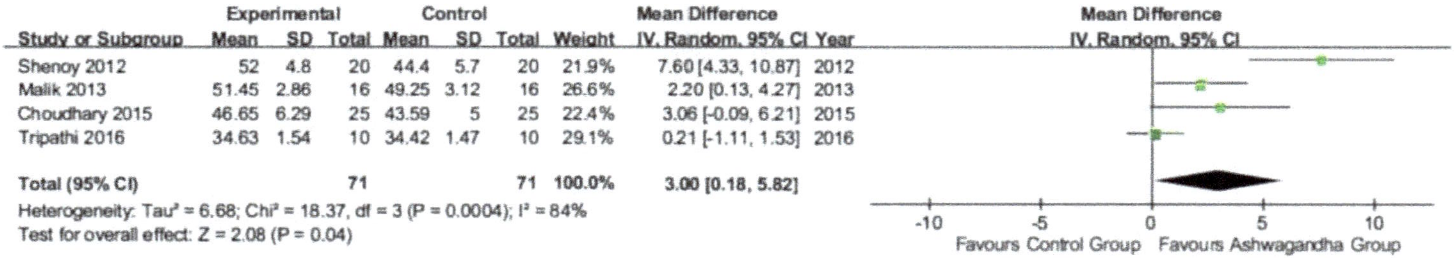

Study or Subgroup	Experimental			Control			Weight	Mean Difference IV, Random, 95% CI	Year
	Mean	SD	Total	Mean	SD	Total			
Shenoy 2012	52	4.8	20	44.4	5.7	20	21.9%	7.60 [4.33, 10.87]	2012
Malik 2013	51.45	2.86	16	49.25	3.12	16	26.6%	2.20 [0.13, 4.27]	2013
Choudhary 2015	46.65	6.29	25	43.59	5	25	22.4%	3.06 [-0.09, 6.21]	2015
Tripathi 2016	34.63	1.54	10	34.42	1.47	10	29.1%	0.21 [-1.11, 1.53]	2016
Total (95% CI)			71			71	100.0%	3.00 [0.18, 5.82]	

Heterogeneity: Tau² = 6.68; Chi² = 18.37, df = 3 (P = 0.0004); I² = 84%
Test for overall effect: Z = 2.08 (P = 0.04)

Figure 3. Meta-analysis results of the effects of Ashwagandha supplementation on VO_{2max}.

4. Discussion

The purpose of this study was to systematically review the scientific literature about the effects of supplementation with Ashwagandha on VO_{2max} and to carry out a meta-analysis to determine the overall effect. After 20 articles were assessed for eligibility, 15 articles were excluded since they did not report $VO_{2\ max}$. A total of 5 articles were included in the systematic review [35–39]. However, one article was excluded from the meta-analysis [35] since the reported mean VO_{2max} was abnormally low for healthy young people and less than half the mean of the rest of the included studies (46.18 mL/kg/min), which may indicate that they were not actually reporting VO_{2max} but VO_2 at rest. The results of this meta-analysis showed that supplementation with Ashwagandha may be useful to improve VO_{2max} in athletes [36,38,39] and healthy adults [37]. Table 2 displayed the amount of Ashwagandha used in each study, which varied from 330 up to 1000 mg/day, which is inside the limits, 750 to 1250 mg/day, found to be well tolerated and safe [40]. In this regard, none of the five articles reported any relevant side effect as a consequence of the treatment, achieving a high compliance with the treatment and very low number of dropouts.

The two studies that achieved the highest treatment effect and effect size [36,39] were those with the highest Ashwagandha intake (>50 g in the whole program). Therefore, it seems like the higher the dose, the higher the improvement in VO_2. However, the study by Tripathi, Shrivastava, Ahmad Mir, Kumar, Govil, Vahedi, and Bisen [14] did not observe any significant difference between the effects of a 330 mg intake and the effects of a 500 mg intake after 2 weeks. Therefore, further studies comparing the effect of different doses, as well as studies with longer duration are needed.

In general terms, the overall effects were better in those studies with a sample comprised of athletes [36,38,39] compared with the studies with healthy adults [14,39]. This is interesting since, as expected, baseline levels were higher in athletes and, consequently, larger improvements were expected in non-athlete healthy adults. It could be that the effects of supplementation with Ashwagandha might be linked to the physical activity levels of the participants, promoting and increasing the physiological adaptations to physical exercise. However, this hypothesis should be explored in future studies. The VO_{2max} defines the body's ability to transport and utilize oxygen, so this physiological parameter is associated with endurance performance. Many factors contribute to the VO_{2max} values, including genetic predisposition [41], enzymes [42], muscle fiber type [43], or training [44]. It is also known that nutritional supplementation can improve the effects of training and reach higher performance [45]. Previous studies with Ashwagandha administration observed improvement in working capacity test in rats by increasing the swimming endurance test [46]. As endurance performance is determined by mitochondrial function, some reasons for the Ashwagandha to improve cardiorespiratory fitness can be the significant effects observed on mitochondrial and energy levels, by reducing the succinate dehydrogenase enzyme activity in the mitochondria and benefiting Mg-ATPase activity [47]. Previous studies showed that Ashwagandha significantly enhanced the hemoglobin concentration and red blood cells in animals [48] and also in humans [38], with the subsequent increase in the capacity to transport oxygen to the muscles. Moreover, it should be considered that Ashwagandha has shown to have anti-fatigue [49,50] and anti-stress [51] actions. This could be connected to the significant improvement in the time to exhaustion of the experimental group that could be observed in the study of Shenoy, Chaskar, Sandhu, and Paadhi [39]. Some of the chemical constituents of *Whitania somnifera* [52] such as flavonoids, alkaloids, and steroidal lactones (withanolides) or the antioxidants (superoxide dismutase, catalase, and glutathione peroxidase) could be behind the improvements of VO_{2max}. Therefore, further studies are needed to explore which are the chemical constituents and mechanism that may explain the potential improvement in the VO_{2max}.

Although all mechanisms by which Ashwagandha can improve the VO_{2max} have not been described yet and future studies are needed to elucidate that improvement, it is known that Ashwagandha exhibits little or no associated toxicity [53], so it seems that this Ayurvedic herb "Ashwagandha" (*Withania somnifera*) can be safely used for improving cardiovascular fitness in healthy adults and also in athletes, offering an additional alternative as a nutritional supplement to enhance VO_{2max}.

Some limitations in the present meta-analysis can be mentioned. The first one is related to the search strategy, only articles published in English were included and a few databases were used. Another limitation can be the large heterogeneity in the included articles. Different doses, levels of physical activity, or the inclusion of both women and men in the protocols make it very difficult to achieve a high level of evidence. In addition, the systematic review and meta-analysis was not prospectively registered in any public database. Furthermore, in order to have a better understanding of long-term ergogenic benefit and potential side effects from Ashwagandha root extract, longer duration studies are needed.

5. Conclusions

Ashwagandha supplementation might improve the VO_{2max} in athlete and non-athlete people. The analyzed studies used oral administration of Ashwagandha which varied between 2 and 12 weeks with intakes between 300 to 1000 mg/day. Due to the limited number of studies included in this systematic review and meta-analysis, further research is needed to confirm the effects and the recommended dose.

Author Contributions: Conceptualization, J.P.-G., J.C.A. and D.C.-M.; methodology, J.P.-G., S.V., E.M.-N. and D.C.-M.; software, J.C.A., and D.C.-M.; formal analysis, J.P.-G., S.V., J.C.A., E.M.-N., and D.C.-M.; investigation, J.P.-G., S.V., J.C.A., E.M.-N., and D.C.-M.; data curation, J.P.-G., J.C.A. and S.V.; writing—original draft preparation, J.P.-G., S.V. and D.C.-M.; writing—review and editing, J.P.-G., S.V., J.C.A., E.M.-N. and D.C.-M.; supervision, J.P.-G., S.V., J.C.A., E.M.-N. and D.C.-M. All authors have read and agreed to the published version of the manuscript.

Funding: S.V. is supported by a grant from the regional Department of Economy and Infrastructure of the Government of Extremadura and European Social Fund (PD16008).

Conflicts of Interest: The authors declare no conflict of interest.

References

1. Dela, F.; Finkenzeller, T.; Ingersen, A.; Potzelsberger, B.; Muller, E. Trajectories of cardio-metabolic health in successful aging. *Scand. J. Med. Sci. Sports* **2019**, *29* (Suppl. 1), 44–51. [CrossRef]
2. Mooses, M.; Hackney, A.C. Anthropometrics and Body Composition in East African Runners: Potential Impact on Performance. *Int. J. Sports Physiol. Perform.* **2017**, *12*, 422–430. [CrossRef] [PubMed]
3. Brandon, L.J. Physiological factors associated with middle distance running performance. *Sports Med.* **1995**, *19*, 268–277. [CrossRef] [PubMed]
4. Helgerud, J.; Engen, L.C.; Wisloff, U.; Hoff, J. Aerobic endurance training improves soccer performance. *Med. Sci. Sports Exerc.* **2001**, *33*, 1925–1931. [CrossRef] [PubMed]
5. Midgley, A.W.; McNaughton, L.R.; Wilkinson, M. Is there an optimal training intensity for enhancing the maximal oxygen uptake of distance runners? Empirical research findings, current opinions, physiological rationale and practical recommendations. *Sports Med.* **2006**, *36*, 117–132. [CrossRef] [PubMed]
6. Steele, J.; Butler, A.; Comerford, Z.; Dyer, J.; Lloyd, N.; Ward, J.; Fisher, J.; Gentil, P.; Scott, C.; Ozaki, H. Similar acute physiological responses from effort and duration matched leg press and recumbent cycling tasks. *PeerJ* **2018**, *6*, e4403. [CrossRef]
7. Myers, J.; Prakash, M.; Froelicher, V.; Do, D.; Partington, S.; Atwood, J.E. Exercise capacity and mortality among men referred for exercise testing. *N. Engl. J. Med.* **2002**, *346*, 793–801. [CrossRef]
8. Blair, S.N.; Kampert, J.B.; Kohl, H.W., 3rd; Barlow, C.E.; Macera, C.A.; Paffenbarger, R.S., Jr.; Gibbons, L.W. Influences of cardiorespiratory fitness and other precursors on cardiovascular disease and all-cause mortality in men and women. *JAMA* **1996**, *276*, 205–210. [CrossRef]
9. Rebollo-Ramos, M.; Velazquez-Diaz, D.; Corral-Perez, J.; Barany-Ruiz, A.; Perez-Bey, A.; Fernandez-Ponce, C.; Garcia-Cozar, F.J.; Ponce-Gonzalez, J.G.; Cuenca-Garcia, M. Aerobic fitness, Mediterranean diet and cardiometabolic risk factors in adults. *Endocrinol. Diabetes Nutr.* **2019**. [CrossRef]

10. Galvez Casas, A.; Rodriguez Garcia, P.L.; Garcia-Canto, E.; Rosa Guillamon, A.; Perez-Soto, J.J.; Tarraga Marcos, L.; Tarraga Lopez, P. Aerobic capacity and quality of life in school children from 8 to 12. *Clin. Investig. Arterioscler.* **2015**, *27*, 239–245. [CrossRef]
11. Dar, N.J.; Hamid, A.; Ahmad, M. Pharmacologic overview of *Withania somnifera*, the Indian Ginseng. *Cell. Mol. Life Sci.* **2015**, *72*, 4445–4460. [CrossRef] [PubMed]
12. Chukwuma, C.I.; Matsabisa, M.G.; Ibrahim, M.A.; Erukainure, O.L.; Chabalala, M.H.; Islam, M.S. Medicinal plants with concomitant anti-diabetic and anti-hypertensive effects as potential sources of dual acting therapies against diabetes and hypertension: A review. *J. Ethnopharmacol.* **2019**, *235*, 329–360. [CrossRef] [PubMed]
13. Sun, G.Y.; Li, R.; Cui, J.; Hannink, M.; Gu, Z.; Fritsche, K.L.; Lubahn, D.B.; Simonyi, A. *Withania somnifera* and Its Withanolides Attenuate Oxidative and Inflammatory Responses and Up-Regulate Antioxidant Responses in BV-2 Microglial Cells. *Neuromol. Med.* **2016**, *18*, 241–252. [CrossRef] [PubMed]
14. Tripathi, N.; Shrivastava, D.; Ahmad Mir, B.; Kumar, S.; Govil, S.; Vahedi, M.; Bisen, P.S. Metabolomic and biotechnological approaches to determine therapeutic potential of *Withania somnifera* (L.) Dunal: A review. *Phytomedicine* **2018**, *50*, 127–136. [CrossRef]
15. Hassannia, B.; Logie, E.; Vandenabeele, P.; Vanden Berghe, T.; Vanden Berghe, W. Withaferin A: From ayurvedic folk medicine to preclinical anti-cancer drug. *Biochem. Pharm.* **2019**. [CrossRef]
16. Kaur, P.; Mathur, S.; Sharma, M.; Tiwari, M.; Srivastava, K.K.; Chandra, R. A biologically active constituent of withania somnifera (ashwagandha) with antistress activity. *Indian J. Clin. Biochem.* **2001**, *16*, 195–198. [CrossRef] [PubMed]
17. Kaur, G.; Singh, N.; Samuel, S.S.; Bora, H.K.; Sharma, S.; Pachauri, S.D.; Dwivedi, A.K.; Siddiqui, H.H.; Hanif, K. *Withania somnifera* shows a protective effect in monocrotaline-induced pulmonary hypertension. *Pharm. Biol.* **2015**, *53*, 147–157. [CrossRef] [PubMed]
18. Yenisetti, S.C.; Manjunath, M.J.; Muralidhara, C. Neuropharmacological Properties of *Withania somnifera* - Indian Ginseng: An Overview on Experimental Evidence with Emphasis on Clinical Trials and Patents. *Recent Pat. CNS Drug Discov.* **2016**, *10*, 204–215. [CrossRef]
19. Ahmed, W.; Mofed, D.; Zekri, A.R.; El-Sayed, N.; Rahouma, M.; Sabet, S. Antioxidant activity and apoptotic induction as mechanisms of action of *Withania somnifera* (Ashwagandha) against a hepatocellular carcinoma cell line. *J. Int. Med. Res.* **2018**, *46*, 1358–1369. [CrossRef]
20. Pradhan, R.; Kumar, R.; Shekhar, S.; Rai, N.; Ambashtha, A.; Banerjee, J.; Pathak, M.; Dwivedi, S.N.; Dey, S.; Dey, A.B. Longevity and healthy ageing genes FOXO3A and SIRT3: Serum protein marker and new road map to burst oxidative stress by *Withania somnifera*. *Exp. Gerontol.* **2017**, *95*, 9–15. [CrossRef]
21. Chandrasekhar, K.; Kapoor, J.; Anishetty, S. A prospective, randomized double-blind, placebo-controlled study of safety and efficacy of a high-concentration full-spectrum extract of ashwagandha root in reducing stress and anxiety in adults. *Indian J. Psychol. Med.* **2012**, *34*, 255–262. [CrossRef] [PubMed]
22. Khan, M.A.; Ahmed, R.S.; Chandra, N.; Arora, V.K.; Ali, A. In vivo, Extract from *Withania somnifera* Root Ameliorates Arthritis via Regulation of Key Immune Mediators of Inflammation in Experimental Model of Arthritis. *Antiinflamm. Antiallergy Agents Med. Chem.* **2019**, *18*, 55–70. [CrossRef] [PubMed]
23. Choudhary, D.; Bhattacharyya, S.; Bose, S. Efficacy and Safety of Ashwagandha (*Withania somnifera* (L.) Dunal) Root Extract in Improving Memory and Cognitive Functions. *J. Diet. Suppl.* **2017**, *14*, 599–612. [CrossRef] [PubMed]
24. Anju, T.R.; Smijin, S.; Jobin, M.; Paulose, C.S. Altered muscarinic receptor expression in the cerebral cortex of epileptic rats: Restorative role of *Withania somnifera*. *Biochem. Cell Biol.* **2018**, *96*, 433–440. [CrossRef]
25. Singh, A.; Naidu, P.S.; Gupta, S.; Kulkarni, S.K. Effect of natural and synthetic antioxidants in a mouse model of chronic fatigue syndrome. *J. Med. Food* **2002**, *5*, 211–220. [CrossRef]
26. Kuboyama, T.; Tohda, C.; Komatsu, K. Effects of Ashwagandha (roots of *Withania somnifera*) on neurodegenerative diseases. *Biol. Pharm. Bull.* **2014**, *37*, 892–897. [CrossRef]
27. Ramakanth, G.S.; Uday Kumar, C.; Kishan, P.V.; Usharani, P. A randomized, double blind placebo controlled study of efficacy and tolerability of Withaina somnifera extracts in knee joint pain. *J. Ayurveda Integr. Med.* **2016**, *7*, 151–157. [CrossRef]
28. Sharma, A.K.; Basu, I.; Singh, S. Efficacy and Safety of Ashwagandha Root Extract in Subclinical Hypothyroid Patients: A Double-Blind, Randomized Placebo-Controlled Trial. *J. Altern. Complement. Med.* **2018**, *24*, 243–248. [CrossRef]

29. Li, W.; Zhang, C.; Du, H.; Huang, V.; Sun, B.; Harris, J.P.; Richardson, Q.; Shen, X.; Jin, R.; Li, G.; et al. Withaferin A suppresses the up-regulation of acetyl-coA carboxylase 1 and skin tumor formation in a skin carcinogenesis mouse model. *Mol. Carcinog.* **2016**, *55*, 1739–1746. [CrossRef]
30. Cakici, N.; van Beveren, N.J.M.; Judge-Hundal, G.; Koola, M.M.; Sommer, I.E.C. An update on the efficacy of anti-inflammatory agents for patients with schizophrenia: A meta-analysis. *Psychol. Med.* **2019**, *49*, 2307–2319. [CrossRef]
31. Durg, S.; Shivaram, S.B.; Bavage, S. *Withania somnifera* (Indian ginseng) in male infertility: An evidence-based systematic review and meta-analysis. *Phytomedicine* **2018**, *50*, 247–256. [CrossRef] [PubMed]
32. Durg, S.; Dhadde, S.B.; Vandal, R.; Shivakumar, B.S.; Charan, C.S. *Withania somnifera* (Ashwagandha) in neurobehavioural disorders induced by brain oxidative stress in rodents: A systematic review and meta-analysis. *J. Pharm. Pharmacol.* **2015**, *67*, 879–899. [CrossRef] [PubMed]
33. Pratte, M.A.; Nanavati, K.B.; Young, V.; Morley, C.P. An alternative treatment for anxiety: A systematic review of human trial results reported for the Ayurvedic herb ashwagandha (*Withania somnifera*). *J. Altern. Complement. Med.* **2014**, *20*, 901–908. [CrossRef] [PubMed]
34. Higgins, J.P.; Thompson, S.G. Quantifying heterogeneity in a meta-analysis. *Stat. Med.* **2002**, *21*, 1539–1558. [CrossRef] [PubMed]
35. Sandhu, J.S.; Shah, B.; Shenoy, S.; Chauhan, S.; Lavekar, G.S.; Padhi, M.M. Effects of *Withania somnifera* (Ashwagandha) and Terminalia arjuna (Arjuna) on physical performance and cardiorespiratory endurance in healthy young adults. *Int. J. Ayurveda Res.* **2010**, *1*, 144–149. [CrossRef] [PubMed]
36. Choudhary, B.; Shetty, A.; Langade, D.G. Efficacy of Ashwagandha (*Withania somnifera* [L.] Dunal) in improving cardiorespiratory endurance in healthy athletic adults. *Ayu* **2015**, *36*, 63–68. [CrossRef]
37. Tripathi, R.; Salve, B.; Petare, A.; Raut, A.; Rege, N. Effect of *Withania somnifera* on physical and cardiovascular performance induced by physical stress in healthy human volunteers. *Int. J. Basic Clin. Pharmacol.* **2016**, *5*, 2510–2516.
38. Malik, A.; Mehta, V.; Dahiya, V. Effect of ashwagandha (withania somnifera) root powder supplementation on the vo2 max. and hemoglobin in hockey players. *Int. J. Behav. Soc. Mov. Sci.* **2013**, *2*, 91–99.
39. Shenoy, S.; Chaskar, U.; Sandhu, J.S.; Paadhi, M.M. Effects of eight-week supplementation of Ashwagandha on cardiorespiratory endurance in elite Indian cyclists. *J. Ayurveda Integr. Med.* **2012**, *3*, 209–214. [CrossRef]
40. Raut, A.A.; Rege, N.N.; Tadvi, F.M.; Solanki, P.V.; Kene, K.R.; Shirolkar, S.G.; Pandey, S.N.; Vaidya, R.A.; Vaidya, A.B. Exploratory study to evaluate tolerability, safety, and activity of Ashwagandha (*Withania somnifera*) in healthy volunteers. *J. Ayurveda Integr. Med.* **2012**, *3*, 111–114. [CrossRef]
41. Williams, C.J.; Williams, M.G.; Eynon, N.; Ashton, K.J.; Little, J.P.; Wisloff, U.; Coombes, J.S. Genes to predict VO2max trainability: A systematic review. *BMC Genom.* **2017**, *18*, 831. [CrossRef]
42. Honig, C.R.; Connett, R.J.; Gayeski, T.E. O2 transport and its interaction with metabolism; a systems view of aerobic capacity. *Med. Sci. Sports Exerc.* **1992**, *24*, 47–53. [CrossRef]
43. Pette, D.; Staron, R.S. Cellular and molecular diversities of mammalian skeletal muscle fibers. *Rev. Physiol. Biochem. Pharmacol.* **1990**, *116*, 1–76.
44. MacInnis, M.J.; Gibala, M.J. Physiological adaptations to interval training and the role of exercise intensity. *J. Physiol.* **2017**, *595*, 2915–2930. [CrossRef]
45. Dominguez, R.; Cuenca, E.; Mate-Munoz, J.L.; Garcia-Fernandez, P.; Serra-Paya, N.; Estevan, M.C.; Herreros, P.V.; Garnacho-Castano, M.V. Effects of Beetroot Juice Supplementation on Cardiorespiratory Endurance in Athletes. A Systematic Review. *Nutrients* **2017**, *9*, 43. [CrossRef]
46. Dhuley, J.N. Adaptogenic and cardioprotective action of ashwagandha in rats and frogs. *J. Ethnopharmacol.* **2000**, *70*, 57–63. [CrossRef]
47. Begum, V.H.; Sadique, J. Effect of *Withania somnifera* on glycosaminoglycan synthesis in carrageenin-induced air pouch granuloma. *Biochem. Med. Metab. Biol* **1987**, *38*, 272–277. [CrossRef]
48. Ziauddin, M.; Phansalkar, N.; Patki, P.; Diwanay, S.; Patwardhan, B. Studies on the immunomodulatory effects of Ashwagandha. *J. Ethnopharmacol.* **1996**, *50*, 69–76. [CrossRef]
49. Mishra, L.C. *Scientific Basis for Ayurvedic Therapies*; CRC Press: Boca Raton, FL, USA, 2003.
50. Biswal, B.M.; Sulaiman, S.A.; Ismail, H.C.; Zakaria, H.; Musa, K.I. Effect of *Withania somnifera* (Ashwagandha) on the development of chemotherapy-induced fatigue and quality of life in breast cancer patients. *Integr. Cancer Ther.* **2013**, *12*, 312–322. [CrossRef] [PubMed]

51. Lopresti, A.L.; Smith, S.J.; Malvi, H.; Kodgule, R. An investigation into the stress-relieving and pharmacological actions of an ashwagandha (*Withania somnifera*) extract: A randomized, double-blind, placebo-controlled study. *Medicine* **2019**, *98*, e17186. [CrossRef] [PubMed]
52. Kumar, V.; Dey, A.; Hadimani, M.B.; Marcović, T.; Emerald, M. Chemistry and pharmacology of *Withania somnifera*: An update. *TANG* **2015**, *5*, 1–13. [CrossRef]
53. Mishra, L.C.; Singh, B.B.; Dagenais, S. Scientific basis for the therapeutic use of *Withania somnifera* (ashwagandha): A review. *Altern. Med. Rev.* **2000**, *5*, 334–346. [PubMed]

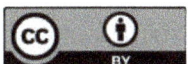

© 2020 by the authors. Licensee MDPI, Basel, Switzerland. This article is an open access article distributed under the terms and conditions of the Creative Commons Attribution (CC BY) license (http://creativecommons.org/licenses/by/4.0/).

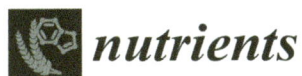

Article

Exogenous Ketone Supplements Improved Motor Performance in Preclinical Rodent Models

Csilla Ari [1,2,*], **Cem Murdun** [3], **Craig Goldhagen** [3], **Andrew P. Koutnik** [3,4], **Sahil R. Bharwani** [1], **David M. Diamond** [1,3], **Mark Kindy** [5,6,7], **Dominic P. D'Agostino** [2,3,4] and **Zsolt Kovacs** [8]

1. Department of Psychology, Behavioral Neuroscience Research Laboratory, University of South Florida, Tampa, FL 33620, USA; sahilbharwani2692@gmail.com (S.R.B.); ddiamond@usf.edu (D.M.D.)
2. Ketone Technologies, Tampa, FL 33612, USA; ddagosti@usf.edu
3. Department of Molecular Pharmacology and Physiology, Laboratory of Metabolic Medicine, Morsani College of Medicine, University of South Florida, Tampa, FL 33612, USA; biocem@gmail.com (C.M.); cgoldhagen@usf.edu (C.G.); akoutnik@usf.edu (A.P.K.)
4. Institute for Human and Machine Cognition, Ocala, FL 34471, USA
5. Department of Pharmaceutical Sciences, College of Pharmacy, University of South Florida, Tampa, FL 33612, USA; kindym@health.usf.edu
6. James A. Haley VA Medical Center, Tampa, FL 33612, USA
7. Shriners Hospital for Children, Tampa, FL 33612, USA
8. Savaria Department of Biology, ELTE Eötvös Loránd University, Savaria University Centre, Károlyi Gáspár tér 4., 9700 Szombathely, Hungary; zskovacsneuro@gmail.com
* Correspondence: cdrari@usf.edu or Csari2000@yahoo.com; Tel.: +1-813-240-9925

Received: 3 July 2020; Accepted: 13 August 2020; Published: 15 August 2020

Abstract: Nutritional ketosis has been proven effective for neurometabolic conditions and disorders linked to metabolic dysregulation. While inducing nutritional ketosis, ketogenic diet (KD) can improve motor performance in the context of certain disease states, but it is unknown whether exogenous ketone supplements—alternatives to KDs—may have similar effects. Therefore, we investigated the effect of ketone supplements on motor performance, using accelerating rotarod test and on postexercise blood glucose and R-beta-hydroxybutyrate (R-βHB) levels in rodent models with and without pathology. The effect of KD, butanediol (BD), ketone-ester (KE), ketone-salt (KS), and their combination (KE + KS: KEKS) or mixtures with medium chain triglyceride (MCT) (KE + MCT: KEMCT; KS + MCT: KSMCT) was tested in Sprague-Dawley (SPD) and WAG/Rij (WR) rats and in GLUT-1 Deficiency Syndrome (G1D) mice. Motor performance was enhanced by KEMCT acutely, KE and KS subchronically in SPD rats, by KEKS and KEMCT groups in WR rats, and by KE chronically in G1D mice. We demonstrated that exogenous ketone supplementation improved motor performance to various degrees in rodent models, while effectively elevated R-βHB and in some cases offsets postexercise blood glucose elevations. Our results suggest that improvement of motor performance varies depending on the strain of rodents, specific ketone formulation, age, and exposure frequency.

Keywords: ketone ester; ketogenic diet; ketone salt; MCT; rotarod; R-βHB

---

1. Introduction

Motor impairment can be caused by injury or degeneration to the motor cortex, premotor cortex, motor tracts, or associated pathways in the cerebrum, cerebellum, or neuromuscular junction. These pathological changes have been observed in a variety of neurological conditions, such as Alzheimer's Disease (AD), Huntington's Disease (HD), Parkinson's Disease (PD), Amyotrophic Lateral Sclerosis (ALS), Glucose 1 Deficiency Syndrome (G1D), or those who have suffered a cerebral vascular accident (CVA) stroke, and in patients with traumatic brain injuries (TBI) [1–6]. These neurological conditions present with metabolic impairment, neuroinflammation, and other related molecular characteristics.

Nutritional ketosis significantly improved outcomes and motor function in HD, PD, ALS, G1D, and AD through various mechanisms, such as reduced proinflammatory cytokines, decreased mitochondrial damage, and preservation of cellular bioenergetics. These results suggest that the mechanism of action for ketone bodies to enhance/preserve motor performance is multifactorial, but has significant overlap between biological pathways [1–9]. However, the predominant mechanism of action of nutritional ketosis on motor performance is largely unknown, as is the optimal method of administration.

The ketogenic diet (KD) was designed to induce nutritional ketosis, initially employed for its metabolic benefits and ability to treat epilepsy [10]. Physiologically, the metabolic response to a KD closely resembles the insulin suppression associated with fasting if total calories and ketogenic ratios (3:1 to 4:1 ratio, by weight, of fat to a combination of protein and carbohydrates) are maintained [5]. Despite the efficacy of the KD clinically, patient compliance can be low due to the strict nutritional requirements, fat intolerance, or potential complications and side effects [11,12]. Subjects report difficulty maintaining ketosis as excess consumption of carbohydrates or protein can rapidly shift the body back towards glycolysis and inhibit ketogenesis [13]. Alternative solutions to achieving nutritional ketosis are needed, and exogenous ketone supplementation has been reported to be an effective alternative to KD in the context of various disease states [11,14–19].

Under normal physiological conditions and when adhering to a "traditional" western diet typically rich in carbohydrate, glucose is the primary metabolic fuel in the CNS and skeletal muscle [20]. However, during low glucose bioavailability and hepatic glycogen depletion, free fatty acids are mobilized from adipose tissue and released into the bloodstream to be used directly as fuel or converted to ketone bodies in the liver through the process of ketogenesis to sustain metabolic demands [21]. The primary ketone bodies produced, acetoacetate (AcAc) and R-β-hydroxybutyrate (R-βHB), are subsequently released into the bloodstream and serve as an alternative fuel for most tissues, but especially the central nervous tissue, as long-chain fatty acids cannot readily be used by the brain [22].

Hyperketonemia is the metabolic state characterized by an elevation of blood ketone bodies and is observed in individuals who adhere to a KD or are fasted for extended periods of time [22]. In this state, a large portion of tissue energetic requirements are met via fatty acid oxidation and ketolysis [23]. Under normal physiological conditions, blood ketone levels rarely exceed 0.01 mmol/L and account for less than 3% of total brain metabolism [24]. However, in periods of nutritional ketosis, characterized by blood ketone levels of 0.5–6 mmol/L, ketone bodies cross the blood–brain barrier (BBB) through monocarboxylate class transporters [25] and serve as supplemental fuel accounting for up to 60% of brain energy metabolism [21,26]. Once inside of the cell's mitochondria, the ketone bodies are converted into Acetyl CoA, enter the TCA cycle, and generate the reduced intermediates (NADH and FADH$_2$) needed to sustain ATP production [22].

Supplementation with ketone (ketogenic) supplements, such as ketone ester (KE), has proven effective in achieving a state of nutritional ketosis independent of carbohydrate restriction [14,17,18,27,28]. Ketone supplementation that contains either KE, ketone salt (KS), medium chain triglycerides (MCTs), or their combinations (e.g., KEKS, KEMCT, and KSMCT) has been studied in both animal models and humans. It has been demonstrated that exogenous ketone supplementation is a safe and effective option to induce nutritional ketosis [16,29–32], and, consequently, evoke alleviating effects of ketosis on motor performance similar to KD [2,4,6,33]. Indeed, it was suggested that administration of KE and MCTs may evoke beneficial effects on motor dysfunction [34,35]. However, it is unknown whether different exogenous ketone supplements and their combinations would increase motor performance in animal models under different conditions associated with motor function impairment. Our previous study also demonstrated that exogenous ketones have a blood glucose lowering effect [27]; however, the hormonal response to exercise can cause stored glucose to be released from the liver and skeletal muscle while temporarily raising blood glucose levels. Thus, the main goal of the present study was to determine if specific ketogenic supplements and/or combinations would improve motor performance in rodents with pathology (Wistar Albino Glaxo/Rijswijk, WAG/Rij/WR rats and Glut1 Deficiency Syndrome/G1D mice) and without pathology (Sprague-Dawley/SPD rats) [36,37] and to test whether they are able to offset the postexercise induced blood glucose elevation. WR rat strain is an accepted model of absence epilepsy with comorbidity of low-grade depression, but without pathological changes in locomotor activity/motor performance [38–40], while G1D mice are models of Glut1 Deficiency Syndrome and show motor dysfunction [37,41]. We hypothesized that nutritional ketosis induced by various ketone therapeutics (KD and exogenous ketone supplements) can improve motor performance in rodent models, as defined by latency to fall from the accelerated rotarod and can offset blood glucose elevation in postexercised states.

2. Materials and Methods

2.1. Animals

Three rodent models were used for the experiments: SPD rats (male, 4 months old and 1 year old, 320–360 g and 540–660 g, respectively, Harlan Laboratories), WR rats (male, 6 months old, 320–360 g, breeding colony, Eötvös Loránd University, Savaria University Centre, Szombathely, Hungary), and G1D mice (male, 3–5 months old, 17–27 g, breeding colony, University of South Florida, Morsani College of Medicine, Tampa, FL, USA) that were housed at either the College of Medicine Animal Facility (Morsani College of Medicine, University of South Florida, Tampa, FL, USA) or at the Savaria Department of Zoology (Eötvös Loránd University, Savaria University Centre, Szombathely, Hungary). Standard laboratory conditions (12:12 h light-dark cycle) were maintained for the animals that were housed in air-conditioned rooms at 22 ± 2 °C in groups of 2–4.

Institutional Animal Care and Use Committee (IACUC; Protocol #0006R) of the University of South Florida (University of South Florida, Tampa, FL, USA) and Hungarian Act of Animal Care and Experimentation (1998. XXVIII. Section 243/1998) and the regulations for animal experimentation in the European Communities Council Directive of 24 November 1986 (86/609/EEC) guidelines were followed during the experimental procedures. Experiments were approved by the Animal Care and Experimentation Committee of the Eötvös Loránd University (Savaria University Centre) and by the National Scientific Ethical Committee on Animal Experimentation (Hungary) under license number VA/ÉBNTF02/85–8/2016. We made all efforts to reduce the number of animals used.

2.2. Ketogenic Compounds

Ad libitum access to water and standard rodent chow (standard diet: SD, NIH-31 Rodent Chow; Envigo), or ketogenic rodent food (KD; TD. 10911; Envigo), or SD with ketone supplements (Table 1, and Supplementary Tables S1 and S2) were provided for the animals. The KD used in this study was modified from TD.10787 (Teklad) to remove maltodextrin to make the diet essentially free of carbohydrate. The KD had a 2:1 ratio of n-3 to n-6 fatty acids and a 1.5:1 ratio of fat to protein + carbohydrate. Compared to TD.10787 (common KD formula), TD.10911 had the same % fat (wt/wt), but it had a higher % kcal from fat, because maltodextrin was removed and replaced with cellulose. KE (R,S 1,3-butanediol-acetoacetate diester) was synthesized by D'Agostino, 2013, as previously described [17]. The KS (Na^+/K^+– R,S βHB mineral salt) was mixed into a 50% solution supplying approximately 375 mg/g of pure βHB and 125 mg/g of Na^+/K^+ in a 1:1 ratio. KE and KS development and synthesis were performed in collaboration with Savind Inc. Human food-grade MCT oil (~60% caprylic triglyceride/40% capric triglyceride, Now Foods, Bloomingdale, IL, USA) was used for the experiments. KS and KE were mixed with MCT in a 1:1 ratio, resulting the KSMCT and KEMCT combinations, respectively. KE was mixed with KS in a 1:1 ratio to make KEKS. R,S-1,3-butanediol (BD) was purchased from Sigma (Milwaukee, WI, USA).

Table 1. Macronutrient information of each diet. (More details about the ingredients of each diet can be found in Supplementary Tables S1 and S2).

	Standard Diet (SD)	Ketogenic Diet (KD)
Protein, % of kcal	24	22.4
Carbohydrate, 5 of kcal	62	0.5
Fat, % by kcal	14	77.1
kcal/g	3.0	4.7

2.3. Exposure Schedule

For the trials involving SPD and WR rats, intragastric delivery by oral gavage was used. To acclimatize the rodents, each animal was orally gavaged with water for five days prior to treatment (Figure 1). After acclimatization and baseline measurements (5th days), the rats were orally gavaged either once with different exogenous ketone supplements (acute treatment on the 6th day; 5 g/kg for SPD rats) and the effects (motor function and blood measurements) were measured after 30 min^{-1} h, or they were gavaged once daily for 7 days (subchronic treatment between 6th and 12th day; 5 g/kg/day for SPD rats and 2.5 g/kg/day for WR rats) and the effects were recorded after 24 h and after 7 days (Figure 1). In relation to G1D mice with chronic exposure, ketone supplements were administered daily for 10 weeks and the effects were measured after 3, 6, and 10 weeks treatment (Figure 1).

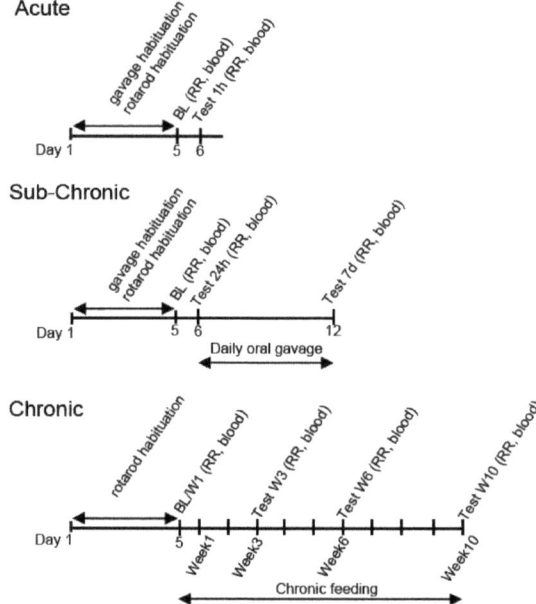

Figure 1. Experimental design for the different exposure schedules (acute, subchronic, and chronic). BL: Baseline measurement; blood: blood draw with glucose and R-βHB measurements; RR: Rotarod test; blood: blood draw with glucose and R-βHB measurements.

2.4. Treatment Groups

One-year-old SPD rats were divided into 6 groups for the acute treatment and were fed with SD and they were administered a single oral gavage. The treatment groups included water (control, $n = 10$), BD ($n = 8$), KE ($n = 12$), KSMCT ($n = 8$), KEKS ($n = 12$), and KEMCT ($n = 8$). Motor performance was evaluated prior to the beginning of dietary treatment (baseline; 5th day of habituation) and 30 min after gavage.

Subchronic experiments used 4-month old SPD rats that were divided into 5 groups and fed with either SD, KD and supplemented with a once-daily oral gavage for 7 days. Treatment groups included control (SD, water gavage, $n = 11$), KD ($n = 10$), KE ($n = 9$), KS ($n = 9$), and KSMCT ($n = 10$). The animals were evaluated for motor performance prior to the beginning of dietary treatment (baseline), 24 h after 1st treatment (KD or gavage), and 1 h after the 7th treatment.

The WR rats with subchronic exposure were divided into 6 groups. They were fed with SD and orally gavaged daily with either water (SD, control; $n = 9$) or KE ($n = 9$), KS ($n = 9$), KSMCT ($n = 9$), KEKS ($n = 9$), KEMCT ($n = 9$) for 7 days. Rotarod test was carried out similarly to subchronically treated SPD rats.

The G1D mice exposed to chronic treatment were split into four groups, SD (control; $n = 12$), KD ($n = 12$), or the SD supplemented with KS ($n = 12$) or KE ($n = 12$) and were treated for 10 weeks. Rotarod test was performed before the beginning of dietary treatment (baseline) and after 3, 6, and 10 weeks of treatment.

2.5. Motor Performance Testing

Motor performance was evaluated using the accelerating rotarod test on a RotaRod Rotamex 5 (rotarod; Columbus Inst., Columbus, OH, USA). The rats were placed on the rods of the accelerating rotarod, and the time the animals remained on the rod was measured. The rotarod was set to accelerate from zero to 40 rpm in 180 s. To acclimate the animals to both the equipment and the task, prior to the administration of a test, animals were trained on the rotarod for 5 consecutive days. Thus, habituation to rotarod test was parallel with habituation to oral gavage (Figure 1). Each day of training consisted of 3 sessions, with a 120 s rest period between trials. Animals were placed on the rotarod and timed until they fell from the rotating rod. Following last trial, the blood measurements were collected within 10 min.

2.6. Blood Glucose and R-βHB

Whole blood (~10 μL) was acquired from saphenous vein (rats) and tail vein (mice) for analysis of blood glucose (mg/dL) and R-βHB (mmol/L) with Precision Xtra™ (Abbott Laboratories, Abbott Park, IL, USA). Note that the Precision Xtra™ measures R-βHB exclusively—not S-βHB, AcAc, or Acetone—therefore, total ketone level may be somewhat underrepresented. R/D and S/L are two stereoisomers, called enantiomers, that are mirror images of each other. While R-βHB is the normal product of human and mouse metabolism, it is metabolized much faster than S-βHB is. S-βHB is not a normal product of human metabolism, however, it is a transient intermediate of β-oxidation of fatty acids, therefore, administration of the same amount of S-βHB may lead to higher level and more sustained blood levels of S-βHB, compared to similar administration of R-βHB [42]. Blood was drawn prior to the beginning of the treatments (5th day of habituation), and this value was used as the established baseline. Treatment-generated changes in glucose and R-βHB were measured (60 min) after the beginning of treatment (acute treatments, SPD rats). Blood was drawn after treatment started, at either 1 h, 24 h, or after 7 daily treatments (subchronic treatments, SPD, and/or WR rats). During chronic treatments (G1D mice), blood was drawn before treatment started (baseline) and at week 3, 6, and 10 after beginning treatment.

2.7. Statistics

Data are presented as the mean ± standard error of the mean (SEM). The effects of ketogenic agents on both R-βHB and glucose, as well as motor performance (latency to fall: rotarod) were compared to experimental controls and respective baseline levels. GraphPad Prism (6.0a) was used for data analysis. Comparisons of data were made using a one or two-way ANOVA with Tukey's multiple comparisons. Results were considered significant when p values were less than 0.05. Results are indicated on figures using the following notations *: $p < 0.05$, **: $p < 0.01$, ***: $p < 0.001$, and ****: $p < 0.0001$ level of significance.

3. Results

3.1. Changes in Motor Performance, Blood Glucose, and R-βHB Levels in SPD Rats with Acute Exposure

In acutely exposed one-year-old SPD rats, the latency to fall from an accelerating rotarod was significantly elevated in KEMCT group, compared to baseline ($p = 0.0011$, Figure 2A). The KEKS group showed a trend of increase, however, the results were nonsignificant, while the BD, KSMCT, and KE groups also showed no significant change in motor performance. The percent change in latency to fall was significantly higher in KEMCT group, compared to control ($p = 0.003$, Figure 2B). Blood R-βHB levels in postexercise state were elevated significantly in KSMCT group, compared to baseline ($p = 0.0099$) and control ($p = 0.0040$), in KEKS group, compared to baseline ($p = 0.0021$) and control ($p = 0.0119$), in KEMCT group, compared to baseline ($p < 0.0001$) and control ($p < 0.0001$), and in KE group, compared to baseline ($p < 0.0001$) and control ($p < 0.0001$, Figure 2C). The BD group displayed a nonsignificant increase in blood R-βHB levels. The blood glucose levels in postexercise state were elevated significantly after 1 h in the control group ($p = 0.0064$), in BD group ($p < 0.0001$), in KSMCT group ($p < 0.0001$), in KEKS group ($p = 0.0048$), and KE group ($p = 0.0255$), compared to their respective baselines (Figure 2D).

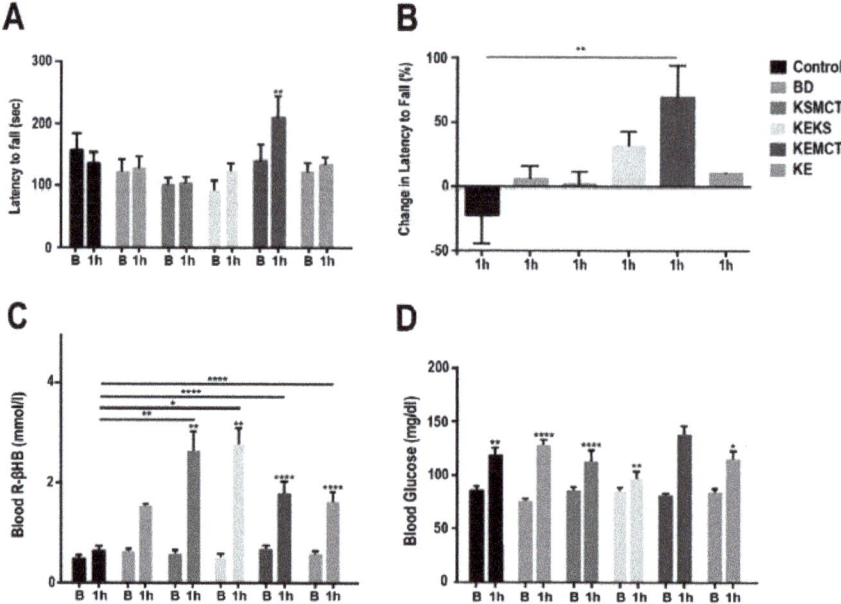

Figure 2. Changes in motor performance and blood parameters from postexercise state for one-year old Sprague-Dawley rats, 1 h following treatment. (**A**) Latency to fall (sec) on accelerating rotarod at each timepoint. (**B**) Percent change in latency to fall on accelerating rotarod at 1 h, compared to baseline. (**C**) Blood R-βHB levels in postexercise state at each timepoint. (**D**) Blood glucose levels in postexercise state at each timepoint. Abbreviations: B: Baseline; 1 h: 1 h timepoint; R-βHB: R-beta-hydroxybutyrate; BD: butanediol; KE: ketone ester; KEKS: combination of ketone ester and ketone salt (KS); KEMCT: ketone ester in combination with medium chain triglyceride (MCT); KSMCT: ketone-salt in combination with medium chain triglyceride (MCT); SPD: Sprague-Dawley rats. *: $p < 0.05$, **: $p < 0.01$, and ****: $p < 0.0001$ level of significance.

3.2. Changes in Motor Performance, Blood Glucose, and R-βHB Levels in SPD Rats with Subchronic Exposure

In the 4-month-old SPD rats after subchronic treatment the latency to fall from the accelerating rotarod was significantly decreased for the KD group at 24 h ($p = 0.0296$) and at 7 days ($p = 0.0133$), compared to baseline (Figure 3A). The latency to fall increased in KE group at 24 h, compared to baseline ($p = 0.0313$), and at 7 days, compared to the control ($p = 0.0413$) and baseline ($p = 0.0106$). The latency to fall increased in KS group at 24 h, compared to the control ($p = 0.0138$) and baseline ($p = 0.039$), and at 7 days, compared to the control ($p = 0.011$). The KSMCT group displayed no significant change in latency to fall. No groups had significantly different percent change in latency to fall, compared to baseline or control (Figure 3B). Blood R-βHB levels increased significantly in the KD group at 24 h, compared to baseline ($p = 0.038$) and control ($p < 0.0001$) and in the KE group at 24 h, compared to control ($p = 0.0325$, Figure 3C). After 7 days the blood R-βHB levels increased significantly in KD and KS groups, compared to the control ($p < 0.0001$ and $p = 0.0194$ respectively), and in KSMCT, compared to baseline ($p < 0.0001$), 24 h ($p < 0.0001$), and control ($p < 0.0001$). Blood glucose level at 24 h was significantly decreased in KD group, compared to control ($p < 0.0001$), and in the KE group, compared to control ($p < 0.0001$) and baseline ($p = 0.0047$, Figure 3D). After 7 days of treatment, the postexercise blood glucose level was decreased in KSMCT group, compared to baseline ($p < 0.0001$), 24 h ($p < 0.0001$), and control ($p < 0.0001$). An increase in blood glucose level was observed in the KE group relative to its 24-h reading ($p = 0.0049$).

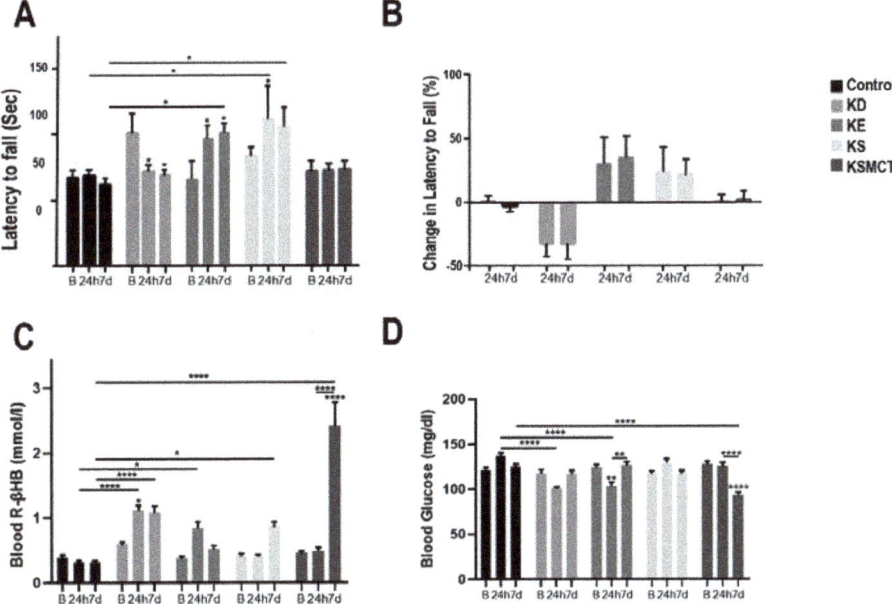

Figure 3. Motor performance and blood parameters in postexercise state for 4-month-old Sprague-Dawley rats after subchronic treatment, measured at baseline, 24 h and at 7 days following treatment. (**A**) The latency to fall (sec) on the accelerating rotarod was presented at each timepoint. (**B**) The percent change in latency to fall on the accelerating rotarod presented at 24 h and at 7 days, compared to baseline. (**C**) Blood R-βHB levels are presented in postexercise state at each timepoint. (**D**) Blood glucose levels are presented in postexercise state at each timepoint. Abbreviations: B: Baseline; 24 h: 24 h timepoint; 7d: 7 days timepoint; R-βHB: R-beta-hydroxybutyrate; KD: ketogenic diet; KE: ketone ester; KS: ketone salt; KSMCT: ketone salt in combination with medium chain triglyceride (MCT); SPD: Sprague-Dawley rats. *: $p < 0.05$, **: $p < 0.01$, and ****: $p < 0.0001$ level of significance.

3.3. Changes in Motor Performance, Blood Glucose, and R-βHB Levels in WR Rats with Acute and Subchronic Exposure

In WR rats with acute and subchronic exposure, the latency to fall on accelerating rotarod was significantly decreased in KSMCT group at 1 h and at 7 days, compared to the baseline ($p < 0.0129$; $p = 0.0078$; respectively, Figure 4A). In KEKS group the latency to fall increased at 1 h, compared to baseline ($p < 0.0001$) and control ($p < 0.0001$), and at 7 days, compared to baseline ($p < 0.0001$), 1 h ($p < 0.0001$), and control ($p < 0.0001$). In the KS group the latency to fall significantly decreased between 1 h and 7 days ($p = 0.0138$). The latency to fall increased in KEMCT group at 1 h, compared to baseline ($p < 0.0001$) and control ($p < 0.0001$), and at 7 days, compared to baseline ($p < 0.0001$) and control ($p < 0.0001$). The percent change in latency to fall on the accelerated rotarod was significantly increased in the KEKS group at 1 h, compared to control ($p = 0.0001$), and at 7 days, compared to control ($p < 0.0001$, Figure 4B). The KEMCT group at 1 h had a significantly increased percent change in latency to fall, compared to control ($p < 0.0001$) and similarly at 7 days, compared to control ($p < 0.0001$).

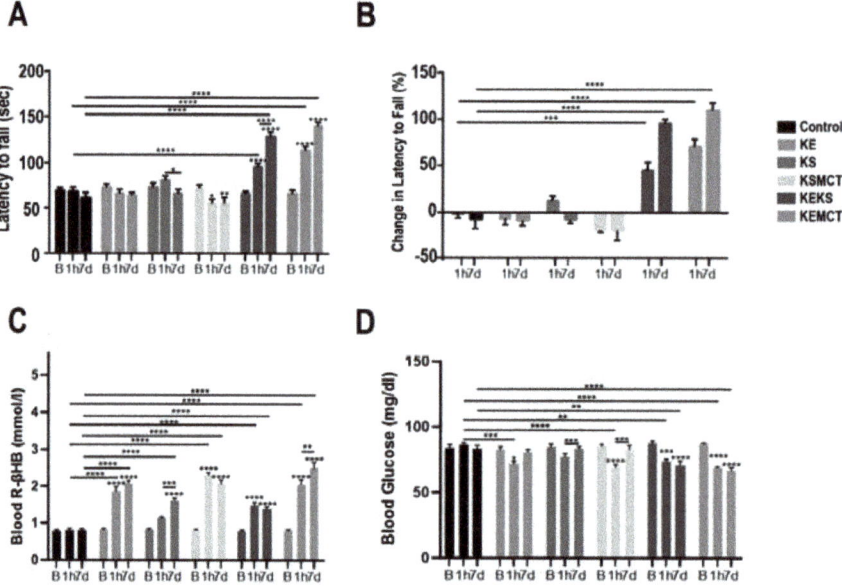

Figure 4. Changes in motor performance and blood parameters in postexercise state for WR rats with acute and subchronic exposure, at baseline, at 1 h and 7 days following treatment. (**A**) The latency to fall (sec) on accelerating rotarod at each timepoint. (**B**) The percent change in latency to fall on accelerated rotarod, compared to baseline at 1 h and 7 days post treatment. (**C**) Blood R-βHB levels are presented in postexercise state at each timepoint. (**D**) Blood glucose levels are presented in postexercise state at each timepoint. Abbreviations: B: Baseline; 1 h: 1 h timepoint; 7d: 7 days timepoint; R-βHB, R-beta-hydroxybutyrate; KE: ketone ester; KEKS: combination of ketone ester and ketone salt (KS); KEMCT: ketone ester in combination with medium chain triglyceride (MCT); KS: ketone salt; KSMCT: ketone-salt in combination with medium chain triglyceride (MCT); WR: WAG/Rij rats. *: $p < 0.05$, **: $p < 0.01$, ***: $p < 0.001$ and ****: $p < 0.0001$ level of significance.

Blood R-βHB levels were increased significantly after 1 h in the KE, KSMCT, KEKS, and KEMCT groups, compared to their respective baselines ($p < 0.0001$) and control ($p < 0.0001$, Figure 4C). All treatment groups at 7 days had elevated blood ketone levels, compared to their baselines ($p < 0.0001$) and the control ($p < 0.0001$). At 7 days, the blood ketone levels in KEMCT and KS groups were significantly increased from their 1-h level ($p = 0.0025$; $p = 0.0007$; respectively). Blood glucose levels decreased significantly at 1 h in the KE group, compared to baseline ($p = 0.0307$) and control ($p = 0.0002$), in the KSMCT group, compared to baseline ($p < 0.0001$) and control ($p < 0.0001$), in the KEKS group, compared to baseline ($p = 0.0003$) and control ($p = 0.0022$), and in KEMCT group, compared to baseline ($p < 0.0001$) and control ($p < 0.0001$, Figure 4D). After 7 days, blood glucose levels decreased in KEKS group, compared to baseline ($p < 0.0001$) and control ($p = 0.0034$), increased in KS and KSMCT groups, compared to 1 h ($p = 0.0006$; $p = 0.0006$), and decreased in KEMCT group, compared to baseline ($p < 0.0001$), and control ($p < 0.0001$).

3.4. Changes in Motor Performance, Blood Glucose, and R-βHB Levels in G1D Mice with Chronic Exposure

In G1D mice after chronic treatment the latency to fall on the accelerating rotarod was significantly increased in the KE group at week 3 ($p < 0.01$), and at week 6 ($p < 0.05$), compared to baseline (Figure 5A). The KD and KS groups were observed to have a trend of nonsignificant increase in latency to fall. The percent change in latency to fall was not significantly elevated in any groups, compared to baseline or control (Figure 5B). KD and KS were observed to have a marginal and nonsignificant increase percent change in latency to fall, while the KE had a larger, but still nonsignificant increase in percent change in latency to fall. Blood R-βHB levels increased significantly in the KD group at week 6, compared to baseline ($p = 0.0157$) and control ($p = 0.0211$, Figure 5C). The KS group had a significant increase in blood R-βHB levels at week 6, compared to baseline ($p = 0.045$). Blood glucose level decreased significantly in the KE group at week 6, compared to baseline ($p = 0.0113$), and in the KD group at week 3, compared to baseline ($p = 0.0393$, Figure 5D).

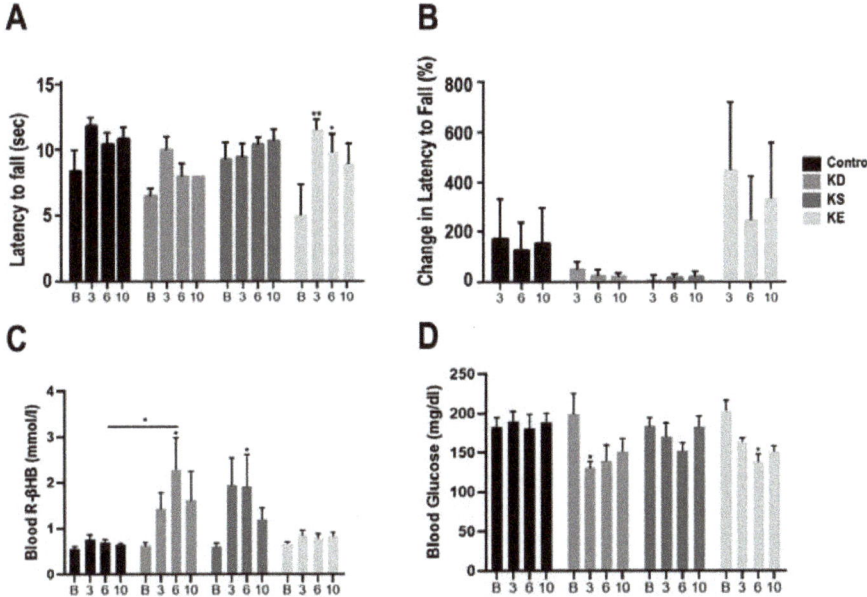

Figure 5. Changes in motor performance and blood parameters in postexercise state for G1D mice with chronic treatment, at baseline, at week 3, at weeks 6, and at week 10. (**A**) The latency to fall (sec) on accelerating rotarod presented, compared to baseline. (**B**) The percent change in latency to fall at each timepoint, compared to baseline. (**C**) Blood R-βHB levels are presented in postexercise state at each timepoint. (**D**) Blood glucose levels are presented in postexercise state at each timepoint. Abbreviations: B: Baseline; 3: Week 3; 6: Week 6; 10: Week 10; R-βHB, R-beta-hydroxybutyrate; G1D, Glucose Transporter Type-1 Deficiency Syndrome mice; KD, ketogenic diet; KE, ketone ester; KS, ketone-salt. *: $p < 0.05$, **: $p < 0.01$ level of significance.

4. Discussion

In this study, we demonstrated the effect of KD and various exogenous ketone formulations on motor performance in different rodent models with (WR rats and G1D mice) and without (SPD rats) pathology after acute, subchronic, or chronic exposures. We reported improvement of motor performance by ketone supplementation, which may depend on the strain of rodents, specific ketone formulation, age, species, and exposure frequency. Moreover, we reported significant changes in blood R-βHB and glucose levels after exercise. Previous experiments have demonstrated that ketogenic diets significantly improved motor function in studies on AD, ALS, HD, PD, stroke, and MS disease models [1–7,9,33]. Our experiments expand upon these previous studies by reporting about the positive effect of exogenous ketone supplementation on motor performance in nonpathological and additional pathological rodent models.

Ketone-based therapies were found to be effective in the treatment of a variety of diseases, including neurological pathologies with motor dysfunction [2,8,25,43–54]. For example, in patients with PD nutritional ketosis decreased neuron degeneration, reduced mitochondrial damage, improved motor outcomes, and reduced proinflammatory cytokine levels [1,4,43–46]. Application of nutritional ketosis attenuated motor dysfunction in mouse models of HD [47]. Ketone-based therapies were reported effective in improving motor function in a model animal of ALS (SOD1-G93A transgenic mice) through neuroprotective outcomes [2,35]. Moreover, in a study on G1D mice (characterized by impaired glucose transportation and motor dysfunction), adherence of a KD improved motor symptoms [41]. Our results demonstrated that exogenous ketone supplement can improve motor dysfunction in G1D mice. While several therapeutic mechanisms for the KD have been explored, its role in disease pathologies is relatively unknown and further research into the physiological and mechanistic effect of ketone-based therapeutics is warranted [1]. It has been demonstrated that exogenous ketone supplementation is a viable and safe method in various animal models of, for example, central nervous system (CNS) diseases and in human CNS disorders when alternative ketone-based therapies are needed that address the limitations with KD [1,14,17,19,31].

We report that the motor performance may improve with KD in disease context, but also with exogenous ketone supplementation even in rodents eating a standard, carbohydrate-rich diet, suggesting that ketone supplementation may be a viable alternative for those unwilling or unable to adhere to a KD. Our data supports that exogenous ketone supplementation was more efficient in improving motor performance than KD, as KD reduced motor performance in SPD rats after 24 h and 7 days (Figure 3A), although the effect was not significant when assessing % change (Figure 3B). On the other hand, exogenous ketones showed more consistent improvement throughout different model systems, illustrating a potentially more translatable therapeutic tool across healthy and disease context.

While our previous study showed that ketone supplementation lowered blood glucose levels [27] in the nonexercised state, we found that in the postexercise state it was elevated at 1 h (Figure 2D), possibly due to exercise augmenting glycogenolysis induced glucose elevation which may offset the blood glucose lowering effect. However, in some cases in SPD and WR rats after 1 h and 7 days the blood glucose levels were lower than control and baseline (Figures 2D, 3D and 4D) and in G1D mice after 6 weeks it was lower than baseline (Figure 5D), suggesting that exogenous ketones may be able to offset the glycogenolysis induced glucose elevation in postexercised state. It has been suggested that alleviating effects of ketone-based therapies, such as KD on motor performance, likely results from carbohydrate restriction (and low glucose levels), but not from increased blood βHB levels [48,49]. However, based on our results it is unclear whether KD- and ketone supplements- evoked alterations in blood glucose level had a major influencing factor on motor performance. For example, both KD and KE decreased blood glucose level at 24 h (Figure 3D), but only KE improved motor performance of SPD rats.

Many different beneficial effects on diseases have been linked to ketone therapies and this is likely due to the resulting decreased production of reactive oxygen species (ROS), improved mitochondrial function, reduction in inflammation, neuroprotective effects, and increased expression of brain-derived neurotrophic factor (BDNF) [1,50–52]. Additionally, ketones have been found to produce changes in post-translational modification of proteins and histone acetylation [53–55]. It has also been reported that ketones may enhance learning in multiple rodent models and may explain the motor performance increase observed in the nonpathological mouse models [56]. Furthermore, ketones may enhance muscle performance or CNS control of muscle contractions/coordination, which could be a contributing factor to the rodent's ability to remain on the rotarod longer, not only in rodents with motor dysfunction, but also rodents without motor impairment, such as SPD rats and WR rats.

Ketogenic diet and exogenous ketone supplementation may also act on cellular homeostasis through various signaling pathways, such as mTOR, AMPK, and neurotransmitter systems. Ketosis has been shown to affect cell proliferation, energetic metabolism, protein biosynthesis, and attenuate muscle wasting [57–62]. KD acts upon specific tyrosine kinase receptors for insulin and insulin growth factor (IGF) and upregulates the phosphatidylinositol-3 kinase (PI3K)-Akt-mammalian target of rapamycin complex 1 (mTORC1). This is counteracted by a lower intracellular ATP/AMP ratio and the subsequent upregulation of liver kinase B1 (LKB1)-AMP-activated protein kinase (AMPK) signaling, which then inhibits the mTORC1 pathway [48,53]. Research also suggests that ketone-based therapies likely have additional therapeutic applications by reduced levels of proinflammatory cytokines, ROS, attenuation of skeletal muscle catabolism, and various neuroprotective effects [15,50,51,62,63]. Moreover, it was also suggested that KD- and exogenous ketone supplements-evoked alleviating effects on different CNS diseases may be modulated by different neurotransmitter/neuromodulator systems, such as GABAergic (e.g., by increased GABA level) and purinergic/adenosinergic (e.g., via increased adenosine concentration) systems [19,31,64–67]. Therefore, studies about the application of ketone metabolic therapies for various neurological conditions suggest that multifactorial mechanisms play a role in improving motor function (e.g., mitochondrial function, neurotransmitter systems, anti-inflammatory processes, and skeletal muscle physiology), but further research is required to fully elucidate pathways and potential therapeutic applications.

While no motor function impairments (motor dysfunction) have been demonstrated in SPD rats and WR rats [39,40], the subchronically administered ketone supplement KE, KS (in SPD rats), KEKS and KEMCT (in WR rats) improved motor performance. These results suggest that exogenous ketone supplements may improve motor performance not only in animal models with neurometabolic pathology, such as motor dysfunction (e.g., G1D mice), but also in animals without pathology (e.g., SPD rats) or with pathology, but without motor dysfunction (e.g., WR rats), likely by enhanced learning and muscle performance [5,44,56,68]. Moreover, exogenous ketone supplements-evoked effects on motor performance may be rat strain dependent. Indeed, it was demonstrated that influences of KD and ketone supplements may be modulated by strain-, age-, and species-dependent changes. For example, it has been demonstrated that expression of monocarboxylate class type 1 transporter on the BBB may be not only age-, but also species-dependent [69–71]. In addition, age- and species-dependent changes in activity of βHB metabolizing enzymes were also demonstrated [39,40,72–75]. It has been revealed that level, uptake, metabolism, as well as utilization, and consequently, effects of ketone bodies may be regionally different in the brain areas implicated not only in physiological, but also in pathophysiological processes in different strains [72,76–78]. All of these factors may result in brain area-, age-, strain-, and species-dependent influences/effectivity of KD and ketone supplements on motor performance in different animal models. Consequently, efficacy of treatments may also be dependent on the various type of ketone supplements (e.g., KSMCT decreased whereas KEKS and KEMCT increased the motor performance in WR rats), on the exposure frequency/time after administration (e.g., acute treatment by KE was not effective on motor performance, but subchronic administration of KE improved the motor performance in SPD rats) and on the interference of different factors.

Limitations and Inconsistencies

One limitation of these results is that we used racemic (R/S) βHB exclusively, because this was the most economical and commercially available product on the market for both experimental purposes and for consumer consumption at the time of the study. Racemic βHB has been used clinically in patients and consumers for years [79], and no serious adverse events from βHB supplement ingestion have been reported (CAERS open-FDA database), even with >1 million estimated servings consumed annually. Thus, our approach was to evaluate molecules, which may be economically feasible to translate to humans and would be accessible to end-users in the near future. However, one consideration with racemic βHB supplements is the potential differences in metabolism of S- βHB and R- βHB, although existing data on this is still limited. Based on previous studies we know that S-βHB and R- βHB from racemic mixtures are naturally metabolized in rats and humans [80], but S-βHB remains elevated in the blood longer after consumption of racemic mixtures. It appears that ketolytic metabolism favors a more rapid catabolism of R- βHB, the predominant form of βHB that is produced endogenously. It is possible that the rate limiting enzymes for S-βHB conversion to acetyl CoA (e.g., S-3-hydroxybutyryl-CoA dehydrogenase) may be in lower quantities since endogenous levels are much lower. Although previous studies suggest that the enzymatic kinetics of S- βHB metabolism is slower, this does not appear to be the case in the rat liver, at least with S-1,3-butanediol. Of potential relevance to our results is the observation that S-1,3-butanediol, a specific S- βHB precursor, has a greater blood glucose lowering effect [81], which could conceivably influence motor function performance. These previous metabolic observations need to be considered when interpreting our data and designing future experiments that test enantiomerically pure forms of both βHB isomers in physiological testing.

Considering these limitations, we can speculate that R-βHB levels may be an important factor in KD/exogenous ketone supplement-evoked positive effects on motor performance, but other factors likely have a modulatory role. Since we could not unambiguously correlate elevated R-βHB levels with augmented motor performance, future dose-response studies can help to identify the optimal range for this specific application. It is also possible that other forms of ketone molecules contributed to the performance enhancing effect that were not directly measured in the present study, but previous studies show their elevation (e.g., KE will elevate acetoacetate levels as well, which was not directly measured here, but may have contributed to the performance enhancing effect, see Figure 5B,C). For example, acute KSMCT and KEKS treatment significantly increased the blood R-βHB level at 1 h, but did not augment motor performance (latency to fall), whereas KEMCT treatment enhanced R-βHB concentration to a lesser degree (compared to KSMCT and KEKS), but significantly increased latency to fall, compared to baseline in one year old SPD rats (Figure 2). Acetoacetate, from KE, may have contributed to the performance enhancing effect here as well, which may have increased efficacy for this application when working synergistically with MCT rather than with KS. In regards to KD treatment, we observed increased blood R-βHB at 24 h and 7 days, but this treatment significantly decreased the latency to fall from rotarod, compared to baseline in 4-months-old SPD rats (Figure 3). It is likely that adaptation (which takes weeks to months) to the KD confers additional beneficial effects, so this outcome was not unexpected after only 24 h and even 7 days, as we would expect to see ketoadaptation and its beneficial effects over longer timeframe. KE treatment significantly increased blood R-βHB level only at 24 h, but improved motor function at both 24 h and 7 days, compared to baseline (24 h and 7 days), and control (at 7 days). KS treatment did not increase blood R-βHB levels at 24 h, however this treatment significantly improved motor function, compared to both control and baseline (Figure 3). It is conceivable that low R-βHB at 24 h is indicative of tissue utilization, leading augmentation of muscle tissue performance. Moreover, KSMCT treatment increased blood R-βHB concentration to high levels at 7 days more than any other treatment, but it did not show a motor performance improving effect (Figure 3), suggesting that higher R-βHB levels may not be as beneficial, or that MCT may be negating the performance benefits (perhaps by reducing R-βHB metabolism). Subchronic treatment of WR rats by KE and KSMCT increased blood R-βHB levels at 1 h and at 7 days, but did not improve motor performance (Figure 4), again suggesting that higher R-βHB levels might not be optimal in this context. Chronic KE treatment improved motor performance at week 3 and week 6 in G1D mice, but blood R-βHB levels were not changed by KE treatment at these time points (Figure 5). Therefore, it is possible that other ketone bodies, such as acetoacetate may contribute to the performance enhancing effect that was associated with chronic KE treatment. Based on these results, we can speculate that a particular range of R-βHB level may be needed to improve motor function, and this may be age-, strain-, and species dependent. It is possible that higher levels of acute (or subchronic) ketosis may induce a mild metabolic acidosis (lower pH), and this could conceivably blunt performance effects. Moreover, other contributing factors should also be considered, e.g., different ketone-based therapies evoke direct and indirect influences on neurotransmission, cell energetics, muscle and nerve regeneration, as well as gastric hormone levels (e.g., ghrelin, which is in connection with muscular trophism) [48,82,83], other modulatory effects, such as mobilization of polyunsaturated fatty acids (PUFAs),which can directly modulate ion channel functioning [84,85], and elevated neurosteroid synthesis resulting in modulation of GABAA receptors [86,87]. These and other, yet unidentified factors may influence the modulatory role of KD/ketone supplements on physiological and pathophysiological processes, as well as CNS diseases. Thus, our results suggest that KD/ketone supplements may be effective to improve motor function in different physiological and pathophysiological conditions by affecting multiple organs.

Given these inconsistencies we need to point out the following: (i) we could not make definitive conclusion about direct correlation between motor performance and R-βHB levels; (ii) our experimental design did not mechanistically elucidate the contributing role of acetoacetate (and perhaps acetone) in augmenting motor performance; (iii) these data do not clarify if ketone supplementation augments performance via enhancing muscular cellular energetics or through some yet to be identified ketone-induced signaling/neuropharmacological change, potentially influencing CNS-control of motor performance. However, we can conclude that (i) positive effects of exogenous ketone supplementation were identified on motor performance in nonpathological and pathological states; (ii) exogenous ketones may be able to offset the glycogenolysis induced glucose elevation in postexercised state; (iii) exogenous ketones may have a specific therapeutic range for various applications; (iv) different forms and formulations can have different effects independently from the level of blood βHB elevation.

In order to address these remaining questions, future experiments will need to focus on: (1) More direct comparisons of the physiological effects between racemic and enantiomerically pure βHB substances; (2) Comprehensively evaluate the dose-dependent effects of both racemic and enantiomerically purified forms of βHB; (3) Investigate acetoacetate-specific effects; (4) Monitoring correlations between blood glucose lowering effect and motor performance; (5) Conduct additional tests focusing on potential differences in efficacy between various motor functions, e.g., endurance, fine motor control, strength, balance; (6) Mechanistically isolate R-βHB signaling effects from ketone-induced changes in cellular energetics and metabolic control, especially focusing on signaling effects that can influence motor performance; (7) Detailed investigation of agent-specific mechanism on not only the brain, but also on other organs (e.g., heart, skeletal muscle, lungs, and liver); (8) Develop and identify optimal ketone formulations (e.g., types, doses, exposure frequency vs. age) to alleviate motor dysfunction in patients with different physiological and pathological conditions.

In light of these inconsistencies in the data we would like to caution end-users to avoid making generalizations about the use of ketone supplements in different contexts and we call to direct more attention to the differences between various forms (racemic and enantiomerically pure) and formulations (combined agents) and their potential positive, negative, or synergistic effect.

5. Conclusions

Our study demonstrates the effects of the KD and ketone supplementation on motor performance in SPD, and WR rats, as well as in G1D mice after acute, subchronic, or chronic administration. We observed that motor performance improved significantly in various pathological and nonpathological rodent models for different exposure schedules and that the effectiveness of the supplements differed according to rodent strain, the schedule of treatment, the specific supplement they were exposed to, and age of the rodents. We found that exogenous ketone supplementation was more efficient in improving motor performance than KD. While KD treatment led to mixed results—demonstrating more efficacy in disease context (G1D)—exogenous ketones showed consistent effect across disease and nondisease states. Furthermore, in certain scenarios, exogenous ketone supplements offset the glycogenolysis-induced glucose elevation in the postexercise state, which might be beneficial when there is a need to keep blood glucose levels low even after exercising. These results also strengthen previous research on the potential of ketone therapies and their ability to improve motor performance in a variety of pathological and nonpathological rodent models. The differences in the efficacy of a given formulation are potentially due to differences in neuronal ketone metabolism between the different rodent strains and species, hepatic metabolism (ketogenesis), or variabilities in skeletal muscle metabolism. However, further studies are needed to explore the safe and effective therapeutic applications of ketone-based therapies and elucidate their exact mechanisms of action on motor performance.

Supplementary Materials: The following are available online at http://www.mdpi.com/2072-6643/12/8/2459/s1, Table S1: NIH-31 Open Formula Mouse/Rat Sterilizable Diet, Table S2: Teklad Custom Research Diet Data Sheet.

Author Contributions: Conceptualization, C.A.; Data curation, C.A.; Formal analysis, C.A.; Funding acquisition, C.A., D.P.D. and Z.K.; Investigation, C.A., C.M., C.G., A.P.K., S.R.B. and Z.K.; Methodology, C.A. and Z.K.; Project administration, C.A. and Z.K.; Resources, D.P.D. and Z.K.; Supervision, C.A.; Writing–original draft, C.A., S.B. and Z.K.; Writing–review and editing, C.A., A.P.K., S.R.B., D.M.D., M.K., D.P.D. and Z.K. All authors have read and agreed to the published version of the manuscript.

Funding: Funding was provided by Quest Nutrition (to Csilla Ari), ONR Grant N000141310062 (to Dominic P. D'Agostino), the Glucose Transporter Type-2 Deficiency Syndrome Foundation (Glut1DS) (to Dominic P. D'Agostino), and the National Development Agency of Hungary (under Grant No. TIOP-1.3.1.-07/2-2F-2009-2008), and OTKA K124558 Research Grant (to Zsolt Kovács).

Acknowledgments: Quest Nutrition provided partial funding to Csilla Ari.

Conflicts of Interest: International Patent # PCT/US2014/031237, University of South Florida for DPD: Compositions and Methods for Producing Elevated and Sustained Ketosis. Patent pending: USF Ref. No: 16A019 for CA and DPD: "Exogenous Ketone Supplementation Improved Motor Function in Sprague-Dawley Rats." DPD and CA are co-owners of the company Ketone Technologies LLC, a company specialized on scientific consulting. DMD is a paid consultant and member of the science advisory board for Axcess Global Sciences and Anutra. These interests have been reviewed and managed by the university in accordance with its Institutional and Individual Conflict of Interest policies. All authors declare that there are no additional conflicts of interest.

References

1. Koppel, S.J.; Swerdlow, R.H. Neuroketotherapeutics: A modern review of a century-old therapy. *Neurochem. Int.* **2018**, *117*, 114–125. [CrossRef] [PubMed]
2. Zhao, Z.; Lange, D.J.; Voustianiouk, A.; MacGrogan, D.; Ho, L.; Suh, J.; Humala, N.; Thiyagarajan, M.; Wang, J.; Pasinetti, G.M. A ketogenic diet as a potential novel therapeutic intervention in amyotrophic lateral sclerosis. *BMC Neurosci.* **2006**, *7*, 29. [CrossRef]
3. Van der Auwera, I.; Wera, S.; Van Leuven, F.; Henderson, S.T. A ketogenic diet reduces amyloid beta 40 and 42 in a mouse model of Alzheimer's disease. *Nutr. Metab. (Lond.)* **2005**, *2*, 28. [CrossRef] [PubMed]
4. Vanitallie, T.; Nonas, C.; Di Rocco, A.; Boyar, K.; Hyams, K.; Heymsfield, S. Treatment of Parkinson disease with diet-induced hyperketonemia: A feasibility study. *Neurology* **2005**, *64*, 728–730. [CrossRef]
5. Paoli, A.; Rubini, A.; Volek, J.S.; Grimaldi, K.A. Beyond weight loss: A review of the therapeutic uses of very-low-carbohydrate (ketogenic) diets. *Eur. J. Clin. Nutr.* **2013**, *67*, 789–796. [CrossRef]
6. Klepper, J. Glucose transporter deficiency syndrome (GLUT1DS) and the ketogenic diet. *Epilepsia* **2008**, *49*, 46–49. [CrossRef]
7. De la Monte, S.M. Insulin resistance and Alzheimer's disease. *BMB Rep.* **2009**, *42*, 475–481. [CrossRef]
8. Henderson, S.T.; Vogel, J.L.; Barr, L.J.; Garvin, F.; Jones, J.J.; Costantini, L.C. Study of the ketogenic agent AC-1202 in mild to moderate Alzheimer's disease: A randomized, double-blind, placebo-controlled, multicenter trial. *Nutr. Metab.* **2009**, *6*, 31. [CrossRef]
9. Yin, J.X.; Maalouf, M.; Han, P.; Zhao, M.; Gao, M.; Dharshaun, T.; Ryan, C.; Whitelegge, J.; Wu, J.; Eisenberg, D.; et al. Ketones block amyloid entry and improve cognition in an Alzheimer's model. *Neurobiol. Aging* **2016**, *39*, 25–37. [CrossRef]
10. Allen, F.M.; Stillman, E.; Fitz, R. *Total Dietary Regulation in the Treatment of Diabetes*; Rockefeller Institute for Medical Research: New York, NY, USA, 1919.

11. Coppola, G.; Veggiotti, P.; Cusmai, R.; Bertoli, S.; Cardinali, S.; Dionisi-Vici, C.; Elia, M.; Lispi, M.L.; Sarnelli, C.; Tagliabue, A.; et al. The ketogenic diet in children, adolescents and young adults with refractory epilepsy: An Italian multicentric experience. *Epilepsy Res.* **2002**, *48*, 221–227. [CrossRef]
12. Hemingway, C.; Freeman, J.M.; Pillas, D.J.; Pyzik, P.L. The Ketogenic Diet: A 3- to 6-Year Follow-Up of 150 Children Enrolled Prospectively. *Pediatrics* **2001**, *108*, 898–905. [CrossRef] [PubMed]
13. Pfeifer, H.H.; Thiele, E.A. Low-glycemic-index treatment: A liberalized ketogenic diet for treatment of intractable epilepsy. *Neurology* **2005**, *65*, 1810–1812. [CrossRef] [PubMed]
14. Ari, C.; Kovács, Z.; Juhasz, G.; Murdun, C.; Goldhagen, C.R.; Koutnik, A.P.; Poff, A.M.; Kesl, S.L.; D'Agostino, D.P. Exogenous Ketone Supplements Reduce Anxiety-Related Behavior in Sprague-Dawley and Wistar Albino Glaxo/Rijswijk Rats. *Front. Mol. Neurosci.* **2016**, *9*. [CrossRef]
15. Ari, C.; Kovács, Z.; Murdun, C.; Koutnik, A.P.; Goldhagen, C.R.; Rogers, C.; Diamond, D.; D'Agostino, D.P. Nutritional ketosis delays the onset of isoflurane induced anesthesia. *BMC Anesthesiol.* **2018**, *18*, 85. [CrossRef] [PubMed]
16. Ari, C.; Koutnik, A.P.; DeBlasi, J.; Landon, C.; Rogers, C.Q.; Vallas, J.; Bharwani, S.; Puchowicz, M.; Bederman, I.; Diamond, D.M.; et al. Delaying latency to hyperbaric oxygen-induced CNS oxygen toxicity seizures by combinations of exogenous ketone supplements. *Physiol. Rep.* **2019**, *7*, e13961. [CrossRef] [PubMed]
17. D'Agostino, D.P.; Pilla, R.; Held, H.E.; Landon, C.S.; Puchowicz, M.; Brunengraber, H.; Ari, C.; Arnold, P.; Dean, J.B. Therapeutic ketosis with ketone ester delays central nervous system oxygen toxicity seizures in rats. *Am. J. Physiol. Regul. Integr. Comp. Physiol.* **2013**, *304*, R829–R836. [CrossRef]
18. Kesl, S.L.; Poff, A.M.; Ward, N.P.; Fiorelli, T.N.; Ari, C.; Van Putten, A.J.; Sherwood, J.W.; Arnold, P.; D'Agostino, D.P. Effects of exogenous ketone supplementation on blood ketone, glucose, triglyceride, and lipoprotein levels in Sprague–Dawley rats. *Nutr. Metab.* **2016**, *13*, 9. [CrossRef]
19. Kovács, Z.; D'Agostino, D.P.; Diamond, D.; Kindy, M.S.; Rogers, C.; Ari, C. Therapeutic Potential of Exogenous Ketone Supplement Induced Ketosis in the Treatment of Psychiatric Disorders: Review of Current Literature. *Front. Psychiatry* **2019**, *10*. [CrossRef]
20. Adlercreutz, H. Western diet and Western diseases: Some hormonal and biochemical mechanisms and associations. *Scand. J. Clin. Lab. Investig.* **1990**, *50*, 3–23. [CrossRef]
21. Cahill, G.F. Fuel Metabolism in Starvation. *Annu. Rev. Nutr.* **2006**, *26*, 1–22. [CrossRef]
22. Lieberman, M.; Peet, A.; Chansky, M. *Marks' Basic Medical Biochemistry: A Clinical Approach, 5e|Medical Education|Health Library*; Wolters Kluwer: Alphen aan den Rijn, The Netherlands, 2018; ISBN 978-1-4963-2481-8.
23. Grabacka, M.; Pierzchalska, M.; Dean, M.; Reiss, K. Regulation of Ketone Body Metabolism and the Role of PPARα. *Int. J. Mol. Sci.* **2016**, *17*, 2093. [CrossRef] [PubMed]
24. Hawkins, R.A.; Williamson, D.H.; Krebs, H.A. Ketone-body utilization by adult and suckling rat brain in vivo. *Biochem. J.* **1971**, *122*, 13–18. [CrossRef] [PubMed]
25. Prins, M.L. Cerebral Metabolic Adaptation and Ketone Metabolism after Brain Injury. *J. Cereb. Blood Flow Metab.* **2008**, *28*, 1–16. [CrossRef]
26. Owen, O.E.; Morgan, A.P.; Kemp, H.G.; Sullivan, J.M.; Herrera, M.G.; Cahill, G.F. Brain Metabolism during Fasting. *J. Clin. Investig.* **1967**, *46*, 1589–1595. [CrossRef] [PubMed]
27. Ari, C.; Murdun, C.; Koutnik, A.P.; Goldhagen, C.R.; Rogers, C.; Park, C.; Bharwani, S.; Diamond, D.M.; Kindy, M.S.; D'Agostino, D.P.; et al. Exogenous Ketones Lower Blood Glucose Level in Rested and Exercised Rodent Models. *Nutrients* **2019**, *11*, 2330. [CrossRef]
28. D'Agostino, D.P.; Putnam, R.W.; Dean, J.B. Superoxide (O_2^-) Production in CA1 Neurons of Rat Hippocampal Slices Exposed to Graded Levels of Oxygen. *J. Neurophysiol.* **2007**, *98*, 1030–1041. [CrossRef]
29. Clarke, K.; Tchabanenko, K.; Pawlosky, R.; Carter, E.; Knight, N.S.; Murray, A.J.; Cochlin, L.E.; King, M.T.; Wong, A.W.; Roberts, A.; et al. Oral 28-day and developmental toxicity studies of (R)-3-hydroxybutyl (R)-3-hydroxybutyrate. *Regul. Toxicol. Pharmacol.* **2012**, *63*, 196–208. [CrossRef]
30. Clarke, K.; Tchabanenko, K.; Pawlosky, R.; Carter, E.; Todd King, M.; Musa-Veloso, K.; Ho, M.; Roberts, A.; Robertson, J.; VanItallie, T.B.; et al. Kinetics, safety and tolerability of (R)-3-hydroxybutyl (R)-3-hydroxybutyrate in healthy adult subjects. *Regul. Toxicol. Pharmacol.* **2012**, *63*, 401–408. [CrossRef]

31. Kovács, Z.; D'Agostino, D.P.; Dobolyi, A.; Ari, C. Adenosine A1 Receptor Antagonism Abolished the Anti-seizure Effects of Exogenous Ketone Supplementation in Wistar Albino Glaxo Rijswijk Rats. *Front. Mol. Neurosci.* **2017**, *10*, 235. [CrossRef]
32. Masino, S.A. *Ketogenic Diet and Metabolic Therapies: Expanded Roles in Health and Disease*; Oxford University Press: Oxford, UK, 2016; ISBN 978-0-19-049800-9.
33. Brownlow, M.L.; Benner, L.; D'Agostino, D.; Gordon, M.N.; Morgan, D. Ketogenic Diet Improves Motor Performance but Not Cognition in Two Mouse Models of Alzheimer's Pathology. *PLoS ONE* **2013**, *8*, e75713. [CrossRef]
34. Ciarlone, S.L.; Grieco, J.C.; D'Agostino, D.P.; Weeber, E.J. Ketone ester supplementation attenuates seizure activity, and improves behavior and hippocampal synaptic plasticity in an Angelman syndrome mouse model. *Neurobiol. Dis.* **2016**, *96*, 38–46. [CrossRef] [PubMed]
35. Zhao, W.; Varghese, M.; Vempati, P.; Dzhun, A.; Cheng, A.; Wang, J.; Lange, D.; Bilski, A.; Faravelli, I.; Pasinetti, G.M. Caprylic Triglyceride as a Novel Therapeutic Approach to Effectively Improve the Performance and Attenuate the Symptoms Due to the Motor Neuron Loss in ALS Disease. *PLoS ONE* **2012**, *7*, e49191. [CrossRef] [PubMed]
36. Coenen, A.M.L.; van Luijtelaar, E.L.J.M. Genetic Animal Models for Absence Epilepsy: A Review of the WAG/Rij Strain of Rats. *Behav. Genet.* **2003**, *33*, 635–655. [CrossRef] [PubMed]
37. Marin-Valencia, I.; Good, L.B.; Ma, Q.; Duarte, J.; Bottiglieri, T.; Sinton, C.M.; Heilig, C.W.; Pascual, J.M. Glut1 deficiency (G1D): Epilepsy and metabolic dysfunction in a mouse model of the most common human phenotype. *Neurobiol. Dis.* **2012**, *48*, 92–101. [CrossRef]
38. Citraro, R.; Iannone, M.; Leo, A.; De Caro, C.; Nesci, V.; Tallarico, M.; Abdalla, K.; Palma, E.; Arturi, F.; De Sarro, G.; et al. Evaluation of the effects of liraglutide on the development of epilepsy and behavioural alterations in two animal models of epileptogenesis. *Brain Res. Bull.* **2019**, *153*, 133–142. [CrossRef]
39. Sarkisova, K.; van Luijtelaar, G. The WAG/Rij strain: A genetic animal model of absence epilepsy with comorbidity of depression [corrected]. *Prog. Neuropsychopharmacol. Biol. Psychiatry* **2011**, *35*, 854–876. [CrossRef]
40. Sarkisova, K.Y.; Midzianovskaia, I.S.; Kulikov, M.A. Depressive-like behavioral alterations and c-fos expression in the dopaminergic brain regions in WAG/Rij rats with genetic absence epilepsy. *Behav. Brain Res.* **2003**, *144*, 211–226. [CrossRef]
41. Friedman, J.R.L.; Thiele, E.A.; Wang, D.; Levine, K.B.; Cloherty, E.K.; Pfeifer, H.H.; Vivo, D.C.D.; Carruthers, A.; Natowicz, M.R. Atypical GLUT1 deficiency with prominent movement disorder responsive to ketogenic diet. *Mov. Disord.* **2006**, *21*, 241–244. [CrossRef]
42. Newman, J.C.; Verdin, E. β-Hydroxybutyrate. *Annu. Rev. Nutr.* **2017**, *37*, 51–76. [CrossRef]
43. Kim, D.Y.; Davis, L.M.; Sullivan, P.G.; Maalouf, M.; Simeone, T.A.; van Brederode, J.; Rho, J.M. Ketone bodies are protective against oxidative stress in neocortical neurons. *J. Neurochem.* **2007**, *101*, 1316–1326. [CrossRef]
44. Paoli, A.; Grimaldi, K.; Toniolo, L.; Canato, M.; Bianco, A.; Fratter, A. Nutrition and acne: Therapeutic potential of ketogenic diets. *Ski. Pharm. Physiol.* **2012**, *25*, 111–117. [CrossRef] [PubMed]
45. Tieu, K.; Perier, C.; Caspersen, C.; Teismann, P.; Wu, D.-C.; Yan, S.-D.; Naini, A.; Vila, M.; Jackson-Lewis, V.; Ramasamy, R.; et al. D-β-Hydroxybutyrate rescues mitochondrial respiration and mitigates features of Parkinson disease. *J. Clin. Investig.* **2003**, *112*, 892–901. [CrossRef] [PubMed]
46. Yang, X.; Cheng, B. Neuroprotective and Anti-inflammatory Activities of Ketogenic Diet on MPTP-induced Neurotoxicity. *J. Mol. Neurosci.* **2010**, *42*, 145–153. [CrossRef]
47. Lim, S.; Chesser, A.S.; Grima, J.C.; Rappold, P.M.; Blum, D.; Przedborski, S.; Tieu, K. D-β-Hydroxybutyrate Is Protective in Mouse Models of Huntington's Disease. *PLoS ONE* **2011**, *6*, e24620. [CrossRef] [PubMed]
48. Veyrat-Durebex, C.; Reynier, P.; Procaccio, V.; Hergesheimer, R.; Corcia, P.; Andres, C.R.; Blasco, H. How Can a Ketogenic Diet Improve Motor Function? *Front. Mol. Neurosci.* **2018**, *11*. [CrossRef] [PubMed]
49. Gano, L.B.; Patel, M.; Rho, J.M. Ketogenic diets, mitochondria, and neurological diseases. *J. Lipid Res.* **2014**, *55*, 2211–2228. [CrossRef]
50. Maalouf, M.; Rho, J.M.; Mattson, M.P. The neuroprotective properties of calorie restriction, the ketogenic diet, and ketone bodies. *Brain Res. Rev.* **2009**, *59*, 293–315. [CrossRef]
51. Marosi, K.; Kim, S.W.; Moehl, K.; Scheibye-Knudsen, M.; Cheng, A.; Cutler, R.; Camandola, S.; Mattson, M.P. 3-Hydroxybutyrate regulates energy metabolism and induces BDNF expression in cerebral cortical neurons. *J. Neurochem.* **2016**, *139*, 769–781. [CrossRef]

52. Sleiman, S.F.; Henry, J.; Al-Haddad, R.; Hayek, L.E.; Haidar, E.A.; Stringer, T.; Ulja, D.; Karuppagounder, S.S.; Holson, E.B.; Ratan, R.R.; et al. Exercise promotes the expression of brain derived neurotrophic factor (BDNF) through the action of the ketone body b- hydroxybutyrate. *Cell Biol.* **2016**, *21*. [CrossRef]
53. Newman, J.C.; Verdin, E. Ketone bodies as signaling metabolites. *Trends Endocrinol. Metab.* **2014**, *25*, 42–52. [CrossRef]
54. Newman, J.C.; Verdin, E. β-hydroxybutyrate: Much more than a metabolite. *Diabetes Res. Clin. Pract.* **2014**, *106*, 173–181. [CrossRef] [PubMed]
55. Stilling, R.M.; Dinan, T.G.; Cryan, J.F. Microbial genes, brain & behaviour—epigenetic regulation of the gut–brain axis. *Genes Brain Behav.* **2014**, *13*, 69–86. [CrossRef] [PubMed]
56. Kim, D.Y.; Hao, J.; Liu, R.; Turner, G.; Shi, F.-D.; Rho, J.M. Inflammation-Mediated Memory Dysfunction and Effects of a Ketogenic Diet in a Murine Model of Multiple Sclerosis. *PLoS ONE* **2012**, *7*, e35476. [CrossRef] [PubMed]
57. Zou, X.; Meng, J.; Li, L.; Han, W.; Li, C.; Zhong, R.; Miao, X.; Cai, J.; Zhang, Y.; Zhu, D. Acetoacetate Accelerates Muscle Regeneration and Ameliorates Muscular Dystrophy in Mice. *J. Biol. Chem.* **2016**, *291*, 2181–2195. [CrossRef] [PubMed]
58. Nair, K.S.; Welle, S.L.; Halliday, D.; Campbell, R.G. Effect of beta-hydroxybutyrate on whole-body leucine kinetics and fractional mixed skeletal muscle protein synthesis in humans. *J. Clin. Investig.* **1988**, *82*, 198–205. [CrossRef] [PubMed]
59. Vandoorne, T.; De Smet, S.; Ramaekers, M.; Van Thienen, R.; De Bock, K.; Clarke, K.; Hespel, P. Intake of a Ketone Ester Drink during Recovery from Exercise Promotes mTORC1 Signaling but Not Glycogen Resynthesis in Human Muscle. *Front. Physiol.* **2017**, *8*, 310. [CrossRef]
60. Thomsen, H.H.; Rittig, N.; Johannsen, M.; Møller, A.B.; Jørgensen, J.O.; Jessen, N.; Møller, N. Effects of 3-hydroxybutyrate and free fatty acids on muscle protein kinetics and signaling during LPS-induced inflammation in humans: Anticatabolic impact of ketone bodies. *Am. J. Clin. Nutr.* **2018**, *108*, 857–867. [CrossRef]
61. Koutnik, A.P.; D'Agostino, D.P.; Egan, B. Anticatabolic Effects of Ketone Bodies in Skeletal Muscle. *Trends Endocrinol. Metab.* **2019**, *30*, 227–229. [CrossRef]
62. Koutnik, A.P.; Poff, A.M.; Ward, N.P.; DeBlasi, J.M.; Soliven, M.A.; Romero, M.A.; Roberson, P.A.; Fox, C.D.; Roberts, M.D.; D'Agostino, D.P. Ketone Bodies Attenuate Wasting in Models of Atrophy. *J. Cachexia Sarcopenia Muscle* **2020**. [CrossRef]
63. Youm, Y.-H.; Nguyen, K.Y.; Grant, R.W.; Goldberg, E.L.; Bodogai, M.; Kim, D.; D'Agostino, D.; Planavsky, N.; Lupfer, C.; Kanneganti, T.D.; et al. The ketone metabolite β-hydroxybutyrate blocks NLRP3 inflammasome–mediated inflammatory disease. *Nat. Med.* **2015**, *21*, 263–269. [CrossRef]
64. Calderón, N.; Betancourt, L.; Hernández, L.; Rada, P. A ketogenic diet modifies glutamate, gamma-aminobutyric acid and agmatine levels in the hippocampus of rats: A microdialysis study. *Neurosci. Lett.* **2017**, *642*, 158–162. [CrossRef] [PubMed]
65. Erecińska, M.; Nelson, D.; Daikhin, Y.; Yudkoff, M. Regulation of GABA level in rat brain synaptosomes: Fluxes through enzymes of the GABA shunt and effects of glutamate, calcium, and ketone bodies. *J. Neurochem.* **1996**, *67*, 2325–2334. [CrossRef] [PubMed]
66. Kovács, Z.; D'Agostino, D.P.; Ari, C. Anxiolytic Effect of Exogenous Ketone Supplementation Is Abolished by Adenosine A1 Receptor Inhibition in Wistar Albino Glaxo/Rijswijk Rats. *Front. Behav. Neurosci.* **2018**, *12*, 29. [CrossRef] [PubMed]
67. Masino, S.A.; Li, T.; Theofilas, P.; Sandau, U.S.; Ruskin, D.N.; Fredholm, B.B.; Geiger, J.D.; Aronica, E.; Boison, D. A ketogenic diet suppresses seizures in mice through adenosine A_1 receptors. *J. Clin. Investig.* **2011**, *121*, 2679–2683. [CrossRef]
68. Paoli, A.; Grimaldi, K.; D'Agostino, D.; Cenci, L.; Moro, T.; Bianco, A.; Palma, A. Ketogenic diet does not affect strength performance in elite artistic gymnasts. *J. Int. Soc. Sports Nutr.* **2012**, *9*, 34. [CrossRef]
69. Gerhart, D.Z.; Enerson, B.E.; Zhdankina, O.Y.; Leino, R.L.; Drewes, L.R. Expression of monocarboxylate transporter MCT1 by brain endothelium and glia in adult and suckling rats. *Am. J. Physiol.* **1997**, *273*, E207–E213. [CrossRef]
70. Ito, K.; Uchida, Y.; Ohtsuki, S.; Aizawa, S.; Kawakami, H.; Katsukura, Y.; Kamiie, J.; Terasaki, T. Quantitative membrane protein expression at the blood-brain barrier of adult and younger cynomolgus monkeys. *J. Pharm. Sci.* **2011**, *100*, 3939–3950. [CrossRef]

71. Uchida, Y.; Ohtsuki, S.; Katsukura, Y.; Ikeda, C.; Suzuki, T.; Kamiie, J.; Terasaki, T. Quantitative targeted absolute proteomics of human blood-brain barrier transporters and receptors. *J. Neurochem.* **2011**, *117*, 333–345. [CrossRef]
72. Achanta, L.B.; Rae, C.D. β-Hydroxybutyrate in the Brain: One Molecule, Multiple Mechanisms. *Neurochem. Res.* **2017**, *42*, 35–49. [CrossRef]
73. Leong, S.F.; Lai, J.C.; Lim, L.; Clark, J.B. Energy-metabolizing enzymes in brain regions of adult and aging rats. *J. Neurochem.* **1981**, *37*, 1548–1556. [CrossRef]
74. Page, M.A.; Williamson, D.H. Enzymes of Ketone-Body Utilisation in Human Brain. *Lancet* **1971**, *298*, 66–68. [CrossRef]
75. Williamson, D.H.; Bates, M.W.; Page, M.A.; Krebs, H.A. Activities of enzymes involved in acetoacetate utilization in adult mammalian tissues. *Biochem. J.* **1971**, *121*, 41–47. [CrossRef] [PubMed]
76. Allen, C.N. Circadian rhythms, diet, and neuronal excitability. *Epilepsia* **2008**, *49*, 124–126. [CrossRef] [PubMed]
77. Blomqvist, G.; Thorell, J.O.; Ingvar, M.; Grill, V.; Widén, L.; Stone-Elander, S. Use of R-beta-[1-11C]hydroxybutyrate in PET studies of regional cerebral uptake of ketone bodies in humans. *Am. J. Physiol.* **1995**, *269*, E948–E959. [CrossRef]
78. Hawkins, R.A.; Biebuyck, J.F. Ketone bodies are selectively used by individual brain regions. *Science* **1979**, *205*, 325–327. [CrossRef]
79. Van Rijt, W.J.; Jager, E.A.; Allersma, D.P.; Aktuğlu Zeybek, A.Ç.; Bhattacharya, K.; Debray, F.-G.; Ellaway, C.J.; Gautschi, M.; Geraghty, M.T.; Gil-Ortega, D.; et al. Efficacy and safety of D,L-3-hydroxybutyrate (D,L-3-HB) treatment in multiple acyl-CoA dehydrogenase deficiency. *Genet. Med.* **2020**, *22*, 908–916. [CrossRef]
80. Stubbs, B.J.; Cox, P.J.; Evans, R.D.; Santer, P.; Miller, J.J.; Faull, O.K.; Magor-Elliott, S.; Hiyama, S.; Stirling, M.; Clarke, K. On the Metabolism of Exogenous Ketones in Humans. *Front. Physiol.* **2017**, *8*, 848. [CrossRef]
81. Desrochers, S.; David, F.; Garneau, M.; Jetté, M.; Brunengraber, H. Metabolism of R- and S-1,3-butanediol in perfused livers from meal-fed and starved rats. *Biochem. J.* **1992**, *285*, 647–653. [CrossRef]
82. Li, R.-J.; Liu, Y.; Liu, H.-Q.; Li, J. Ketogenic diets and protective mechanisms in epilepsy, metabolic disorders, cancer, neuronal loss, and muscle and nerve degeneration. *J. Food Biochem.* **2020**, *44*, e13140. [CrossRef]
83. Marchiò, M.; Roli, L.; Giordano, C.; Trenti, T.; Guerra, A.; Biagini, G. Decreased ghrelin and des-acyl ghrelin plasma levels in patients affected by pharmacoresistant epilepsy and maintained on the ketogenic diet. *Clin. Nutr.* **2019**, *38*, 954–957. [CrossRef]
84. Rogawski, M.A.; Löscher, W.; Rho, J.M. Mechanisms of Action of Antiseizure Drugs and the Ketogenic Diet. *Cold Spring Harb. Perspect. Med.* **2016**, *6*. [CrossRef] [PubMed]
85. Vreugdenhil, M.; Bruehl, C.; Voskuyl, R.A.; Kang, J.X.; Leaf, A.; Wadman, W.J. Polyunsaturated fatty acids modulate sodium and calcium currents in CA1 neurons. *Proc. Natl. Acad. Sci. USA* **1996**, *93*, 12559–12563. [CrossRef] [PubMed]
86. Mazier, M.; Jones, P. Diet fat saturation and feeding state modulate rates of cholesterol synthesis in normolipidemic men. *J. Nutr.* **1997**, *127*, 332–340. [CrossRef] [PubMed]
87. Hartman, A.L.; Gasior, M.; Vining, E.P.G.; Rogawski, M.A. The Neuropharmacology of the Ketogenic Diet. *Pediatr. Neurol.* **2007**, *36*, 281–292. [CrossRef] [PubMed]

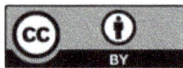
© 2020 by the authors. Licensee MDPI, Basel, Switzerland. This article is an open access article distributed under the terms and conditions of the Creative Commons Attribution (CC BY) license (http://creativecommons.org/licenses/by/4.0/).

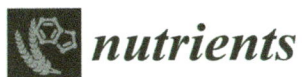

Review

Effects of Beta-Alanine Supplementation on Physical Performance in Aerobic–Anaerobic Transition Zones: A Systematic Review and Meta-Analysis

Álvaro Huerta Ojeda [1,*], Camila Tapia Cerda [2], María Fernanda Poblete Salvatierra [2], Guillermo Barahona-Fuentes [1] and Carlos Jorquera Aguilera [3]

1. Grupo de Investigación en Salud, Actividad Física y Deporte ISAFYD, Escuela de Educación Física, Universidad de Las Américas, sede Viña del Mar 2531098, Chile; danielbarahonaf@gmail.com
2. Facultad de Ciencias, Escuela de Nutrición y Dietética, Magíster en Nutrición para la Actividad Física y Deporte, Universidad Mayor, Santiago 8580745, Chile; camitapiac@hotmail.com (C.T.C.); mariafernandapoblete@gmail.com (M.F.P.S.)
3. Facultad de Ciencias, Escuela de Nutrición y Dietética, Universidad Mayor, Santiago 8580745, Chile; carlos.jorquera@mayor.cl
* Correspondence: achuertao@yahoo.es; Tel.: +56-9-77980432

Received: 13 July 2020; Accepted: 13 August 2020; Published: 19 August 2020

Abstract: Beta-alanine supplementation (BA) has a positive impact on physical performance. However, evidence showing a benefit of this amino acid in aerobic–anaerobic transition zones is scarce and the results controversial. The aim of this systematic review and meta-analysis is to analyze the effects of BA supplementation on physical performance in aerobic–anaerobic transition zones. At the same time, the effect of different dosages and durations of BA supplementation were identified. The search was designed in accordance with the PRISMA® guidelines for systematic reviews and meta-analyses and performed in Web of Science (WOS), Scopus, SPORTDiscus, PubMed, and MEDLINE between 2010 and 2020. The methodological quality and risk of bias were evaluated with the Cochrane Collaboration tool. The main variables were the Time Trial Test (TTT) and Time to Exhaustion (TTE) tests, the latter separated into the Limited Time Test (LTT) and Limited Distance Test (LDT). The analysis was carried out with a pooled standardized mean difference (SMD) through Hedges' g test (95% CI). Nineteen studies were included in the systematic review and meta-analysis, revealing a small effect for time in the TTT (SMD, −0.36; 95% CI, −0.87–0.16; I^2 = 59%; p = 0.010), a small effect for LTT (SMD, 0.25; 95% CI, −0.01–0.51; I^2 = 0%; p = 0.53), and a large effect for LDT (SMD, 4.27; 95% CI, −0.25–8.79; I^2 = 94%; p = 0.00001). BA supplementation showed small effects on physical performance in aerobic–anaerobic transition zones. Evidence on acute supplementation is scarce (one study); therefore, exploration of acute supplementation with different dosages and formats on physical performance in aerobic–anaerobic transition zones is needed.

Keywords: beta-alanine; ergogenic aid; physical performance; aerobic–anaerobic transition zone

1. Introduction

A proper diet is one of the main factors in the improvement of physical performance. However, sometimes it is not enough to meet the energetic demands of training sessions [1]. For this reason and with the aim of maximizing physical performance, the use of nutritional supplements is widespread in sport [2], even more in younger athletes [3]. Nutritional supplements, such as protein and carbohydrates, are concentrated nutrient sources that substitute or complement the use of certain foods, while ergogenic aids, such as caffeine, creatine, or beta-alanine (BA), are pharmacological agents used with the aim of enhancing physical performance [4]. In this regard, one study showed that

48% of athletes use nutritional supplements and ergogenic aids [3], claiming that certain components, such as creatine, caffeine, sodium bicarbonate, and BA, contribute to an improvement in their physical performance [5–7].

Specifically, BA is a non-essential amino acid synthesized in the liver and found in products of animal origin [8]. Evidence shows that poultry, beef, and fish are products with a large BA content [9]. BA has been consistently shown to increase levels of carnosine (CA) in human skeletal muscle [9–12]. This last substance is synthesized by CA synthase when bonding BA with L-histidine [13]; CA is found in the muscular tissue and acts as a buffer of hydrogen protons (H^+) in high-intensity physical exercises of short duration [11,14]. This is why athletes who follow a vegetarian diet will have lower muscular CA concentrations than those who follow an omnivorous diet [15].

When performing high-intensity exercises, due to the predominant energetic system (anaerobic metabolism of carbohydrates), a high release of H^+ takes place, which leads to a decrease in pH [12]. This pH decrease can negatively affect the metabolic processes of phosphocreatine resynthesis, inhibit contractile processes, and diminish the glycolytic rate—all these factors contribute to the onset of muscular fatigue [14]. Some studies have concluded that an elevated muscular CA concentration could buffer between 8–15% of H^+, opening the possibility of maximizing physical effort for a longer period of time [1]. On the other hand, other studies have shown that CA and L-histidine supplementation do not increase the bioavailability of intramuscular CA [5,14]. For this reason, and considering BA as a precursor in CA formation, several studies have shown an increase between 40–80% of intramuscular CA post BA supplementation [1,9–11,16]. In this regard, the acute effect of BA supplementation has been tested in doses of 30 mg·kg^{-1} of body mass and prolonged supplementation with doses ranging from 2.0 to 6.4 g/day for periods of time between 4 and 10 weeks [12,17]. At the same time, BA can be found as the main ingredient in multi-ingredient pre-workout supplements, although it is worth mentioning that these products have a lower dosage than that studied clinically [18]. Specifically, lower pH values have been measured after 4 min of high-intensity exercise [19] and the drop of pH is one of the factors responsible for the increase in ventilatory responses [20]. In parallel, the background shows that BA supplementation reported only one secondary effect, paresthesia [21,22]; this is a sensation of flushing associated with an irritant tingling in the ears, scalp, hands, and torso [23].

Related to pH stabilization, there are several studies that have used ergogenic aids to improve physical performance in aerobic–anaerobic transition zones [8,24]. The aerobic–anaerobic transition zone corresponds to an intensity range between aerobic threshold and anaerobic threshold [25] and may serve as a basis for assessing endurance performance individually as well as for prescribing intensities in endurance training [26]. In this regard, BA is among the ergogenic aids used to increase performance in aerobic–anaerobic transition zones [8,9,27]. One study has evaluated the effect of BA supplementation on physical performance, showing an improvement of 13.9% in ventilatory threshold [20]. In addition, another study reported that BA supplementation for 28 days enhanced sub-maximal endurance performance by delaying the onset of blood lactate accumulation (OBLA) [8]. However, other investigations have not found significant results in athletic performance [12], specifically in rowers [28], and trained cyclists [29] with BA supplementation.

The existing evidence shows controversial results that make it impossible to categorize or ensure that BA supplementation improves physical performance in aerobic–anaerobic transition zones (performance mainly connected to ventilator parameters). Hence, the primary aim of this systematic review and meta-analysis was to analyze the effects of BA supplementation on physical performance in aerobic–anaerobic transition zones. Likewise, the effects of different doses and supplementation times with BA were identified.

2. Materials and Methods

2.1. Literature Search Strategies

In order to perform this review, a thorough electronic search was carried out in several databases and search engines. Articles published in Web of Science (WOS), Scopus, SPORTDiscus, PubMed, and MEDLINE were included. A search limit was established from January 2010 to February 2020.

The bibliographic search was performed in accordance with the PRISMA® statement guidelines for systematic reviews and meta-analyses [30]. In each of the aforementioned databases, the search included hits in the title, abstract, and key words search fields. The following key words were combined with Boolean operators AND/OR: [("b-alanine" OR "beta-alanine" OR "b-alanine supplementation" OR "beta-alanine supplementation") AND ("maximal aerobic speed" OR "maximal oxygen uptake" OR "maximal aerobic consumption" OR "endurance")]. One of the authors performed the search, and two reviewed the studies. Together, they decided whether the studies were appropriate for inclusion.

2.2. Inclusion and Exclusion Criteria

The importance of each study was assessed according to the following inclusion criteria: (1) BA supplementation, either acute or chronic supplementation, (2) experimental design studies, (3) healthy adults, (4) studies that included physical performance evaluation in the aerobic–anaerobic transition zone (60–100% VO_2max), (5) studies that included Time Trial Tests (TTT), or Time to Exhaustion (TTE) tests for physical performance evaluation, (6) studies that stated a baseline and control group, (7) studies showing negative and positive changes in TTT or TTE tests, and (8) studies published in English and Spanish. The studies that failed to fulfill the inclusion criteria were not considered in the systematic review nor the meta-analysis. Possible discrepancies were resolved through discussion until a consensus was reached.

2.3. Chronic and Acute Supplementation

Regarding the classification of the supplementation protocols assessed in this systematic review, acute supplementation was considered to be the one in which a unique dose of BA was used between 0 min and 24 h prior to physical exercise, while chronic supplementation was considered those protocols that used repeated dosages of BA for more than one day and up to 10 weeks [31].

2.4. Outcome Measures

The articles were examined regarding the effect of BA supplementation on physical performance in aerobic–anaerobic transition zones (60–100% VO_2max) [26,32]. The primary outcome used for the systematic review and meta-analysis were (a) TTT and (b) TTE tests (Limited Time Test (LTT) and Limited Distance Test (LDT)). In order to establish the upper limit in the aerobic–anaerobic transition zone (100% VO_2max), the minimum time used on the TTT and TTE test (LTT) was 300 s (the literature sets this as the minimum amount of time needed to determine VO_2max) [33,34], while the minimum lower limit in the aerobic–anaerobic transition zone was 60% of VO_2max [32]. These limits were set in order to include studies showing results of 5–63 min [21,35]. The systematic review and meta-analysis also included secondary outcomes stated in the studies. These secondary variables were (a) capillary lactate (mmol·L^{-1}), (b) absolute VO_2max ($LO_2·min^{-1}$), (c) HR (bpm), and (d) ratings of perceived exertion (RPE) according to the Borg scale [36]. It is important to mention that studies were excluded from the systematic review and meta-analysis if they only showed secondary results in the in extenso reading. Median values, standard deviations (SD), and sample sizes were included for the statistical analysis of the meta-analysis, for both the primary and secondary outcomes. If the selected studies did not include numerical data, it was requested of the authors, or if the data were plotted as figures, the values were estimated based on the pixel count. Additionally, the studies that declared paresthesia symptoms in their subjects were also included.

2.5. Publication Bias

Publication bias was assessed using Egger's statistical test. This test determined the presence of bias at $p \leq 0.05$ [37]. Funnel plots were created to interpret the general effect, followed by an Egger's statistic to confirm or refute publication bias. Egger's analysis suggested that the primary variables did not show publication bias: (a) TTT: $z = 1.35$, $p = 0.18$; (b) LTT: $z = 1.90$, $p = 0.06$; (c) LDT: $z = 1.85$, $p = 0.06$ (Figure 1).

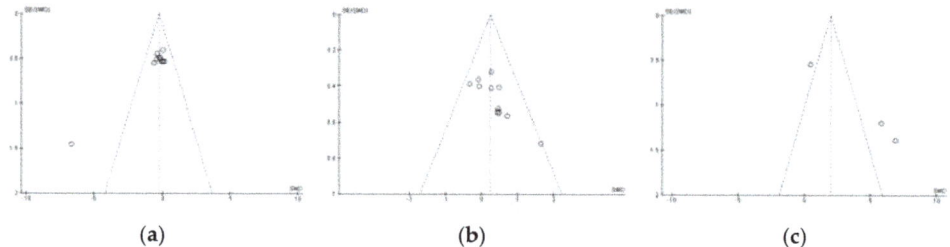

Figure 1. Standard error for Times Trial Test (**a**), Limited Time Test (**b**), and Limited Distance Test (**c**). SE: standard error; SMD: standardized median difference.

2.6. Quality Assessment of the Experiments

The methodological quality and risk of bias for each selected study were assessed through a Cochrane Collaboration guideline [38]. The list was divided into six different domains: selection bias (random sequence generation, allocation concealment), performance bias (blinding of participants and personnel), detection bias (blinding of outcome assessment), attrition bias (incomplete outcome data), reporting bias (selective reporting), and other types of bias (declaration of conflict of interest). For each item, the answer to a question was considered; when the question was answered with a "Yes", the bias was low; when it was "No", the bias was high; when it was "Unclear", the possible bias was connected to a lack of information or uncertainty. The full details of each study and domains are presented in Figures 2 and 3.

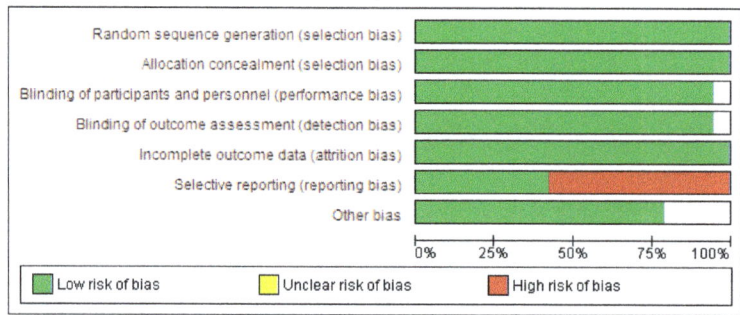

Figure 2. Risk of bias graph: review authors' judgements about each risk of bias item presented as percentages across all included studies.

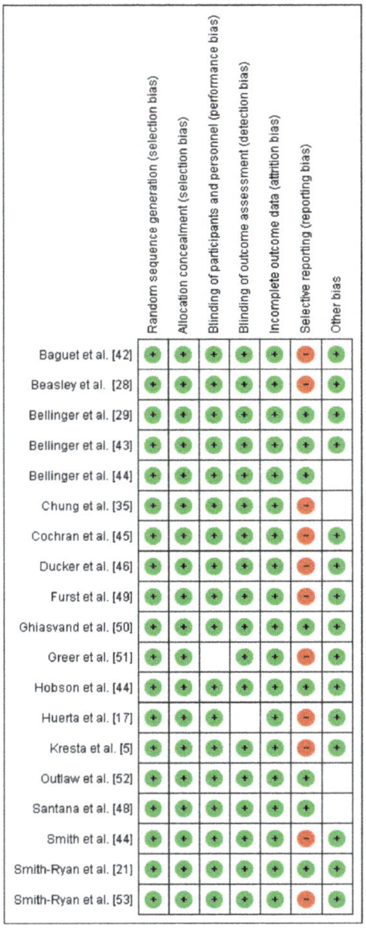

Figure 3. Risk of bias summary: review authors' judgements about each risk of bias item for each included study.

2.7. Statistical Analysis

In order to evaluate the quality of the experiments and interpret the risk of bias values, Review Manager version 5.4 was used (Copenhagen: The Nordic Cochrane Centre, The Cochrane Collaboration, 2014). The same software was used to perform a descriptive and statistical analysis of the meta-analysis. To compare the supplementation of BA versus the placebo (PL), the number of participants, standardized mean difference (SMD), and standard error of SMD were analyzed for each study. Hedges' g test was used to calculate the SMD of each study [39]. The overall effect and its 95% confidence interval (CI) were calculated by weighting the SMD by the inverse of the variance. Additionally, the SMD of both the BA supplemented and PL groups were subtracted to obtain the net effect size (ES), which was used together with the pooled SD of change to calculate the variance (ES = [mean BA − mean PL]/SD); to interpret the magnitude of the ES, Cohen's criteria were followed: <0.2, trivial; 0.2–0.5, small; 0.5–0.8, moderate; and >0.8, large [40].

The I^2 statistic was calculated as an indicator of the percentage of observed total variation within studies due to real heterogeneity rather than chance. I^2 values are included from 0 to 100%, representing a small amount of inconsistency between 25% and 50%, a medium amount of heterogeneity between

50% and 75%, and a large amount of heterogeneity when the I^2 value was higher than 75%. In this sense, low, moderate, and high adjectives would be accepted referring to I^2 values of 25%, 50%, and 75%, respectively, although a restrictive categorization would not be adequate in all circumstances [41].

3. Results

3.1. Main Search

The literature search through electronic databases identified 323 articles of which 177 were duplicates. The remaining 146 articles were filtered by title and abstract, and 57 studies remained to be read and analyzed. After a review of those 57 studies, 40 were eliminated because they did not meet the inclusion criteria. In the search for articles oriented by bibliographic references, two extra studies were added. As a result, 19 articles were included for the systematic review and meta-analysis. The search strategy and study selection are shown in Figure 4. Out of 19 studies, eight considered time in a TTT to assess the effect of BA supplementation on physical performance [29,42–48], nine used time (LTT) on a TTE test to assess the same effect [5,21,22,35,49–53], one considered the distance (LDT) on a TTE test [28], while one considered both the time (LTT) and the distance (LDT) on a TTE test [17] (Table 1).

3.2. Effect of BA on Time Trial Tests

Eight studies were considered for this analysis [29,42–48]. However, two of them included two TTTs in the research design [29,44]. For the meta-analysis, the study by Bellinger et al. [29] was considered as two independent designs (TTT of 4 and 10 km on a cycle ergometer, respectively). In the same way, the study by Bellinger et al. [44] was considered as two independent designs (TTT of 4 and 10 km on a cycle ergometer, respectively). Thus, 10 studies were included in the meta-analysis that calculated the effect of BA supplementation on time in TTT. Figure 5 shows that BA supplementation generates a small and non-significant effect on physical performance in TTT (SMD, −0.36; 95% CI −0.87–0.16; $p = 0.18$). The meta-analysis showed moderate heterogeneity among the studies reviewed ($I^2 = 59\%$; $p = 0.01$). Out of the 10 studies analyzed, seven of them declared a beneficial effect of supplementation with BA on physical performance in TTT [29,42,43,46–48]. Out of these studies, the research of Santana et al. [48] presented a large ES (−6.70). On the other hand, three of the 10 studies showed a neutral or prejudicial effect after BA supplementation [44,45].

3.3. Effect of BA on the Limited Time Test

Ten studies were considered for this analysis [5,17,21,22,35,49–53]. However, one of them included two experimental groups for the LTT in their research design [21]. For the meta-analysis, two experimental groups presented by Smith-Ryan et al. [21] were considered as two independent studies (LTT at 90% of VO_2max on a treadmill for women and LTT at 90% of VO_2max on a treadmill for men). This way, 11 studies were included in the meta-analysis that calculated the effect of BA supplementation on the TTE test. Figure 6 shows that BA supplementation generated a small and non-significant effect for time on the TTE test (SMD, 0.25; 95% CI −0.01–0.51; $p = 0.06$). A meta-analysis showed low heterogeneity among the reviewed studies ($I^2 = 0\%$; $p = 0.53$). Out of the 11 studied and analyzed, eight showed a positive effect of BA on time in the LTT [5,17,21,22,49–52]. Out of these studies, Furst et al. [49] showed a large ES (1.64). On the other hand, three of the 11 studies showed an unbeneficial effect after BA supplementation [21,35,53].

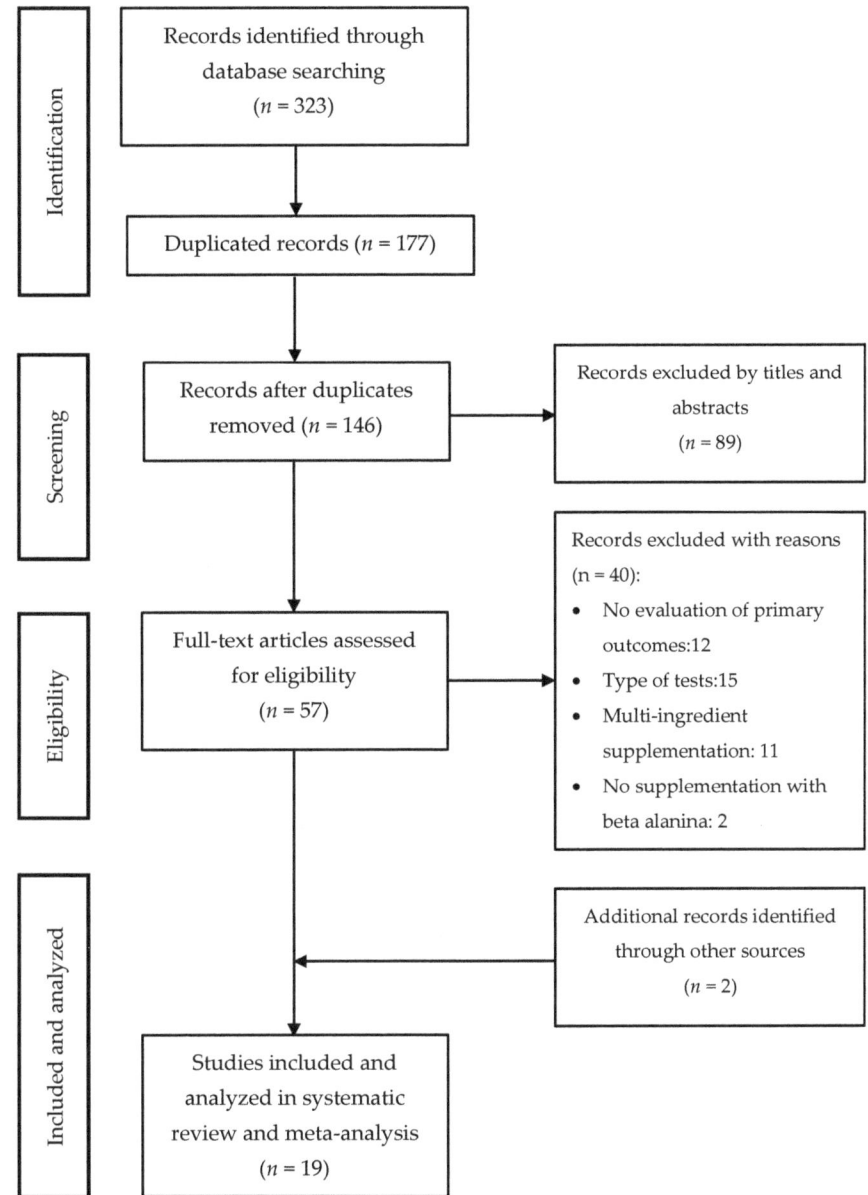

Figure 4. Studies included in the systematic review and meta-analysis.

Table 1. Characteristics of the studies that connect BA supplementation with physical performance in aerobic–anaerobic transition zone.

Author	Objective	Subjects	Variables	Test	Supplementation Protocol	Results	Performance in PO
					Chronic effect of BA supplementation in aerobic–anaerobic transition zone		
Baguet et al. [42]	To investigate if performance is related to the muscle CA content and if BA suppl improves performance in highly trained rowers.	C/A: Rowers M = 16; F = 1 (EG = 8; CG = 9) A: 22.9 ± 4.2 years	I: EG: BA + training CG: PL + training D: PO: TTT	TTT: 2000 m rowing ergometer	Oral suppl of 7 w Total dose 7 w: 245 g EG: BA 5 g/day (5 doses of 1 g, c/2 h) CG: maltodextrin	Time (s) post test: EG = 386.5 vs. CG = 391.5; $p > 0.05$ The authors declared paresthesia: no	↔
Beasley et al. [28]	To investigate the effect of two BA dosing strategies on 30 min rowing and subsequent sprint performance.	RA: Rowers M = 27 (EG$_1$ = 9; EG$_2$ = 9; CG = 9) A: 24.0 ± 5.0 years	I: EG: BA + training CG: PL + training D: PO: LDT SO: VO$_2$max, [La], RPE, HR	LDT: 30 min rowing ergometer	Oral suppl of 28 d Total dose 28 d: 67.2 g EG$_1$: BA 2.4 g/day (1 dose of 2.4 g, e/24 h) EG$_2$: BA 4.8 g/day (1 dose of 4.8 g, e/48 h) CG: corn flour	Distance (m) post test: GE$_1$ = 7579 vs. CG = 7228; $p > 0.05$ GE$_2$ = 7575 vs. CG = 7228; $p > 0.05$ VO$_2$max (LO$_2 \cdot$min^{-1}) post test: GE$_1$ = 3.63 vs. CG = 3.33; $p > 0.05$ GE$_2$ = 3.50 vs. CG = 3.33; $p > 0.05$ [La] (mmol·L^{-1}) post test: GE$_1$ = 10.0 vs. CG = 9.1; $p > 0.05$ GE$_2$ = 8.8 vs. CG = 9.1; $p > 0.05$ RPE (1–10) post test: GE$_1$ = 9.7 vs. CG = 9.6; $p > 0.05$ GE$_2$ = 9.3 vs. CG = 9.6; $p > 0.05$ HR (bpm) post test: GE$_1$ = 190 vs. CG = 185; $p > 0.05$ GE$_2$ = 182 vs. CG = 185; $p > 0.05$ The authors declared paresthesia: no	↔
Bellinger et al. [43]	To investigate the effects of BA suppl on the resultant blood acidosis, lactate accumulation, and energy provision during supramaximal-intensity cycling, as well as the aerobic and anaerobic contribution to power output during a 4000 m cycling time trial.	C/A: Cyclists M = 17 (EG = 9; CG = 8) A: 24.5 ± 6.2 years	I: EG: BA + training CG: PL + training D: PO: TTT SO: VO$_2$max, [La], RPE	TTT 4000 m cycle ergometer	Oral suppl of 28 d Total dose of 28 d: 179.2 g EG: BA 6.4 g/day (4 dose of 1.6 g, in every meal) CG: dextrose monohydrate	Time (s) post test: EG = 355.6 vs. CG = 360.4; $p < 0.05$ VO$_2$max (LO$_2 \cdot$min^{-1}) post test: EG = 4.45 vs. CG = 4.44; $p > 0.05$ [La] (mmol·L^{-1}) post test: EG = 15.1 vs. CG = 15.2; $p > 0.05$ RPE (6–20) post test: EG = 18.8 vs. CG = 18.8; $p > 0.05$ The authors declared paresthesia: no	↑

Table 1. Cont.

Author	Objective	Subjects	Variables	Test	Supplementation Protocol	Results	Performance in PO
Chronic effect of BA supplementation in aerobic–anaerobic transition zone							
Bellinger et al. [29]	To assess the efficacy of BA suppl on cycling time trial of different length in the same group of trained cyclists and to contrast the effects of BA supply on a supramaximal time to fatigue test.	C/A: Cyclists M = 14 (EG = 7; CG = 7) A: 24.8 ± 6.7 years	I: EG: BA + training CG: PL + training D: PO: TTT SO: [La]	TTT 4 km and 10 km cycle ergometer	Oral suppl of 28 d Total dose 28 d: 179.2 g EG: BA 6.4 g/day (4 dose of 1.6 g, with every meal) CG: dextrose monohydrate	4 km Time (s) post test: EG = 356.6 vs. CG = 357.8; $p > 0.05$ [La] (mmol·L^{-1}) post test: EG = 15.3 vs. CG = 15.4; $p > 0.05$ 10 km Time (s) post test: EG = 938.1 vs. CG = 929.9; $p > 0.05$ [La] (mmol·L^{-1}) post test: EG = 11.0 vs. CG = 12.9; $p > 0.05$ The authors declared paresthesia: yes	4 km ↔ 10 km ↔
Bellinger et al. [44]	To investigate the effects of BA suppl only, and in combination with sprint-interval training, on training intensity, and energy provision and performance during exhaustive supramaximal-intensity cycling and a 4 and 10 km time trial.	C/A: Cyclists M = 14 (EG = 7; CG = 7) A: 25.4 ± 7.2 years	I: EG: BA + training CG: PL + training D: PO: TTT	TTT 4 km and 10 km cycle ergometer	Oral suppl of 9 w Total dose 9 w: 221.2 g EG: BA 6.4 g/day for 4 w (4 doses of 1.6 g w/every meal) + BA 1.2 g/day for 5 w (3 doses of 400 mg, every 3 to 4 h) CG: dextrose monohydrate	4 km Time (s) post test: EG = 339.7 vs. CG = 350.1; $p > 0.05$ 10 km Time (s) post test: EG = 918.5 vs. CG = 916.6; $p > 0.05$ The authors declared paresthesia: no	4 km ↔ 10 km ↔
Chung et al. [35]	To investigate whether BA suppl can increase muscle CA stores in endurance-trained athletes, and whether CA loading can improve their endurance performance.	C/A: Cyclists and triathletes M = 27 (EG = 14; CG = 13) A: 30.9 ± 7.9 years	I: EG: BA + training CG: PL + training D: PO: LTT SO: [La], RPE, HR	LTT incremental cycle ergometer (from 50 W, ≥60 rpm until exhaustion)	Oral suppl of 6 w Total dose 6 w 268.8 g EG: BA 6.4 g/day (4 doses of 1.6 g, with every meal) CG: maltodextrin	Time (s) post test: EG = 3696 vs. CG = 3780; $p > 0.05$ [La] (mmol·L^{-1}) post test: EG = 9.7 vs. CG = 7.3; $p > 0.05$ RPE: (6–20) post test: EG = 19.0 vs. CG = 18.8; $p > 0.05$ HR (bpm) post test: EG = 181 vs. CG = 180; $p > 0.05$ The authors declared paresthesia: no	↔

Table 1. Cont.

Author	Objective	Subjects	Variables	Test	Supplementation Protocol	Results	Performance in PO
Chronic effect of BA supplementation in aerobic-anaerobic transition zone							
Cochran et al. [45]	To increase skeletal-muscle CA and augment muscle buffering capacity during a 6 week sprint interval training intervention.	PA: Healthy subjects M = 24 (EG = 12; CG = 12) A: 22.5 ± 2.0 years	I: EG: BA + training CG: PL + training D: PO: TTT SO: VO$_2$max	TTT 250 KJ cycle ergometer	Oral suppl of 10 w Total dose 10 w: 224 g EG: BA 3.2 g/day (2 doses of 1.6 g, every 12 h) CG: dextrose	Time (s) post test: EG = 1130 vs. CG = 1125; $p > 0.05$ VO$_2$max (mL O$_2$·kg^{-1}·min^{-1}) post test: EG = 52.2 vs. CG = 55.4; $p > 0.05$ The authors declared paresthesia: no	↔
Ducker et al. [46]	To assess if beta-alanine suppl could improve 2000 m rowing-ergometer performance in well-trained male rowers.	C/A: Rowers M = 16 (EG = 7; CG = 9) A: 26.0 ± 9.0 years	I: EG: BA + training CG: PL + training D: PO: TTT SO: [La]	TTT 2000 m rowing ergometer	Oral suppl of 28 d Total dose 28 d: ~168 a 196 g (80 mg·kg^{-1}·d^{-1}) EG: BA ~6-7 g/day (4 doses of 1.5-1.75 g, with every meal) CG: glucose	Time (s) post test: EG = 391.0 vs. CG = 393.4; $p > 0.05$ [La] (mmol·L^{-1}) post test: EG = 12.5 vs. CG = 12.4; $p > 0.05$ The authors declared paresthesia: no	↔
Furst et al. [49]	To investigate the effect of BA suppl on exercise endurance and executive function in a middle-aged human population.	N/T: Healthy subjects M = 8; F = 4 (EG = 7; CG = 5) A: 60.5 ± 8.6 years	I: EG: BA + training CG: PL + training D: PO: LTT SO: [La]	LTT at 70% VO$_2$peak cycle ergometer	Oral suppl of 28 d Total dose 28 d: 67.2 g EG: BA 2.4 g/day (3 doses of 800 mg, with every meal) CG: microcrystalline cellulose	Time (s) post test: EG = 876 vs. CG = 522; $p > 0.05$ [La] (mmol·L^{-1}) post test: EG = 6.6 vs. CG = 4.2; $p > 0.05$ The authors declared paresthesia: no	↔
Ghiasvand et al. [50]	To assess the effects of alanine suppl on VO$_2$max, time to exhaustion, and lactate concentrations in physical education male students.	RA: Healthy college students M = 39 (EG = 20; CG = 19) A: 21.5 ± 1.1 years	I: EG: BA + training CG: PL + training D: PO: LTT SO: VO$_2$max, [La]	LTT incremental cycle ergometer (from 30 W, ≥70 rpm to exhaustion)	Oral suppl of 6 w Total dose 6 w: 84 g EG: BA 2 g/day (5 doses of 400 mg, with every meal) CG: dextrose	Time (s) post test: EG = 992.4 vs. CG = 926.5; $p < 0.05$ VO$_2$max (L O$_2$·min^{-1}) post test: EG = 2.79 vs. CG = 2.81; $p < 0.05$ [La] (mg·dL^{-1}) post test: EG = 27.9 vs. CG = 36.0; $p < 0.05$ The authors declared paresthesia: no	↑
Greer et al. [51]	To determine the effect of 30 days of BA suppl on peak aerobic power and ventilatory threshold in aerobically fit males.	C/A: Aerobically fit males M = 14 A: 28.8 ± 9.8 years	I: EG: BA + training CG: PL + training D: PO: LTT SO: VO$_2$max	LTT cycle ergometer	Oral suppl of 30 d Total dose 30 d: 159 g EG: BA 3 g/day for 7 d (2 doses of 1.5 g, every 12 h) + BA 6 g/day for 23 d (4 doses of 1.5 g, with every meal) CG: maltodextrin	Time (s) post test: EG = 1304 vs. CG = 1125; $p > 0.05$ VO$_2$max (L O$_2$·min^{-1}) post test: EG = 4.14 vs. CG = 3.97; $p > 0.05$ The authors declared paresthesia: yes	↔
Hobson et al. [47]	To examine the effect of BA only and BA with sodium bicarbonate suppl on 2000 m rowing performance.	C/A: Rowers M = 20 (EG = 10; CG = 10) A: 23.0 ± 4.0 years	I: EG: BA + training CG: PL + training D: PO: TTT SO: [La]	TTT 2000 m rowing ergometer	Oral suppl of 30 d Total dose 30 d: 192 g EG: BA 6.4 g/day (4 doses of 1.6 g, every 3-4 h) CG: maltodextrin	Time (s) post test: EG = 410.3 vs. CG = 416.4; BA probability on PL: 96% effect (+) [La] (mmol·L^{-1}) post test: EG = 14.7 vs. CG = 14.5; $p > 0.05$ The authors declared paresthesia: no	↑

Table 1. Cont.

Author	Objective	Subjects	Variables	Test	Supplementation Protocol	Results	Performance in PO
					Chronic effect of BA supplementation in aerobic–anaerobic transition zone		
Kresta et al. [5]	To examine the short-term and chronic effects of BA suppl with and without creatine monohydrate on body composition, aerobic, and anaerobic exercise performance and muscle CA and creatine levels in college-aged recreationally active females.	FA: Healthy college students F = 15 (EG = 8; CG = 7) A: 21.5 ± 2.8 years	I: EG: BA + training CG: PL + training D: PO: LIT SO: VO$_2$max	LIT incremental cycle ergometer (from 50 W, ≥70 rpm to exhaustion)	Oral suppl of 28 d Total dose 28 d: ~ 170.8 g (0.1 g·kg^{-1}·d^{-1}) EG: BA ~ 6.1 g/day (around 4 doses of 800 mg, every 4 h) CG: dextrose and maltodextrin	Time (s) post test: EG = 1293 vs. CG = 1083; $p > 0.05$ VO$_2$max (mL O$_2$·kg^{-1}·min^{-1}) post test: EG = 41.53 vs. CG = 37.90; $p > 0.05$ The authors declared paresthesia: no	↔
Outlaw et al. [32]	To evaluate the cumulative effect of resistance training and BA suppl on aerobic and anaerobic performance markers, as well as body composition, in collegiate females.	S/E: Untrained collegiate females F = 15 (EG = 7; CG = 8) A: 21.0 ± 2.2 years	I: EG: BA + training CG: PL + training D: PO: LIT SO: VO$_2$max	LIT treadmill	Oral suppl of 8 w Total dose 8 w: 108.8 g (32 doses) EG: BA 3.4 g/day (1 single dose before training) CG: maltodextrin	Time (s) post test: EG = 629.1 vs. CG = 591.1; $p > 0.05$ VO$_2$max (mL O$_2$·kg^{-1}·min^{-1}) post test: EG = 41.2 vs. CG = 38.6; $p > 0.05$ The authors declared paresthesia: no	↔
Santana et al. [48]	To investigate the effects of BA suppl on a 10 km running time trial and lactate concentration in physically active adults.	PA: Healthy subjects M = 16 (EG = 8; CG = 8) A: 29.4 ± 3.9 years	I: EG: BA + training CG: PL + training D: PO: TTT SO: [La]	TTT 10 km treadmill	Oral suppl of 23 d Total dose 23 d: 115 g EG: BA 5 g/day (around 3 doses of 1.6 g, every 3 h) CG: resistant starch	Time (s) post test: EG = 3210 vs. CG = 3480; $p < 0.05$ [La] (mmol·L^{-1}) post test: EG = 6.8 vs. CG = 10.8; $p < 0.05$ The authors declared paresthesia: no	↑
Smith et al. [22]	To evaluate the effects of 28 days of BA suppl on markers of oxidative stress.	RA: Healthy women F = 24 (EG = 13; CG = 11) A: 21.7 ± 2.1 years	I: EG: BA + training CG: PL + training D: PO: LIT SO: VO$_2$max	LIT incremental in treadmill (from 10 km·h^{-1} to exhaustion)	Oral suppl of 28 d Total dose 28 d: 134.4 g EG: BA 4.8 g/day (3 doses of 1.6 g, in intervals) CG: maltodextrin	Time (s) post test: EG = 405 vs. CG = 388; $p > 0.05$ VO$_2$max (L·O$_2$·min^{-1}) post test: EG = 2.71 vs. CG = 2.64; $p > 0.05$ The authors declared paresthesia: yes	↔

Table 1. Cont.

Author	Objective	Subjects	Variables	Test	Supplementation Protocol	Results	Performance in PO
Chronic effect of BA supplementation in aerobic–anaerobic transition zone							
Smith-Ryan et al. [21]	To evaluate the effects of BA suppl on high-intensity running performance and critical velocity anaerobic running capacity.	RA: Healthy subjects M and F = 50 (EG = 26; CG = 24) A: 21.9 ± 2.7 years	I: EG: BA + training CG: PL + training D: PO: LTT SO: [La]	LTT at 90% V_{max} treadmill	Oral suppl of 28 d Total dose 28 d: 134.4 g EG: BA 4.8 g/day (3 doses of 1.6 g, in intervals) CG: maltodextrin	Women Time (s) post test: EG = 313.8 vs. CG = 240.5; $p > 0.05$ [La] (mmol·L^{-1}) post test: EG = 13.15 vs. CG = 13.8; $p > 0.05$ Men Time (s) post test: EG = 317.0 vs. CG = 322.6; $p > 0.05$ [La] (mmol·L^{-1}) post test: EG = 15.7 vs. CG = 13.8; $p > 0.05$ The authors declared paresthesia: yes	↔
Smith-Ryan et al. [53]	To determine the effect of 28 days of BA suppl on work physical capacity test in heart rate threshold.	FA: Healthy subjects M and F = 30 (EG = 15; CG = 15) A: 21.0 ± 2.1 years	I: EG: BA + training CG: PL + training D: PO: LTT SO: VO$_2$max	LTT incremental cycle ergometer (from 20 W, ≥60 rpm until exhaustion)	Oral suppl of 28 d Total dose 28 d: 1792 g EG: BA 6.4 g/day (4 dose of 1.6 g, every 3–4 h) CG: maltodextrin	Time (s) post test: EG = 690.5 vs. CG = 703.6; $p > 0.05$ VO$_2$max (mL O$_2$·kg^{-1}·min^{-1}) post test: EG = 39.1 vs. CG = 43.4; $p > 0.05$ The authors declared paresthesia: no	↔
Acute effect of BA supplementation on aerobic–anaerobic transition zone							
Huerta et al. [17]	To determine the acute effect of BA suppl on a limited time test at maximum aerobic speed on endurance athletes.	C/A: High-level athletes M and F = 7 (EG = 7; CG = 7) A: 24.2 ± 4.4 years	I: EG: BA + training CG: PL + training D: PO: TTE (LDT and LTT) SO: [La], RPE, HR	TTE (LTT and LDT) at maximum aerobic speed in athletic track	Oral suppl Total dose: 30 mg·kg^{-1} body mass EG: BA from 1.5–2.1 g/day 60 min before TTE (LDT and LTT) CG: simple carbohydrates	Time (s): EG = 366.5 vs. CG = 326.0; $p < 0.05$ Distance (m): EG = 1828.6 vs. CG = 1651.4; $p > 0.05$ [La] (mmol·L^{-1}): EG = 14.80 vs. CG = 13.84; $p > 0.05$ RPE (1–10): EG = 8.28 vs. CG = 7.60; $p > 0.05$ HR (bpm): EG = 185.4 vs. CG = 178.8; $p > 0.05$ The authors declared paresthesia: no	Time ↑ Distance ↔

A: age; BA: beta-alanine; bpm: beat per minute; C/A: competitive athlete; CA: carnosine; CG: control group; d: days; D: dependent variable; e/: every; EG: experimental group; EG$_1$: experimental group 1; EG$_2$: experimental group 2; g/day: grams per day; g: grams; h: hours; HR: heart rate; I: independent variable; kg: kilograms; KJ: Kilo Joule; km: kilometers; L: liters; LDT: limited distance test; LTT: limited time test; M: male; F: female; m: meters; mg: milligrams; mg·dL^{-1}: milligrams per deciliter; mg·kg^{-1}: milligrams per kilogram; min: minutes; mmol·L^{-1}: millimole per liter; N/T: no training; PA: physically active; PL: placebo; PO: primary outcome; RA: recreational athlete; RPE: ratings of perceived exertion; s: seconds; SO: secondary outcome; suppl: supplementation; T: time; TTE: time to exhaustion; TTT: time trial test; Vmax: maximum velocity; VO$_2$: oxygen uptake; VO$_2$max: maximal oxygen uptake; vs: versus; VT: ventilatory threshold; W: watt; w: weeks; [La]: blood lactate concentration; $p < 0.05$: significant change; $p > 0.05$: non-significant change; ~: approximate; ↑: positive effect; ↔: no effect.

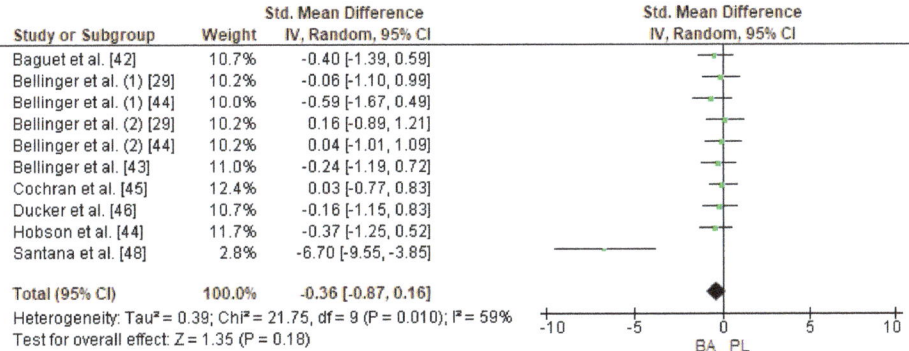

Figure 5. Forest plot comparing the effects of BA supplementation on Time Trial Tests. BA: beta-alanine; PL: placebo.

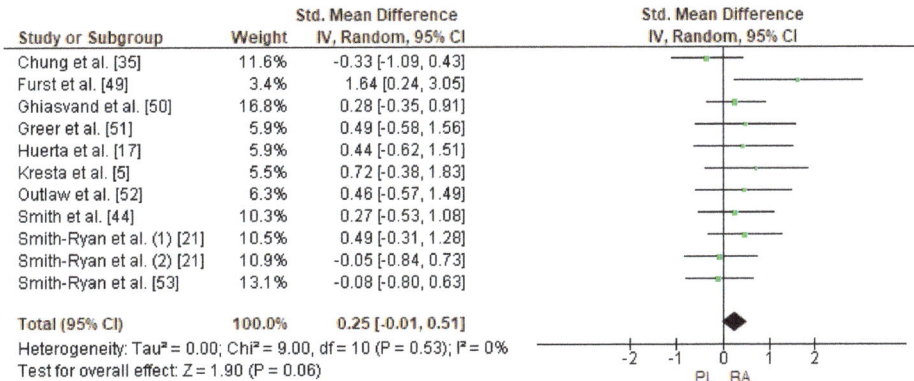

Figure 6. Forest plot comparing the effect of BA on Limited Time Test. BA: beta-alanine; PL: placebo.

3.4. Effect of BA on the Limited Distance Test

Two studies were considered for this analysis [17,28]. However, the study of Baesley et al. [28] included two experimental groups for the LDT in their research design (30 min on a rowing ergometer with 2.4 g/day of BA supplementation every 24 h and 30 min on a rowing ergometer with 4.8 g/day of BA supplementation every 48 h). In this way, three studies were included in the meta-analysis that calculated the effect of BA supplementation on the TTE test. Figure 7 shows that BA supplementation generates a large and non-significant effect on distance in the TTE test (SMD, 4.27; 95% CI −0.25–8.79; $p = 0.06$). The meta-analysis showed high heterogeneity among the studies reviewed ($I^2 = 94\%$; $p = 0.00001$). All studies analyzed declared a beneficial effect of supplementation with BA on physical performance in LDT [17,28].

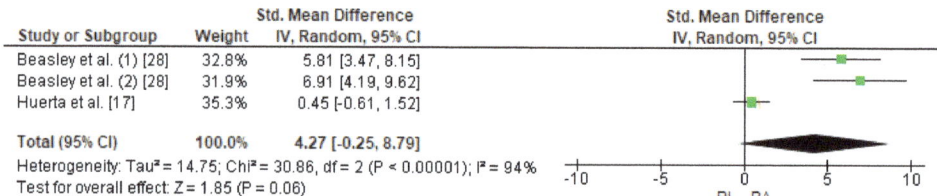

Figure 7. Forest plot comparing the effect of BA on Limited Distance Test. BA: beta-alanine; PL: placebo.

3.5. Effect of BA Supplementation on Secondary Outcomes

Of the total of 19 studies included in the systematic review and meta-analysis, 17 of them reported on different parameters of physical performance. These parameters were defined as secondary outcomes and included blood lactate concentration ([La]), VO_2max, RPE, and HR [32].

The meta-analysis of [La] (mmol·L^{-1}) included 11 studies [5,17,21,28,29,35,43,46–49]. The total number of cases supplemented with BA included 128 participants, while 121 participants were supplemented with PL. The meta-analysis showed that BA supplementation generated a trivial and non-significant effect on [La] post effort (SMD, 0.16; 95% CI −0.35–0.67; $p = 0.53$), while moderate heterogeneity was present among the reviewed studies ($I^2 = 71\%$; $p = 0.0001$). A meta-analysis of absolute VO_2max (LO$_2$·min^{-1}) included nine studies [5,22,28,43,45,50–53]. The total number of cases supplemented with BA included 109 participants, while the PL group comprised 104 participants. The meta-analysis showed that BA supplementation generated a trivial and non-significant effect on absolute VO_2max (SMD, 0.17; 95% CI −0.11–0.45; $p = 0.24$), and low heterogeneity was observed among the studies ($I^2 = 6\%$; $p = 0.39$). The meta-analysis of RPE [36] included four studies [17,28,35,43]: the total number of cases supplemented with BA included 48 participants, while those supplemented with PL comprised 46. The meta-analysis showed that BA supplementation generated a trivial and non-significant effect on RPE (SMD, 0.03; 95% CI −0.52–0.58; $p = 0.92$), and low heterogeneity was observed in the studies ($I^2 = 42\%$; $p = 0.14$). Finally, the meta-analysis for HR included three studies [17,28,35], and the total of number of cases supplemented with BA included 39 participants, while those supplemented with PL comprised 38. The meta-analysis showed that BA supplementation generates a small and non-significant effect on HR (SMD, 0.30; 95% CI −0.66 to −1.26; $p = 0.54$), and a high heterogeneity was observed among the studies reviewed ($I^2 = 75\%$; $p = 0.008$).

3.6. Paresthesia

At the end of this review, out of the 19 studies included in the systematic review and meta-analysis, four of them reported paresthesia [21,22,29,51] (Table 1).

4. Discussion

In connection with the studies included in the systematic review and meta-analysis, the results showed that BA supplementation presents an ES ranging from a small (0.2–0.5) to a large magnitude (>0.8) in aerobic–anaerobic transition zones. At the same time, the results showed that changes in physical performance are associated with both acute and chronic BA supplementation, while the administered doses ranged from 1.5–6.4 g/day in periods ranging from 1 h before physical tests (acute supplementation) to 10 weeks with one or several doses during the day (chronic supplementation).

At the end of this review, several studies concluded that the increase in physical performance after BA supplementation is due to an increase in muscular CA concentrations [21,42,53]. The ergogenic effect that generates increased CA is associated with intracellular regulation of pH (buffer), an increase in Calcium (Ca^{2+}) sensitivity in type I and II muscle fibers, and an increase in Ca^{2+}/H^+ ion exchange; as a consequence, these events showed an increase in muscular contractility [1]. For this reason, direct supplementation with CA has been studied with inconclusive results [14,54,55], since CA is degraded into BA and L-histidine in the stomach [5]. Specifically, the low effectiveness of direct supplementation with CA is related to the fact that L-histidine has a larger presence in plasma than BA [1]. Because of this, BA supplementation shows better results than CA supplementation [44,50].

At the end of this review, the only secondary effect reported and associated with BA supplementation was paresthesia [21,22]. This is a sensation of flushing associated with an irritant tingling in the ears, scalp, hands, and torso [23]. The process responsible for paresthesia is the release of L-histidine to form CA [9,12,27]. Paresthesia is transitory and can be avoided by dosing and ingesting BA in smaller portions throughout the day [9,12,27].

4.1. Effect of BA on the Time Trial Test and Time to Exhaustion Test

BA supplementation and the subsequent increase in CA could diminish H^+ circulation and prevent the drop in intracellular pH during high-intensity exercise [50]. In fact, CA has been described as the main buffering substance of H^+ at the muscular level [56]. Previous studies have stated that blood and muscular acidosis limit muscular contractility, which would favor the onset of fatigue [17,29,47,50]. At the same time, due to an increase in Ca^{2+} sensitivity to type I fibers, it has been mentioned that BA supplementation can improve muscular contractile properties, delaying fatigue onset [17,57].

As mentioned above, the performance increase in aerobic–anaerobic transition zones is associated with greater availability of muscular CA [20,50]. This way, evidence has shown that prolonged BA supplementation in doses ranging from 2.0–6.4 g/day for 4–10 weeks can increase CA concentrations between 64–80% [9]. In connection with acute supplementation in aerobic–anaerobic transition zones, evidence is scarce [17]. In this regard, Huerta et al. [17] performed supplementation with 30 $mg \cdot kg^{-1}$ body mass (1.5–2.1 g/day) of BA 60 min prior to a TTE test. These researchers obtained an average increase of 40.5 s at the end of the study ($p < 0.05$). Despite that, and due to the limited evidence relating acute supplementation with BA on physical performance in aerobic–anaerobic transition zones, it is impossible to guarantee a real effect in this physiological zone. However, the increase in physical performance observed in this review is supported by greater bioavailability of CA, an increase that is observed shortly after the intake of BA [58]. This raises the possibility of studying the acute effects of BA using different protocols and observing the real effects in aerobic–anaerobic transition zones.

The ES for distance on the TTE test was large (ES = 4.27), while TTT and time on the TTE test was small (ES = −0.36 and 0.25, respectively). In light of these results, these last values show a small effect of BA supplementation on physical performance in aerobic–anaerobic transition zones. However, considering that an elite athlete's performance is bound by extremely tight margins (probably difficult to measure statistically), in real practice, a small ES could be of great importance, since it has been proven that in world finals, differences lower than 3% can be found between first and last place [1].

4.2. Effect of BA on Secondary Outcomes

BA supplementation could prevent the drop in intracellular pH during high-intensity exercise (due to an increase in muscular CA bioavailability) and, as a consequence, generate less lactate accumulation with the same intensity of physical exercise [48,50]. Regarding lactate accumulation, it is important to mention that this is not the cause of H^+ accumulation, but a high intensity of exercise produces a decrease in pH and an increase in intramuscular and blood [La] simultaneously, transforming lactate in a good marker of physical effort [8]. Despite the theoretical background, the meta-analysis showed a trivial effect on [La] post effort (ES = 0.16).

The influence of BA supplementation on aerobic performance has been widely studied [14,20,27,59]; however, the meta-analysis showed a trivial effect of BA on VO_2 (ES = 0.17) [51,60]. Apparently, the increase in VO_2 is less dependent on the buffer qualities that BA supplementation produces [20]. It is possible that the improvement in VO_2 reported in some studies included in the meta-analysis is more connected to physical training in aerobic–anaerobic transition zones than to BA supplementation [61,62].

In connection to RPE, some studies have shown a good correlation between RPE and HR during physical exercise in healthy subjects (1 point of RPE equals approximately 10 bpm). More so, the metabolic thresholds have been associated with specific values on the Borg scale [36]. Likewise, it has been shown that a lower value of RPE for the same workload entails a metabolic adaptation after the training process [63]. Despite these lines of theoretical evidence, the studies included in the meta-analysis showed a trivial effect on RPE reported by the participants (ES = 0.03). This value can be derived from the level of demand experienced by the participant; it is also possible that they exerted themselves to the maximum effort in all tests, reaching the upper limits of the RPE scales used [36].

As a consequence improved cardiac contractility, it has been described that CA can increase HR [53]. In addition, intracellular pH has proven to be a modulator of cardiac function, increasing the entrance of Ca^{2+} during action potentials, facilitating cardiac contraction [64]. This information makes it possible to anticipate an increase in HR after BA supplementation [53]. However, HR is dependent on the intensity of physical effort; hence, if the participants exerted themselves to the maximum in all tests, it is likely that post-effort HR values would not show major variations when supplementing with BA (ES = 0.30).

Finally, due to a limited number of studies, only the secondary outcomes mentioned above were used. Subdividing the 10 TTT studies and 11 TTL studies to perform a meta-analysis by gender, age, exercise modalities, or physical activity level would have generated a bias in the information obtained [38].

4.3. Limitations

The main limitations of this research were the access to information and unspecific data reported by some studies included in the systematic review and meta-analysis. However, the limitations were solved by contacting the authors of each study. Only one document was not included because no answer was received. Another important limitation in this review was the limited number of studies that used TDL as a primary outcome [17,28].

5. Conclusions

Both acute and chronic supplementation with BA in doses of 1.5–6.4 g/day showed a small and non-significant effect on physical performance in aerobic–anaerobic transition zones. Physiologically, this positive change is due to the buffer effects generated by the larger bioavailability of intracellular CA, which allows for a delay in the onset of fatigue in the TTT and TTE tests within this specific physiologic zone. That is why small changes in individual performance must be considered, since they can be the difference between success and failure among high-level and elite athletes.

Furthermore, the findings showed evidence that acute supplementation with BA is scarce, generating alternatives for researchers to study the effect of this form of supplementation with different BA doses and formats on performance in aerobic–anaerobic transition zones.

6. Practical Applications

Coaches and athletes looking for an ergogenic aid to enhance physical performance in aerobic–anaerobic transition zones should consider both acute and chronic supplementation with BA. The dosage can range from 30 mg·kg^{-1} of body mass in acute supplementation to 6.4 g/day in chronic supplementation. The latter may be administered in several doses per day. However, it is advisable to check the dosage and supplementation formats with qualified professionals.

Finally, in order to avoid the presence of paresthesia after supplementation with BA, it is recommended that BA be dosed and ingested in small portions throughout the day (the amount suggested for these doses is 1.6 g of BA per dose) [9]. The second recommendation to avoid paresthesia is to also ingest a large amount of carbohydrates 60 min before ingesting BA (the suggested carbohydrate load is 2 g·kg^{-1} of body mass) [17].

Author Contributions: Á.H.O., C.T.C., and M.F.P.S.: conception, methodology, investigation, data curation, writing—original draft preparation, writing—review and editing. G.B.-F.: visualization and writing—review and editing. C.J.A.: supervision and project administration. All authors have read and agreed to the published version of the manuscript.

Funding: The authors declare no funding sources.

Conflicts of Interest: The authors declare no conflict of interests.

References

1. Santesteban, V.; Ibáñez, J. Ayudas ergogénicas en el deporte. *Nutr. Hosp.* **2017**, *34*, 204–215. [CrossRef] [PubMed]
2. Derave, W.; Tipton, K.D. Dietary supplements for aquatic sports. *Int. J. Sport Nutr. Exerc. Metab.* **2014**, *24*, 437–449. [CrossRef] [PubMed]
3. Frączek, B.; Warzecha, M.; Tyrała, F.; Pięta, A. Prevalence of the use of effective ergogenic aids among professional athletes. *Rocz. Panstw. Zakl. Hig.* **2016**, *67*, 271–278. [PubMed]
4. López-Samanes, Á.; Moreno, V.; Kovacs, M.S.; Pallarés, J.G.; Mora, R.; Ortega, J. Use of nutritional supplements and ergogenic aids in professional tennis players. *Nutr. Hosp.* **2017**, *34*, 1463–1468. [PubMed]
5. Kresta, J.Y.; Oliver, J.M.; Jagim, A.R.; Fluckey, J.; Riechman, S.; Kelly, K.; Meininger, C.; Mertens-Talcott, S.U.; Rasmussen, C.; Kreider, R.B. Effects of 28 days of beta-alanine and creatine supplementation on muscle carnosine, body composition and exercise performance in recreationally active females. *J. Int. Soc. Sports Nutr.* **2014**, *11*, 55. [CrossRef]
6. Galdames, S.; Huerta, Á.; Pastene, A. Efecto de la suplementación aguda con bicarbonato sódico sobre el rendimiento en la cancha con obstáculos en pentatletas militares profesionales. *Arch. Med. del Deport.* **2020**, in press.
7. Maughan, R.J.; Burke, L.M.; Dvorak, J.; Larson-Meyer, D.E.; Peeling, P.; Phillips, S.M.; Rawson, E.S.; Walsh, N.P.; Garthe, I.; Geyer, H.; et al. IOC consensus statement: Dietary supplements and the high-performance athlete. *Int. J. Sport Nutr. Exerc. Metab.* **2018**, *28*, 104–125. [CrossRef]
8. Jordan, T.; Lukaszuk, J.; Misic, M.; Umoren, J. Effect of beta-alanine supplementation on the onset of blood lactate accumulation (OBLA) during treadmill running: Pre/post 2 treatment experimental design. *J. Int. Soc. Sports Nutr.* **2010**, *7*, 20. [CrossRef]
9. Trexler, E.T.; Smith-Ryan, A.E.; Stout, J.R.; Hoffman, J.R.; Wilborn, C.D.; Sale, C.; Kreider, R.B.; Jäger, R.; Earnest, C.P.; Bannock, L.; et al. International society of sports nutrition position stand: Beta-Alanine. *J. Int. Soc. Sports Nutr.* **2015**, *12*. [CrossRef]
10. Stegen, S.; Bex, T.; Vervaet, C.; Vanhee, L.; Achten, E.; Derave, W. β-Alanine dose for maintaining moderately elevated muscle carnosine levels. *Med. Sci. Sports Exerc.* **2014**, *46*, 1426–1432. [CrossRef]
11. Bex, T.; Chung, W.; Baguet, A.; Achten, E.; Derave, W. Exercise Training and Beta-Alanine-Induced Muscle Carnosine Loading. *Front. Nutr.* **2015**, *2*, 13. [CrossRef] [PubMed]
12. Peeling, P.; Binnie, M.J.; Goods, P.S.R.; Sim, M.; Burke, L.M. Evidence-based supplements for the enhancement of athletic performance. *Int. J. Sport Nutr. Exerc. Metab.* **2018**, *28*, 178–187. [CrossRef] [PubMed]
13. Blancquaert, L.; Everaert, I.; Missinne, M.; Baguet, A.; Stegen, S.; Volkaert, A.; Petrovic, M.; Vervaet, C.; Achten, E.; De Maeyer, M.; et al. Effects of histidine and β-alanine supplementation on human muscle carnosine storage. *Med. Sci. Sports Exerc.* **2017**, *49*, 602–609. [CrossRef] [PubMed]
14. Jagim, A.R.; Wright, G.A.; Brice, A.G. Effects of Beta Alanine supplementation on sprint endurance. *J. Strength Cond. Res.* **2013**, *27*, 526–532. [CrossRef] [PubMed]
15. Harris, R.C.; Wise, J.A.; Price, K.A.; Kim, H.J.; Kim, C.K.; Sale, C. Determinants of muscle carnosine content. *Amino Acids* **2012**, *43*, 5–12. [CrossRef]
16. Artioli, G.; Gualano, B.; Smith, A.; Stout, J.; Lancha, A.H. Role of β-alanine supplementation on muscle carnosine and exercise performance. *Med. Sci. Sports Exerc.* **2010**, *42*, 1162–1173. [CrossRef]
17. Huerta, Á.; Contreras-Montilla, O.; Galdames, S.; Jorquera-Aguilera, C.; Fuentes-Kloss, R.; Guisado-Barrilao, R. Efectos de la suplementación con beta alanina sobre una prueba de tiempo límite a velocidad aeróbica máxima en atletas de resistencia. *Nutr. Hosp.* **2019**, *36*, 698–705. [CrossRef]
18. Jagim, A.R.; Harty, P.S.; Camic, C.L. Common ingredient profiles of multi-ingredient pre-workout supplements. *Nutrients* **2019**, *11*, 254. [CrossRef]
19. Osnes, J.B.; Hermansen, L. Acid-base balance after maximal exercise of short duration. *J. Appl. Physiol.* **1972**, *32*, 59–63. [CrossRef]

20. Stout, J.R.; Cramer, J.T.; Zoeller, R.F.; Torok, D.; Costa, P.; Hoffman, J.R.; Harris, R.C.; O'Kroy, J. Effects of β-alanine supplementation on the onset of neuromuscular fatigue and ventilatory threshold in women. *Amino Acids* **2007**, *32*, 381–386. [CrossRef]
21. Smith-Ryan, A.E.; Fukuda, D.H.; Stout, J.R.; Kendall, K.L. High velocity intermittent running: Effects of Beta alanine Supplementation. *J. Strength Cond. Res.* **2012**, *26*, 2798–2805. [CrossRef]
22. Smith, A.E.; Stout, J.R.; Kendall, K.L.; Fukuda, D.H.; Cramer, J.T. Exercise-induced oxidative stress: The effects of β-alanine supplementation in women. *Amino Acids* **2012**, *43*, 77–90. [CrossRef]
23. Décombaz, J.; Beaumont, M.; Vuichoud, J.; Bouisset, F.; Stellingwerff, T. Effect of slow-release β-alanine tablets on absorption kinetics and paresthesia. *Amino Acids* **2012**, *43*, 67–76. [CrossRef]
24. Domínguez, R.; Lougedo, J.H.; Maté-Muñoz, J.L.; Garnacho-Castaño, M.V. Efectos de la suplementación con ß-alanina sobre el rendimiento deportivo. *Nutr. Hosp.* **2015**, *31*, 155–169. [CrossRef]
25. Kindermann, W.; Simon, G.; Keul, J. The significance of the aerobic-anaerobic transition for the determination of work load intensities during endurance training. *Eur. J. Appl. Physiol.* **1979**, *42*, 25–34. [CrossRef] [PubMed]
26. Faude, O.; Kindermann, W.; Meyer, T. Lactate threshold concepts: How valid are they? *Sports Med.* **2009**, *39*, 469–490. [CrossRef]
27. Wilson, J.M.; Wilson, G.J.; Zourdos, M.C.; Smith, A.E.; Stout, J. Beta-alanine supplementation improves aerobic and anaerobic indices of performance. *Strength Cond. J.* **2010**, *32*, 71–78. [CrossRef]
28. Beasley, L.; Smith, L.; Antonio, J.; Gordon, D.; Johnstone, J.; Roberts, J. The effect of two β-alanine dosing strategies on 30-minute rowing performance: A randomized, controlled trial. *J. Int. Soc. Sports Nutr.* **2018**, *15*, 1–11. [CrossRef]
29. Bellinger, P.M.; Minahan, C.L. The effect of β-alanine supplementation on cycling time trials of different length. *Eur. J. Sport Sci.* **2016**, *16*, 829–836. [CrossRef]
30. Moher, D.; Liberati, A.; Tetzlaff, J.; Altman, D.G.; Altman, D.; Antes, G.; Atkins, D.; Barbour, V.; Barrowman, N.; Berlin, J.A.; et al. Preferred reporting items for systematic reviews and meta-analyses: The PRISMA statement. *PLoS Med.* **2009**, *6*. [CrossRef]
31. Huerta, Á.; Dominguez, A.; Barahona-Fuentes, G. The effect of supplementation with L-arginine and L-citrulline on physical performance: A systematic review. *Nutr. Hosp.* **2019**, *36*, 1389–1402. [CrossRef] [PubMed]
32. Chicharro, J.; Vicente, D.; Cancino, J. *Fisiología del Entrenamiento Aeróbico. Una Visión Integrada*, 1st ed.; Editorial Medicap Panamericana: Barcelona, España, 2013; ISBN 978-84-9835-279-5.
33. Berthon, P.; Fellmann, N.; Bedu, M.; Beaune, B.; Dabonneville, M.; Coudert, J.; Chamoux, A. A 5-min running field test as a measurement of maximal aerobic velocity. *Eur. J. Appl. Physiol. Occup. Physiol.* **1997**, *75*, 233–238. [CrossRef] [PubMed]
34. Tong, T.K.; Fu, F.H.; Chow, B.C. Reliability of a 5-min running field test and its accuracy in VO_2max evaluation. *J. Sports Med. Phys. Fitness* **2001**, *41*, 318. [PubMed]
35. Chung, W.; Baguet, A.; Bex, T.; Bishop, D.J.; Derave, W. Doubling of muscle carnosine concentration does not improve laboratory 1-Hr cycling time-trial performance. *Int. J. Sport Nutr. Exerc. Metab.* **2014**, *24*, 315–324. [CrossRef] [PubMed]
36. Borg, G. Psychophysical scaling with applications in physical work and the perception of exertion. *Scand. J. Work. Environ. Health* **1990**, *16*, 55–58. [CrossRef]
37. Egger, M.; Smith, G.D.; Schneider, M.; Minder, C. Bias in meta-analysis detected by a simple, graphical test. *Br. Med. J.* **1997**, *315*, 629–634. [CrossRef]
38. Higgins, J.; Green, S. *Cochrane Handbook for Systematic Reviews of Interventions*; Version 5; London, U., Ed.; Cochrane: Chichester, UK, 2011.
39. Hedges, L. V Distribution theory for Glass's estimator of e ect size and related estimators. *J. Educ. Stat.* **1981**, *6*, 107–128. [CrossRef]
40. Cohen, J. *Statistical Power Analysis for the Behavioral Sciences*; Cambridge, A.P., Ed.; Associated Press: Cambridge, MA, USA, 2013; ISBN 1483276481.
41. Higgins, J.; Thompson, S.; Deeks, J.; Altman, D. Measuring inconsistency in meta-analyses. *BMJ* **2003**, *327*, 557–560. [CrossRef]
42. Baguet, A.; Bourgois, J.; Vanhee, L.; Achten, E.; Derave, W. Important role of muscle carnosine in rowing performance. *J. Appl. Physiol.* **2010**, *109*, 1096–1101. [CrossRef]

43. Bellinger, P.M.; Minahan, C.L. Metabolic consequences of β-alanine supplementation during exhaustive supramaximal cycling and 4000-m time-trial performance. *Appl. Physiol. Nutr. Metab.* **2016**, *41*, 864–871. [CrossRef]
44. Bellinger, P.M.; Minahan, C.L. Additive benefits of β-Alanine supplementation and sprint-interval training. *Med. Sci. Sports Exerc.* **2016**, *48*, 2417–2425. [CrossRef] [PubMed]
45. Cochran, A.J.R.; Percival, M.E.; Thompson, S.; Gillen, J.B.; MacInnis, M.J.; Potter, M.A.; Tarnopolsky, M.A.; Gibala, M.J. β-Alanine supplementation does not augment the skeletal muscle adaptive response to 6 weeks of sprint interval training. *Int. J. Sport Nutr. Exerc. Metab.* **2015**, *25*, 541–549. [CrossRef] [PubMed]
46. Ducker, K.J.; Dawson, B.; Wallman, K.E. Effect of beta-alanine supplementation on 2000-m rowing-ergometer performance. *Int. J. Sport Nutr. Exerc. Metab.* **2013**, *23*, 336–343. [CrossRef] [PubMed]
47. Hobson, R.M.; Harris, R.C.; Martin, D.; Smith, P.; Macklin, B.; Gualano, B.; Sale, C. Effect of β-alanine, with and without sodium bicarbonate on 2000 m Rowing Performance. *Int. J. Sport Nutr. Exerc. Metab.* **2013**, *23*, 480–487. [CrossRef]
48. Santana, J.O.; Freitas, M.C.; dos Santos, D.M.; Rossi, F.E.; Lira, F.S.; Rosa-Neto, J.C.; Caperuto, E.C. Beta-alanine supplementation improved 10-km running time trial in physically active adults. *Front. Physiol.* **2018**, *9*, 1105. [CrossRef] [PubMed]
49. Furst, T.; Massaro, A.; Miller, C.; Williams, B.T.; LaMacchia, Z.M.; Horvath, P.J. β-Alanine supplementation increased physical performance and improved executive function following endurance exercise in middle aged individuals. *J. Int. Soc. Sports Nutr.* **2018**, *15*, 32. [CrossRef]
50. Ghiasvand, R.; Askari, G.; Malekzadeh, J.; Hajishafiee, M.; Daneshvar, P.; Akbari, F.; Bahreynian, M. Effects of six weeks of β-alanine administration on VO_2max, time to exhaustion and lactate concentrations in physical education students. *Int. J. Prev. Med.* **2012**, *3*, 559.
51. Greer, B.K.; Katalinas, M.E.; Shaholli, D.M.; Gallo, P.M. β-alanine supplementation fails to increase peak aerobic power or ventilatory threshold in aerobically trained males. *J. Diet. Suppl.* **2014**, *13*, 165–170. [CrossRef]
52. Outlaw, J.J.; Smith-Ryan, A.E.; Buckley, A.L.; Urbina, S.L.; Hayward, S.; Wingfield, H.L.; Campbell, B.; Foster, C.; Taylor, L.W.; Wilborn, C.D. Effects of β-alanine on body composition and performance measures in collegiate women. *J. Strenght Cond. Res.* **2016**, *30*, 2627–2637. [CrossRef]
53. Smith-Ryan, A.E.; Woessner, M.N.; Melvin, M.N.; Wingfield, H.L.; Hackney, A.C. The effects of beta-alanine supplementation on physical working capacity at heart rate threshold. *Clin. Physiol. Funct. Imaging* **2014**, *34*, 397–404. [CrossRef]
54. Harris, R.C.; Tallon, M.J.; Dunnett, M.; Boobis, L.; Coakley, J.; Kim, H.J.; Fallowfield, J.L.; Hill, C.A.; Sale, C.; Wise, J.A. The absorption of orally supplied β-alanine and its effect on muscle carnosine synthesis in human vastus lateralis. *Amino Acids* **2006**, *30*, 279–289. [CrossRef] [PubMed]
55. Asatoor, A.M.; Bandoh, J.K.; Lant, A.F.; Milne, M.D.; Navab, F. Intestinal absorption of carnosine and its constituent amino acids in man. *Gut* **1970**, *11*, 250–254. [CrossRef] [PubMed]
56. Kerksick, C.M.; Wilborn, C.D.; Roberts, M.D.; Smith-Ryan, A.; Kleiner, S.M.; Jäger, R.; Collins, R.; Cooke, M.; Davis, J.N.; Galvan, E.; et al. ISSN exercise & sports nutrition review update: Research & recommendations. *J. Int. Soc. Sports Nutr.* **2018**, *15*, 38. [CrossRef]
57. Dutka, T.L.; Lamboley, C.R.; McKenna, M.J.; Murphy, R.M.; Lamb, G.D. Effects of carnosine on contractile apparatus Ca^{2+} sensitivity and sarcoplasmic reticulum Ca^{2+} release in human skeletal muscle fibers. *J. Appl. Physiol.* **2012**, *112*, 728–736. [CrossRef] [PubMed]
58. Invernizzi, P.L.; Benedini, S.; Saronni, S.; Merati, G.; Bosio, A. The acute administration of carnosine and beta-alanine does not improve running anaerobic performance and has no effect on the metabolic response to exercise. *Adv. Phys. Educ.* **2013**, *03*, 169–174. [CrossRef]
59. Saunders, B.; Elliott-Sale, K.; Artioli, G.G.; Swinton, P.A.; Dolan, E.; Roschel, H.; Sale, C.; Gualano, B. β-Alanine supplementation to improve exercise capacity and performance: A systematic review and meta-Analysis. *Br. J. Sports Med.* **2017**, *51*, 658–669. [CrossRef]
60. Derave, W.; Everaert, I.; Beeckman, S.; Baguet, A. Muscle carnosine metabolism and β-alanine supplementation in relation to exercise and training. *Sports Med.* **2010**, *40*, 247–263. [CrossRef]
61. Quesnele, J.J.; Laframboise, M.A.; Wong, J.J.; Kim, P.; Wells, G.D. The effects of beta-alanine supplementation on performance: A systematic review of the literature. *Int. J. Sport Nutr. Exerc. Metab.* **2014**, *24*, 14–27. [CrossRef]

62. Gross, M.; Boesch, C.; Bolliger, C.S.; Norman, B.; Gustafsson, T.; Hoppeler, H.; Vogt, M. Effects of beta-alanine supplementation and interval training on physiological determinants of severe exercise performance. *Eur. J. Appl. Physiol.* **2014**, *114*, 221–234. [CrossRef]
63. Ekblom, B.; Golobarg, A.N. The influence of physical training and other factors on the subjective rating of perceived exertion. *Acta Physiol. Scand.* **1971**, *83*, 399–406. [CrossRef]
64. Bountra, C.; Vaughan-Jones, R. Effect of intracellular and extracellullar pH on contraction in isolated, mammalian cardiac muscle. *J. Physiol.* **1989**, *418*, 163–187. [CrossRef] [PubMed]

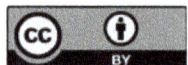

© 2020 by the authors. Licensee MDPI, Basel, Switzerland. This article is an open access article distributed under the terms and conditions of the Creative Commons Attribution (CC BY) license (http://creativecommons.org/licenses/by/4.0/).

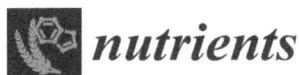

Article

Can Creatine Supplementation Interfere with Muscle Strength and Fatigue in Brazilian National Level Paralympic Powerlifting?

Carlos Rodrigo Soares Freitas Sampaio [1], Felipe J. Aidar [1,2,3,4,*], Alexandre R. P. Ferreira [5], Jymmys Lopes dos Santos [6], Anderson Carlos Marçal [1,3], Dihogo Gama de Matos [1], Raphael Fabrício de Souza [1,2], Osvaldo Costa Moreira [7], Ialuska Guerra [8], José Fernandes Filho [9], Lucas Soares Marcucci-Barbosa [10], Albená Nunes-Silva [10], Paulo Francisco de Almeida-Neto [11], Breno Guilherme Araújo Tinoco Cabral [11] and Victor Machado Reis [12]

1. Group of Studies and Research of Performance, Sport, Health and Paralympic Sports (GPEPS), Federal University of Sergipe (UFS), São Cristovão 49100-000, Sergipe, Brazil; rodrigosfsampaio@hotmail.com (C.R.S.F.S.); acmarcal@yahoo.com.br (A.C.M.); dihogogmc@hotmail.com (D.G.d.M.); raphaelctba20@hotmail.com (R.F.d.S.)
2. Department of Physical Education, Federal University of Sergipe (UFS), São Cristovão 49100-000, Sergipe, Brazil
3. Program of Physical Education, Federal University of Sergipe (UFS), São Cristovão 49100-000, Sergipe, Brazil
4. Program of Physiological Science, Federal University of Sergipe (UFS), São Cristovão 49100-000, Sergipe, Brazil
5. College of Physical Education and Exercise Science, University of Brasília (UnB), Brasília 70910-900, Brazil; alexandreispf@gmail.com
6. Program in Biotechnology, Northeast Network in Biotechnology (RENORBIO), Federal University of Sergipe (UFS), São Cristovão 49100-000, Sergipe, Brazil; jymmyslopes@yahoo.com.br
7. Institute of Biological Sciences and Health, Federal University of Viçosa, Campus Florestal, Minas Gerais 35690-000, Brazil; ocostamoreira@gmail.com
8. Federal Institute of Education, Science and Technology of Ceará (IFCE), Campus of Juazeiro do Norte, Ceará 63040-540, Brazil; ialuskaguerra@gmail.com
9. Brazilian Paralympic Academy, Brazilian Paralympic Committee, São Paulo 04329-000, SP, Brazil; jffbepe@gmail.com
10. Laboratory of Inflammation and Exercise Immunology, Sports Center, Physical Education Scholl, Federal University of OuroPreto (UFOP), OuroPreto, Minas Gerais 35400-000, Brazil; lucasmarcucci@gmail.com (L.S.M.-B.); albenanunes@hotmail.com (A.N.-S.)
11. Department of Physical Education, Federal University of Rio Grande do Norte (UFRN), Natal, Rio Grande do Norte 59078-970, Brazil; paulo220911@hotmail.com (P.F.d.A.-N.); brenotcabral@gmail.com (B.G.A.T.C.)
12. Research Center in Sports Sciences, Health Sciences and Human Development (CIDESD), Trásos Montes and Alto Douro University, 5001-801 Vila Real, Portugal; victormachadoreis@gmail.com
* Correspondence: fjaidar@gmail.com; Tel.: +55-799-9685-7777

Received: 6 July 2020; Accepted: 14 August 2020; Published: 19 August 2020

Abstract: The aim of the present study was to analyze the effect of creatine (Cr) supplementation on peak torque (PT) and fatigue rate in Paralympic weightlifting athletes. Eight Paralympic powerlifting athletes participated in the study, with 25.40 ± 3.30 years and 70.30 ± 12.15 kg. The measurements of muscle strength, fatigue index (FI), peak torque (PT), force (kgf), force (N), rate of force development (RFD), and time to maximum isometric force (time) were determined by a Musclelab load cell. The study was performed in a single-blind manner, with subjects conducting the experiments first with placebo supplementation and then, following a 7-day washout period, beginning the same protocol with creatine supplementation for 7 days. This sequence was chosen because of the lengthy washout of creatine. Regarding the comparison between conditions, Cr supplementation did not show effects on the variables of muscle force, peak torque, RFD, and time to maximum isometric force ($p > 0.05$). However, when comparing the results of the moments with the use of Cr and placebo, a difference was observed for the FI after seven days (U^3: 1.12; 95% CI: (0.03, 2.27); $p = 0.02$); therefore, the FI was higher for placebo. Creatine supplementation has a positive effect on the performance of Paralympic powerlifting athletes, reducing fatigue index, and keeping the force levels as well as PT.

Keywords: Paralympic powerlifting; supplementation; creatine; performance

1. Introduction

Powerlifting (PL) is an international sport where competitors attempt to lift a maximum amount of weight in threeprimary lifts: the bench press, the squat, and the deadlift. These threelifts provide widely accepted measures of upper-body, lower-body, and total body strength [1–3]. At all levels of PL, each competing athlete is ranked based on the best of the threevalid attempts afforded for the bench press, squat, and deadlift [1–3]. The threeare then "totaled," providing a measure of the total weight lifted and determining each athlete's overall place in the competition. The skillful execution of each of the threeafforded lifts for the bench press, squat, and deadlift during competitions can be influenced by the subjects' strength and muscle fatigue [1–3].

In this sense, many of these athletes have used ergogenic aids to keep body conditioning, enhancing recovery, and physiological adaptations during training programs and between competitions [3,4]. The efficacy of ergogenic has always attracted great attention, and numerous researchers have sought to combine ergogenic and exercise training programs to reinforce the benefits of training. Creatine (Cr) is a popular ergogenic aid among athletes at all levels [5,6]. Cr is a non-protein nitrogenous compound—methyl-guanidine-acetic acid—composed of three amino acids (arginine, glycine, and methionine). It is found mainly in skeletal muscle (95%) and plays an important role in rapid energy provision during muscle contraction through the ATP-PCr system [7].

Cr supplementation tends to potentiate the effect of strength training that would promote physiological responses and adaptations that positively interfere with the increase in muscle strength, power, hypertrophy, and local muscle endurance [8]. On the other hand, observing variables related to muscle recovery, there areindications that Cr supplementation could reduce muscle damage after exercise via sarcolemma stabilizing mechanisms [9] and regulate mitochondrial permeability [10]. Studies have demonstrated the beneficial effects of Cr supplementation on performance following resistance training [9–11].

Although the literature has shown the positive impacts of creatine supplementation [8–11], there is a lack of strong evidence about the efficacy of creatine supplementation on elite powerlifting athletes. More evidence is required to testing the efficacy of creatine to minimize fatigue index, which might enhance muscle strength, considering the need for new approaches that contribute to better performance.

Therefore, this was the first study to investigate the effects of creatine supplementation in elite Paralympic powerlifting athletes. We hypothesized that creatine might affect positively the muscle strength and reduce fatigue during high-intensity resistance training used in Paralympic powerlifting training. Thus, the aim of the present study was to analyze the effects of Cr supplementation on indicators of torque, force, time, and fatigue index in Paralympic powerlifting athletes.

2. Materials and Methods

2.1. Sample

The sample consisted of eight Paralympic powerlifting athletes participating in the extension project of the Federal University of Sergipe Brazil. All participants were Brazilian level competitors, eligible for the sport [12], and ranked among the ten best in their respective categories. Among the deficiencies, two athletes presented spinal cord injury due to accidents with an injury below the eighth thoracic vertebra; two with sequelae due to polio; two had lower limb malformation (arthrogryposis); two had cerebral palsy. The sampling power was calculated based on previous results of our studies [2,3], with an effect size of 0.98 that combined with a standard of α < 0.05 and β = 0.80. Thus, it was possible to estimate a sample power of 0.88, suggesting that the sample size has sufficient statistical strength to answer the research approach.

The characterization of the sample is shown in Table 1.

Table 1. Characterization of subjects.

	(Mean ± SD)
Age (years)	25.40 ± 3.30
Weight (Kg)	70.30 ± 12.15
Experience (years)	2.45 ± 0.21
1RM Adapted Bench press (Kg)	119.99 ± 12.14 *
1RM/weight	1.71 ± 0.27 **

* All athletes with loads that keep them in the top 10 of their categories nationwide. ** Values above 1.4 on bench press would be considered elite athletes, according to Ball and Weidman. 1RM: 1 repetition maximum.

The athletes voluntarily participated in the study and signed a free and informed consent form in accordance with Resolution 466/2012 of the National Commission for Research Ethics (CONEP) of the National Health Council and the ethical principles of the latest version of the Declaration of Helsinki (and the World Medical Association). The project was submitted to the Research Ethics Committee of the Federal University of Sergipe and approved with the following opinion 2,637,882.

This study was carried out at the Federal University of Sergipe, from 09:00 h to 13:00 h, and was developed in four weeks, the first one aimed at familiarization and testing of 1 repetition maximum (1RM), force (force (Kgf) and force (N)), peak torque (PT), rate of force development (RFD), time to maximum isometric force (time), and fatigue index (FI), according to the items Section 2.4. Force Measurements and Section 2.5. Load Determination, respectively.

The experimental design of the study is provided in Figure 1.

	Day 1 (Monday)	Day 2 (Wednesday)	Day3 (Friday)	Other days
Week 1 (familiarization) Tests: 1 RM, Time, peak torque (PT), fatigue index (FI), rate of force development (RFD), and force	Tests: 1RM, PT, RFD, Time, Force, and FI Familiarization	Training Familiarization	Tests: PT, RFD, Time, Force, and FI Familiarization	Recovery
Week 2 (maltodextrin)	Training	Training	Post Tests PT, RFD, Time, Force, and FI	Recovery
Week 3 (washout of placebo)	Off	Off	Off	Recovery
Week 4 (creatine)	Training	Training	Post Tests PT, RFD, Time, Force, and FI	Recovery

Figure 1. Experimental design—weekly schedule of tests and washout. 1RM: 1 repetition maximum. Training carried out three times a week, and the remaining days weredestined to rest [2].

2.2. Instruments

Weighing of the athletes was performed on a digital platform-type Michetti (Micheletti, São Paulo, SP, Brazil) electronic scale, with a maximum supported weight capacity of 3000 kg and a size of 1.50 × 1.50 m. For the bench press exercise, an official straight bench (Eleiko Sport AB, Halmstad, Sweden), approved by the International Paralympic Committee [12], with a total length of 210 cm was used. The IPC-approved powerlifting Olympic bar is serrated and has grooves in its material, has a total length of 220 cm, weighing 20 kg. On the bar, there is a marking for the narrowest and widest footprint, according to the International Paralympic Committee [12] official rules 2016–2017, ranging from 42 cm to 81 cm.

2.3. Supplementation

We chose to use a single-blind method with a treatment order that was not counterbalanced due to the lengthy washout time required for muscle creatine to return to pre-supplementation values [13]. Therefore, initially, participants ingested 20 g maltodextrin (placebo, Max Titanium®, Supley, Matão, SP, Brazil), followed by 7 days of washout period. Subsequently, 20 g of creatine monohydrate (Max Titanium®, Supley, Matão, SP, Brazil; 99.9% purity) was administered for another 7 days. The total daily amount of supplement was divided into four equal portions and consumed with food throughout the day. Creatine and placebo were identical in taste, color, texture, and appearance.

2.4. Force Measurements

Measurementsof muscle strength, fatigue index (FI), peak torque (PT), force (Kgf), force (N), rate of force development (RFD), and time to maximum isometric force (time) were determined by a Musclelab load cell (Model PFMA 3010e MuscleLab System; Ergotest, Langesund, Norway), attached to the adapted bench press, using 21 HN Simplex carabiners Spider HMS Simond (Simond, Chamonix, France), approved for climbing by *Union InternationaledesAssociations d'Alpinisme* (UIAA). A steel chain with a breaking load of 2300 kg was used to secure the load cell to the seat. The perpendicular distance between the load cell and joint center was determined and used to calculate joint torques and fatigue index [14].

Isometric peak torque (PT) was measured by the maximum torque generated by the upper limb muscles. The PT was determined by the product of the isometric force peak, measured between the load cell cable attachment point and the adapted bench press bench, which was adjusted so that an elbow angle was close to 90° and at a distance 15 cm from the starting point (chest to bar), verified with an apparatus for measuring the amplitude of angular movement, Model FL6010 (Sanny, São Bernardo do Campo, SP, Brazil). Participants were instructed to perform a single maximal movement, seeking elbow extension (as soon as possible) and relaxing for PT assessment.

For the fatigue index (FI) evaluation, the same exercise was performed, and the subjects determined to maintain the maximum contraction for 10 s, where the index was determined by dividing the initial PT in relation to the final PT, subtracted from one. FI = ((final PT-initial PT/final PT) × 100). Thus, the results in Newton (N) were conceived by the formula N = (M) × (C) × (H), where M = body mass in Kg, C = 9.81 (m·s^{-2}), H = bar height relative to load (45.0 cm), corresponding to the height at which the equipment was fixed, adopting an angle of the forearm with the arm of 90°, adapted from the methodology from Milner-Brown et al. [15].

2.5. Load Determination

To determine the training load, the 1RM test was performed, on the adapted bench press [12], where each subject started the attempts with a weight that he believed could be lifted only once using the maximum effort. Weight increments were then added until the maximum load that could be lifted once was reached. If the practitioner could not perform a single repetition, 2.4 to 2.5% of the load used in the test was subtracted [16]. The subjects rested for 3–5 min between the attempts. The 1RM test was performed within two weeks at least 72 h prior to the intervention.

For the PT, force, RFD, time, and FI tests, three attempts were made in the PT test, where subjects were evaluated with the bar at 15 cm from the chest, and with an elbow angle of 90°, where they made the greatest force possible once, and this procedure was repeated three times after a rest of five minutes between the attempts. For the evaluation of the FI, the subjects remained to dothe maximum isometric contraction for one minute, with the bar 15 cm from the chest, and the loss of PT was verified between the 10 s and the initial moment of the test. The 10 s time was adopted in view of that shown in a study with Paralympic powerlifting [17], where the execution of 1RM, the target of the competition, would not amount to more than 10 s. All subjects underwent the test before and after training with a minimum interval of 10 min between the tests and the training session [18].

2.6. Intervention

The intervention protocol consisted of warm-up for upper limbs, using three exercises (abduction of the shoulders with dumbbells, elbow extension in the pulley, and rotation of the shoulders with dumbbells) with three sets of 10 to 20 repetitions [19]. Soon after, a specific warm-up was performed on the bench press with a 30% load of 1RM, 10 slow repetitions (3:1 s, eccentric:concentric), and 10 fast repetitions (1:1 s, eccentric:concentric),followed with five sets of bench press of five maximum repetitions (5 sets–85 at 90% RM with 3–5 min of rest), using a fixed load. During the test, athletes received verbal encouragement in order to achieve maximum performance [19]. To perform the bench press, an official straight bench (Eleiko Sport AB, Halmstad, Sweden), approved by the International Paralympic Committee, was used [12].

2.7. Statistic

The normality of the data was verified by the Shapiro Wilk and Z-score tests for asymmetry and kurtosis (−1.96 to 1.96). The assumption of normality was denied, and subsequently, the transformation of the data by the square root (i.e., from non-parametric to parametric) was not successful, and subsequently, the attempt to the logarithmic transformation of the data by the log on the basis of 10 was also unsuccessful. In this sense, comparisons between the medians of the same intervention (creatine × creatine; placebo × placebo) in the different conditions of the study (before, after training, after 7 days) were performed using the Kruskal–Wallis test. When differences were found, the Mann–Whitney U test was used to identify the different data set and, subsequently, Bonferroni correction. The differences between interventions (creatine × placebo) in the different conditions of the study (before, after training, after 7 days) were analyzed by the Mann–Whitney U test. The effect size between the median differences and their respective 95% confidence intervals was analyzed using the Cohen's U^3 index test, so the magnitude used was the one proposed by Espirito Santo and Daniel [20]: insignificant: <0.19; small: 0.20–0.49; average: 0.50–0.79; large: 0.80–1.29; very large: <1.30. All analyses were performed using open-source software R (version 3.6.2, R Foundation for Statistical Computing, Vienna, Austria), considering the significance of $p < 0.05$.

3. Results

Figure 2 shows the results of the effect of creatine supplementation (intra-conditions) in relation to the variables studied.

Regarding the use of creatine, Figure 2 shows that, for the RFD variable, significant differences were identified in the after training and after 7 days conditions in relation to the before condition (U^3 = 1.33; CI 95%: [0.15]–[2.52]; p = 0.02), while for the use of placebo, there was no significant difference. Regarding thetime to maximum isometric force, there was a difference during the use of creatine for the after training condition compared to the before condition (U^3 = 1.54; CI 95%: [0.32]–[2.76]; p = 0.01). In relation to the placebo, there was a significant difference in the conditions after training and after 7 days in relation to the before condition for the variable time to maximum isometric force (U^3 = 0.76; CI 95%: [−0.34]–[1.87]; p = 0.04). There were significant differences in the after training condition in relation to the before and after 7 days conditions, and from the after 7 days condition to the before condition when using creatine for the fatigue index (U^3 = 7.97; CI 95%: [4.76]–[11.1]; p = 0.0009). In relation to the use of placebo, significant differences were found in the conditions after training and after 7 days in relation to the before condition for the fatigue index (U^3 = −12.9; CI 95%: [−17.9]–[−7.91]; p = 0.04).

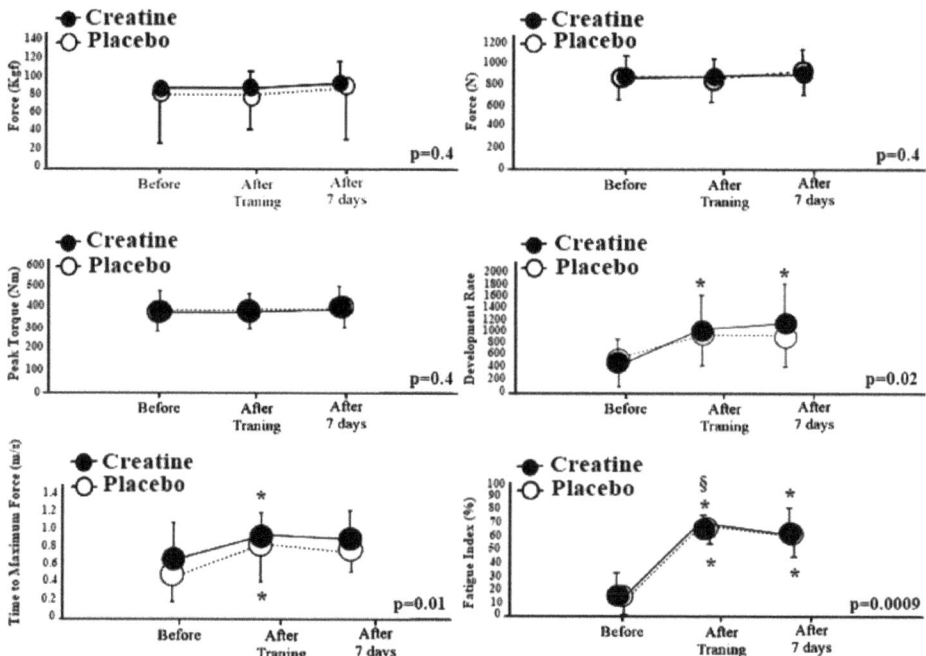

Figure 2. Intra-condition comparisons regarding force indicator at different times. Kgf = Kilograms force. N = Newtons. Nm = Nanometer. p = Value of the degree of statistical significance. m/s = Meters per Second. % = Percentage. * = Significant differences for the before condition. § = Significant difference for the after 7 days condition. p = Value of the degree of statistical significance.

Table 2 reports that the only statistical difference between interventions with the use of creatine and placebo was in the fatigue index (%) in the condition after 7 days (U^3: 1.12; 95% CI: [−0.03]–[2.27]; p = 0.02), where the fatigue index (%) was higher for the intervention using the placebo.

Table 2. Comparison of moments using creatine and using placebo in the different conditions of the study.

Tests	Before				After Training				After 7 Days			
	Creatine		Placebo		Creatine		Placebo		Creatine		Placebo	
	MD	IIQ	MD	IIQ	MD	IIQ	MD	IIQ	MD	IIQ	MD	IIQ
Force (Kgf)	96.4	1.50	92.1	14.6	95.5	9.00	89.8	23.1	99.6	16.60	94.9	11.0
Force (N)	945.2	122.1	902.5	143.4	935.9	109.5	880.6	225.1	976.2	161.2	930.0	162.8
Peak torque (Nm)	425.3	54.9	406.1	64.5	421.1	48.9	396.2	101.6	439.3	73.30	418.5	73.4
Rate of force development	629.0	233.3	674.2	331.8	1.137	472.5	956.5	595.8	1.239	578.5	845.0	513.2
Time (m/s)	0.708	0.317	0.433	0.622	1.000	0.205	1.130	0.850	0.950	0.275	0.987	0.170
Fatigue index (%)	21.9	8.80	24.7	4.1	72.1	4.80	76.1	7.0	66.2	14.70	77.9 *	11.8

MD = Median; IIQ = Interquartile range. Kgf = Kilo grams force. N = Newtons. Nm = Nanometer. m/s = Meters per Second. % = Percentage, Time = Time to maximum isometric force. * = Significant statistical difference p = 0.02. p = Value of the degree of statistical significance.

Figure 3 shows graphically the behavior of the peak torque (Nm) and the percentage of the fatigue index (%) during the moments of the study (before, after training, and after 7 days), showing that in relation to the peak torque (Nm), the behavior was similar for creatine and placebo conditions. Whereas for the fatigue index (%), at the moment after 7 days, a lower percentage was demonstrated in the creatine condition in relation to the placebo condition.

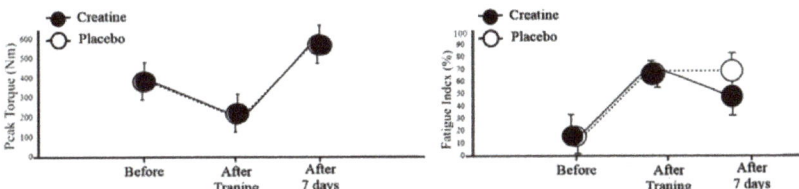

Figure 3. The behavior of peak torque (Nm) and fatigue index (%) at different times.

4. Discussion

The objective of the present study was to analyze the effects of Cr supplementation on the indicators of torque, force, and muscle fatigue in athletes of Paralympic powerlifting. The main results were: (1) Cr supplementation did not show effects on the variables of muscle strength, peak torque, RFD, and time to maximum isometric force. (2) Cr supplementation reduced FIafter 7 days of use.

In the present study, when comparing Cr results with placebo, no significant differences were identified in relation to variables related to muscle strength. In this context, Zuniga et al. [21] examined the effects of 7 days of Cr supplementation on the strength of upper and lower limbs of 22 men and concluded that there was no statistically significant difference between the placebo condition and the Cr condition in all the muscle strength variables analyzed. In addition, Hamilton et al. [22] concluded that Cr supplementation combined with resistance training when relative loads and volumes were the same as a placebo condition did not result in a training advantage in absolute or relative strength performance. Syrotuik et al. [23] did not observe significant differences in the strength of the upper limbs when comparing two conditions after an intervention with Cr and placebo for 5 days.

Buts et al. [24] showed in a systematic review the scientific information from the years 1980 to 2017, stating that the data on the improvement of sports performance through creatinewere inconsistent. In addition, a meta-analysis made up of 100 different studies has shown that in the short term, Cr supplementation does not have significant effects on specific sports performance [25]. Moreover, in previous studies, Cr supplementation, in the short term, hasnot demonstratedeffects on specific strength levels related to different sports [26,27].

The results of the present research also showed that FIof the supplemented condition was approximately 16% lower when compared to placebo. In contradiction to the present study, Bazzucchiet al. [28] evaluated 16 trained men with daily supplementation of 5 g of Cr + 15 g of maltodextrin or 20 g of maltodextrin and evaluated the maximum voluntary isometric contraction and dynamic contractions and fatigue for the flexor muscles of the elbow. The authors concluded that creatinecouldimprove neuromuscular function during voluntary contractions. In addition, they indicated that, according to the electromyography analysis, no significant differences were found between the conditions regarding muscle fatigue.

Possible explanations for the improvement of the Cr condition's FI can be speculated, in addition to neuromuscular adaptation, by the increase in glycogen storage. An increase in glucose transporter type 4 (GLUT4) expression is suggested when Cr supplementation is combined with exercise [29]; positive effects of Cr supplementation are seen at initial levels and also by maintaining high levels of muscle glycogen for up to 2 h [30]. In addition, training tends to promote central and peripheral fatigue, along with other endocrine, immunological, inflammatory, and oxidative stress [31]. Moreover, training tends to modulate physiological adaptation and improve physical performance indicators [32].

In this context, supplementation can be used as a nutritional strategy for athletes to improve their physiological adaptation and performance [33].

Resistance to fatigue and the ability of the muscle to regenerate during intermittent high-intensity exercise are important qualities of neuromuscular function [34]. In addition, Cr can help protect against injury and muscle damage induced by strenuous contractile activities [35]. In athletes, who performed ultra-resistance tests, supplemented with 20 g/d of maltodextrin plus 50 g of Cr for 5 precompetitive days, decreased plasma creatine kinase activities, lactate dehydrogenase, preventing the increase in plasma oxaloacetic glutamic acid and glutamic pyruvic acid, activities have been observed [36].

In subjects with spinal cord injury, Cr levels improve muscle strength parameters, and this has a positive effect on the performance of daily activities and body health [37]. In Paralympic weightlifting athletes, who have suffered spinal cord injury, creatine can help to maximize the performance of the upper limbs by reducing the FI and providing a faster recovery during the practices provided by the sport [38].

In addition, it has been shown in the literature that creatine supplementation appears to reduce the spread of secondary injuries and improves the quality of the neuromotor system's fitness [39]. However, caution is recommended regarding the water balance during the consumption of the supplement [24].

However, despite the relevance of the results, the present study had some limitations: (1) The evaluation was done in an acute way. (2) The improvement in FI might have been a result of the Cr supplementation time phase, that is, due to the fact of the time/order effect in which the study was carried out. Cr supplementation was performed in a second moment, and because of that, there might have been an adaptation to training, which might have influenced the athletes' FI reduction. (3) Athletes' diets were not changed during the study. Therefore, new studies should be carried out with a long washout period as well as other research designs.

5. Conclusions

It was concluded that creatine supplementation has a positive effect on the performance of elite Paralympic powerlifting athletes, reducing fatigue in the execution of the exercise, and keeping the force levels.

Author Contributions: Conceptualization, F.J.A., R.F.d.S., O.C.M., I.G., L.S.M.-B., A.N.-S., P.F.d.A.-N., B.G.A.T.C. and V.M.R.; Data curation, A.R.P.F., J.L.d.S. and D.G.d.M.; Formal analysis, J.L.d.S and A.C.M.; Investigation, C.R.S.F.S., F.J.A., R.F.d.S. and I.G.; Methodology, C.R.S.F.S., F.J.A., A.C.M., A.N.-S., P.F.d.A.-N., B.G.A.T.C. and V.M.R.; Project administration, A.C.M. and J.F.F.; Writing—original draft, F.J.A., J.L.d.S., D.G.d.M., R.F.d.S., O.C.M., I.G., J.F.F. and V.M.R.; Writing—review & editing, A.R.P.F., D.G.d.M., J.F.F., L.S.M.-B., A.N.-S., P.F.d.A.-N., B.G.A.T.C. and V.M.R. All authors have read and agreed to the published version of the manuscript.

Funding: This work received funding from FCT—Fundação para a Ciência e Tecnologia (UID04045/2020). We thank the support of the Foundation for Support to Research and Technological Innovation of the State of Sergipe-FAPITEC/SE for granting research and to Brazilian National Council for Scientific and Technological Development (CNPq).

Conflicts of Interest: The authors declare no conflict of interest.

References

1. Brown, P.; Venables, H.; Liu, H.; de-Witt, J.; Brown, M.; Faghy, M. Ventilatory muscle strength, diaphragm thickness and pulmonary function in world-class powerlifters. *Eur. J. Appl. Phys.* **2013**, *113*, 2849–2855. [CrossRef]
2. Paz, Â.D.A.; Aidar, F.J.; de Matos, D.G.; de Souza, R.F.; da Silva-Grigoletto, M.E.; van den Tillaar, R.; Costa e Silva, A.D.A. Comparison of Post-Exercise Hypotension Responses in Paralympic Powerlifting Athletes after Completing Two Bench Press Training Intensities. *Medicina* **2020**, *56*, 156. [CrossRef]
3. Fraga, G.S.; Aidar, F.J.; Matos, D.G.; Marçal, A.C.; Santos, J.L.; Souza, R.F.; van den Tillaar, R.; Reis, V.M. Effects of Ibuprofen Intake in Muscle Damage, Body Temperature and Muscle Power in Paralympic Powerlifting Athletes. *Int. J. Environ. Res. Public Health* **2020**, *17*, 5157. [CrossRef] [PubMed]

4. Law, Y.L.L.; Ong, W.S.; GillianYap, T.L.; Lim, S.C.J.; Von Chia, E. Effects of two and five days of creatine loading on muscular strength and anaerobic power in trained athletes. *J. Strength Cond. Res.* **2009**, *23*, 906–914. [CrossRef] [PubMed]
5. Close, G.L.; Hamilton, D.L.; Philp, A. New strategies in sport nutrition to increase exercise performance. *Free Radic. Biol. Med.* **2016**, *98*, 144–158. [CrossRef] [PubMed]
6. Lanhers, C.; Pereira, B.; Naughton, G. Creatine supplementation and upper limb strength performance: A systematic review and meta-analysis. *Sports Med.* **2017**, *47*, 163–173. [CrossRef]
7. Bemben, M.G.; Lamont, H.S. Creatine supplementation and exercise performance: Recent findings. *Sports Med.* **2005**, *35*, 107–125. [CrossRef]
8. Schoenfeld, B.J.; Ogborn, D.; Krieger, J.W. Dose-response relationship between weekly resistance training volume and increases in muscle mass: A systematic review and meta-analysis. *J. Sports Sci.* **2017**, *35*, 1073–1082. [CrossRef]
9. Rosene, J.; Matthews, T.; Ryan, C.; Belmore, K.; Love, R.; Marrone, M.; Ward, K. Short and longer-term effects of creatine supplementation on exercise induced muscle damage. *J. Sports Sci. Med.* **2009**, *8*, 89–96.
10. Dolder, M.; Walzel, B.; Speer, O.; Schlattner, U.; Wallimann, T. Inhibition of the mitochondrial permeability transition by creatine kinase substrates. Requirement for microcompartmentation. *J. Biol. Chem.* **2003**, *278*, 17760–17766. [CrossRef]
11. Rosene, J.M.; Matthews, T.D.; Mcbride, K.J.; Galla, A.; Haun, M.; McDonald, K.; Farias, C. The effects of creatine supplementation on thermoregulation and isokinetic muscular performance following acute (3-day) supplementation. *J. Sports Med. Phys. Fit.* **2015**, *55*, 1488–1496. [CrossRef]
12. International Paralympic Comite (IPC). Rules Official Website of IPC Powerlifting. Available online: http://www.paralympic.org/powerlifting/about (accessed on 10 January 2020).
13. Hultman, E.; Söderlund, K.; Timmons, J.A.; Cederblad, G.; Greenhaff, P.L. Muscle creatine loading in men. *J. Appl. Physiol.* **1996**, *81*, 232–237. [CrossRef] [PubMed]
14. Bento, P.C.B.; Pereira, G.; Ugrinowitsch, C.; Rodacki, A.L.F. Peak torque and rate of torque development in elderly with and without fall history. *Clin. Biomech.* **2010**, *25*, 450–454. [CrossRef] [PubMed]
15. Milner-Brown, H.S.; Mellenthin, M.; Miller, R.G. Quantifying human muscle strength, endurance and fatigue. *Arch. Phys. Med. Rehabil.* **1986**, *67*, 530–535. [PubMed]
16. Fleck, S.J.; Kraemer, W.J. *Designing Resistance Training Programs*, 4th ed.; Human Kinetics: Champaign, IL, USA, 2004.
17. Loturco, I.; Pereira, L.A.; Winckler, C.; Santos, W.L.; Kobal, R.; McGuigan, M. Load-speed relationship in national Paralympic powerlifters: A case study. *Int. J. Sports Physiol. Perform.* **2019**, *14*, 531–535. [CrossRef]
18. Bonsu, B.; Terblanche, E. The training and detraining effect of high-intensity interval training on post-exercise hypotensionin young overweight/obese women. *Eur. J. Appl. Physiol.* **2016**, *116*, 77–84. [CrossRef]
19. Austin, D.; Mann, B. *Powerlifting: The Complete Guide to Technique, Training, and Competition*; Human Kinetics: Champaign, IL, USA, 2012.
20. Espirito-Santo, H.; Daniel, F. Calculating and Reporting Effect Sizes on Scientific Papers (1): $p < 0.05$ Limitations in the Analysis of Mean Differences of Two Conditions. *Rev. Port. Invest. Comp. Soc.* **2017**, *1*, 3–16.
21. Zuniga, J.M.; Housh, T.J.; Camic, C.L.; Hendrix, C.R.; Mielke, M.; Johnson, G.O.; Housh, D.J.; Schmidt, R.J. The effects of creatine monohydrate loading on anaerobic performance and one-repetition maximum strength. *J. Strength Cond. Res.* **2012**, *26*, 1651–1656. [CrossRef]
22. Hamilton, K.L.; Meyers, M.C.; Skelly, W.A.; Marley, R.J. Oral creatine supplementation and upper extremity anaerobic response in females. *Int. J. Sport Nutr.* **2000**, *10*, 277–289. [CrossRef]
23. Syrotuik, D.G.; Berll, G.J.; Burnham, R.; Sim, L.L.; Calvert, R.A.; Maclean, I.M. Absolute and relative strength performance following creatine monohydrate supplementation combined with periodized resistance training. *J. Strength Cond. Res.* **2000**, *14*, 182–190.
24. Butts, J.; Jacobs, B.; Silvis, M. Creatine use in sports. *Sports Health* **2018**, *10*, 31–34. [CrossRef] [PubMed]
25. Branch, J.D. Effect of creatine supplementation on body composition and performance: A meta-analysis. *Int. J. Sport Nutr. Exerc. Metabol.* **2003**, *13*, 198–226. [CrossRef]
26. Claudino, J.G.; Mezêncio, B.; Amaral, S.; Zanetti, V.; Benatti, F.; Serrão, J.C. Creatine monohydrate supplementation on lower-limb muscle power in Brazilian elite soccer players. *J. Int. Soc. Sports Nutr.* **2014**, *11*, 1–6. [CrossRef] [PubMed]

27. Aedma, M.; Timpmann, S.; Lätt, E.; Ööpik, V. Short-term creatine supplementation has no impact on upper-body anaerobic power in trained wrestlers. *J. Int. Soc. Sports Nutr.* **2015**, *12*, 45. [CrossRef] [PubMed]
28. Bazzucchi, I.; Felici, F.; Sacchetti, M. Effect of short-term creatine supplementation on neuromuscular function. *Med. Sci. Sports Exerc.* **2009**, *41*, 1934–1941. [CrossRef]
29. Nelson, A.; Arnall, D.; Kokkonen, J.; Day, R.; Evans, J. Muscle glycogen supercompensation is enhanced by prior creatine supplementation. *Med. Sci. Sports Exerc.* **2001**, *33*, 1096–1100. [CrossRef]
30. Hickner, R.; Dyck, D.; Sklar, J.; Hatley, H.; Byrd, P. Effect of 28 days of creatine ingestion on muscle metabolism and performance of a simulated cycling road race. *J. Int. Soc. Sports. Nutr.* **2010**, *7*, 26. [CrossRef]
31. Magherini, F.; Fiaschi, T.; Marzocchini, R.; Mannelli, M.; Gamberi, T.; Modesti, P.; Modesti, A. Oxidative stress in exercise training: The involvement of inflammation and peripheral signals. *Free Radic. Res.* **2019**, *53*, 1–11. [CrossRef]
32. Baranauskas, M.; Jablonskienė, V.; Abaravičius, J.A.; Samsonienė, L.; Stukas, R. Dietary Acid-Base Balance in High-Performance Athletes. *Int. J. Environ. Res. Public Health* **2020**, *17*, 5332. [CrossRef]
33. Huang, W.C.; Hsu, Y.J.; Huang, C.C.; Liu, H.C.; Lee, M.C. Exercise Training Combined with Bifidobacterium Longum OLP-01 Supplementation Improves Exercise Physiological Adaption and Performance. *Nutrients* **2020**, *12*, 1145. [CrossRef]
34. Di Filippo, E.S.; Mancinelli, R.; Marrone, M.; Doria, C.; Verratti, V.; Toniolo, L.; Pietrangelo, T. Neuromuscular electrical stimulation improves skeletal muscle regeneration through satellite cell fusion with myofibers in healthy elderly subjects. *J. Appl. Physiol.* **2017**, *123*, 501–512. [CrossRef] [PubMed]
35. Cooper, R.; Naclerio, F.; Allgrove, J.; Jimenez, A. Creatine supplementation with specific view to exercise/sports performance: An update. *J. Int. Soc. Sports Nutr.* **2012**, *9*, 1–11. [CrossRef] [PubMed]
36. Bassit, R.A.; Pinheiro, C.H.; Vitzel, K.F.; Sproesser, A.J.; Silveira, L.R.; Curi, R. Effect of short-term creatine supplementation on markers of skeletal muscle damage after strenuous contractile activity. *Eur. J. Appl. Physiol.* **2010**, *108*, 945–955. [CrossRef] [PubMed]
37. Amorim, S.; Teixeira, V.H.; Corredeira, R.; Cunha, M.; Maia, B.; Margalho, P.; Pires, J. Creatine or vitamin D supplementation in individuals with a spinal cord injury undergoing resistance training: A double-blinded, randomized pilot trial. *J. Spinal Cord Med.* **2018**, *41*, 471–478. [CrossRef] [PubMed]
38. Jacobs, P.L.; Mahoney, E.T.; Cohn, K.A.; Sheradsky, L.F.; Green, B.A. Oral creatine supplementation enhances upper extremity work capacity in persons with cervical-level spinal cord injury. *Arch. Phys. Med. Rehabil.* **2002**, *83*, 19–23. [CrossRef]
39. Hausmann, O.; Fouad, K.; Wallimann, T. Protective effects of oral creatine supplementation on spinal cord injury in rats. *Spinal Cord* **2002**, *40*, 449–456. [CrossRef]

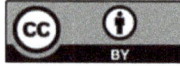

© 2020 by the authors. Licensee MDPI, Basel, Switzerland. This article is an open access article distributed under the terms and conditions of the Creative Commons Attribution (CC BY) license (http://creativecommons.org/licenses/by/4.0/).

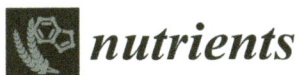

Review

Effects of Dietary Nitrates on Time Trial Performance in Athletes with Different Training Status: Systematic Review

Tomáš Hlinský *, Michal Kumstát and Petr Vajda

Faculty of Sports Studies, Masaryk University, Kamenice 5, 625 00 Brno, Czech Republic; kumstat@fsps.muni.cz (M.K.); vajda@fsps.muni.cz (P.V.)
* Correspondence: hlinsky.tomas@mail.muni.cz; Tel.: +420-732-579-697

Received: 25 August 2020; Accepted: 4 September 2020; Published: 8 September 2020

Abstract: Much research has been done in sports nutrition in recent years as the demand for performance-enhancing substances increases. Higher intake of nitrates from the diet can increase the bioavailability of nitric oxide (NO) via the nitrate–nitrite–NO pathway. Nevertheless, the increased availability of NO does not always lead to improved performance in some individuals. This review aims to evaluate the relationship between the athlete's training status and the change in time trial performance after increased dietary nitrate intake. Articles indexed by Scopus and PubMed published from 2015 to 2019 were reviewed. Thirteen articles met the eligibility criteria: clinical trial studies on healthy participants with different training status (according to VO_{2max}), conducting time trial tests after dietary nitrate supplementation. The PRISMA guidelines were followed to process the review. We found a statistically significant relationship between VO_{2max} and ergogenicity in time trial performance using one-way ANOVA ($p = 0.001$) in less-trained athletes ($VO_2 < 55$ mL/kg/min). A strong positive correlation was observed in experimental situations using a chronic supplementation protocol but not in acute protocol situations. In the context of our results and recent histological observations of muscle fibres, there might be a fibre-type specific role in nitric oxide production and, therefore, supplement of ergogenicity.

Keywords: nitric oxide; dietary supplements; oxygen consumption; muscle fibres; physical activity

1. Introduction

Nitric oxide (NO) plays a crucial role in signalling and physiological regulatory functions of the human body which are crucial to exercise economy and performance (i.e., vasodilatation, mitochondrial respiration, glucose and calcium (Ca^{2+}) homeostasis, skeletal muscle contractility and fatigue development). Because the NO molecule is highly unstable, there is a constant need for its regeneration [1–4].

Interestingly the substrates for NO syntheses (L-arginine and nitrates) come from our daily diet and therefore can be manipulated [5]. Increased availability of NO via diet has been linked to ergogenic effects [6,7]. However, not all athletes can benefit from these nutritional strategies [8,9]. It seems the effectiveness of NO inducing foods and supplements is limited by an athlete's training status (aerobic fitness) and muscle fibre type ratio [10].

1.1. NO Metabolism and Physiological Importance

Nitric oxide synthesis in the human body is carried out via two pathways: the NO synthase (NOS)-dependent pathway and nitrate–nitrite–NO (NO_3^-–NO_2^-–NO) pathway [11]. Formation of NO via the NOS-dependent pathway is carried out through the utilisation of L-arginine and oxygen (O_2). Thus, this reaction relies on the delivery of O_2 [12]. Insufficient O_2 delivery during high-intensity exercise may cause this pathway to become dysfunctional [13]. Therefore, the O_2-independent pathway can substitute NO production [14] via the reduction of NO_3^- from the diet (e.g., green leafy vegetables, beetroot, radish) [15]. Nitrates are reduced by oral anaerobic bacteria to NO_2^- [16]. Subsequently, part of the total NO_2^- is reduced to NO in the acidic environment of the stomach where it protects the organism from some pathogens [17]. The rest of the NO_2^- is then transported via the upper gastrointestinal tract into the blood reaching its plasma peak level 2–3 h postprandially [18]. The reduction of NO_2^- to NO substitutes the O_2-dependent NOS pathway in various tissues under hypoxic or acidic conditions [19]. These are conditions that typically occur in working muscles during vigorous exercise [20].

Increased NO bioavailability via food or supplements may increase exercise performance, as it is the critical factor in three physiological mechanisms related to physical exercise. Firstly, NO increases skeletal muscle O_2 delivery via vasodilatation [21]. Secondly, it reduces the O_2 cost of mitochondrial ATP resynthesis via an increased number of ATP molecules (P) formed per O_2 molecules consumed (O) in the electron transport chain (P/O ratio) [22], possibly via the interaction with five-coordinated cytochrome C oxidase [23,24]. Lastly, it improves the efficiency of muscle contractility via reduced creatine phosphate (PCr) cost of force production [25] and changes in Ca^{2+} metabolism within the muscle cells [26]. Enhancing these physiological mechanisms leads to more efficient energy metabolism, lower O_2 demands of the working muscles and higher muscle contractility [26] and therefore an increase in exercise economy and performance [1,22,25].

1.2. The Role of Dietary Nitrates in Exercise Physiology

Dietary nitrates (DN) have become a trendy topic in sports nutrition as even minor enhancement of human physiology may positively affect high-intensity exercise and, therefore, competition results. For example, there may be a decrease in the time of time-trial (TT) physical activities [27]. It is also important to note that these changes seem to be highly related to the dosage and supplementation protocol where exercise economy can be improved after a single dose of DN [28–33], but exercise performance is more likely augmented after chronic use of DN [34–36]. Interestingly, it seems ergogenicity is somehow related to the fibre-type ratio in muscles, augmenting the exercise economy and performance more likely via type II muscle fibres (MFs) than type I [37].

During high-intensity exercise, oxidative phosphorylation is diminished as the O_2 supply is inadequate, and reliance on the anaerobic metabolic pathway of ATP regeneration is favoured [38]. Long-duration high-intensity exercise and intermittent high-intensity exercise lead to exercise-induced hypoxemia causing the muscles to become hypoxic and acidic [39]. This impairment in homeostasis may also disrupt the functioning of the NOS-dependent pathway, and continuation of exercise is highly dependent on the activity of type II MFs [40,41]. Therefore, the reliance on the substitutional NO_3^-–NO_2^-–NO pathway independent of O_2 supply is increased [40,42]. Moreover, type II MFs have a lower blood supply which affects the partial pressure of O_2 within the microvasculature ($P_{mv}O_2$) causing a lower O_2 supply compared to type I MFs [43–45]. This phenomenon underlines the reliance on the NO_3^-–NO_2^-–NO pathway in type II MFs and even more under hypoxia [24,46]. Lastly, most recent studies suggest improvement in muscle force production and mitochondrial oxidative phosphorylation are more likely observed in type II MFs than in type I MFs after DN supplementation [47,48].

Furthermore, it has already been suggested in earlier studies that neither acute nor chronic DN supplementation can improve performance in highly trained cyclists [49–51], runners [52,53] or cross-country skiers [54]. These groups of endurance-trained athletes tend to have a higher type I MF ratio [55–57]. In contrast, high doses of DN (8.4–9.6 mmol) improved performance in highly trained kayakers and rowers [29,58] but not low doses (~4–5 mmol) [29,59]. In this context, the upper body muscles (e.g., biceps brachii, triceps brachii, deltoid, trapezius or latissimus dorsi) are well described as muscles with a higher type II MF ratio [60–62]. Moreover, as highly trained athletes develop specific adaptation to rowing [63] and kayaking [64], increased type II MF ratio or MF hypertrophy is more likely [65]. This exercise modality, which mostly involves muscle groups with a higher type II MF ratio [65], can be another example of the fibre-type specific effects of DN [37,66].

1.3. Training Status as a Limiting Factor

Nutritional strategies to increase the bioavailability of NO and possibly physical performance have been under the scope of research for many years, and there are some crucial variables (e.g., muscle fibre-type ratio, physiological limitations) which can influence their effectiveness [8,67]. Consumption of dietary NO_3^- (DN) in the form of either nitrate-rich foods or supplements generally increases plasma levels of NO_2^- [28] which interestingly does not always lead to improvement in exercise performance especially in well-trained endurance and elite endurance athletes [68].

Fibre-type specific effects of DN supplementation have been demonstrated in animal experiments where muscle force development increased in type II (fast-twitch glycolytic fibres type IIx) but not in type I MFs (slow-twitch oxidative fibres) [34]. Reliance on the NO_3^-–NO_2^-–NO pathway is higher in type II MFs due to the lower O_2 tension (pO_2) than in type I [43]. Therefore, an increase in the bioavailability of NO mainly affects type II MFs [37]. Endurance-trained athletes are likely to have a higher ratio of slow oxidative type I MFs compared to non-trained and recreationally active athletes [69] or the inactive population and the elderly [70]. This phenomenon also relates to higher aerobic fitness in highly and elite trained athletes which cannot be augmented any further [68]. These seem to be possible explanations for the lower ergogenicity of DN supplementation in highly trained or elite athletes, as some studies failed to enhance the performance of the participants [52,71]. It has been suggested that the efficiency of DN supplementation is related to an athlete's training status, especially in high-intensity endurance exercises, e.g., time trial (TT) performance, where O_2 delivery is impaired and reliance on type II MFs is higher [68].

1.4. Aim and Purpose of the Review

This article reviews the relationship between VO_{2max} and DN ergogenicity in TT performance, defined as the athlete's training status. We further discuss the relationship between simulated high altitude and DN ergogenicity in the context of increased reliance on type II MFs under hypoxic conditions, as it has been proposed that the DN ergogenicity is fibre-type related. Additionally, we wanted to stress the importance of inclusion of certain methodological tools in the evaluation of the results of experiments (e.g., smallest worthwhile change and typical error of measurement).

2. Materials and Methods

A review of the literature was carried out using articles indexed by Scopus and PubMed published from 1 January 2015 to 31 December 2019. The PRISMA guidelines were followed to process the review [72].

2.1. Search Strategy, Data Extraction and Analysis

The following terms were used for the search: dietary nitrates, physical performance and physical exercise. All descriptors were searched using the Boolean operators to maximise the search quality as follows: *((dietary AND nitrates) AND ((physical AND exercise) OR (physical AND performance)))*. The title and abstract of each article were assessed for eligibility. After that, full-text articles were reviewed to determine their suitability for inclusion or exclusion. The inclusion criteria were: (i) studies on healthy human subjects, (ii) original, English-language research articles, (iii) inclusion of the training status of participants (VO_{2max}, training load or other affiliation to training status group), (iv) experimental protocol consisting of time-trial testing, (v) results showing a change in time trial performance, (iv) supplementation protocol is described. The exclusion criteria were: (i) the above inclusion criteria were not met and (ii) the experimental test was combined with environmental modification (e.g., high-altitude simulation and high temperature). No restrictions were made on age, sample size, supplementation protocol or supplement form. Figure 1 describes the process of selecting the articles presented in this review using the PRISMA Flow Diagram.

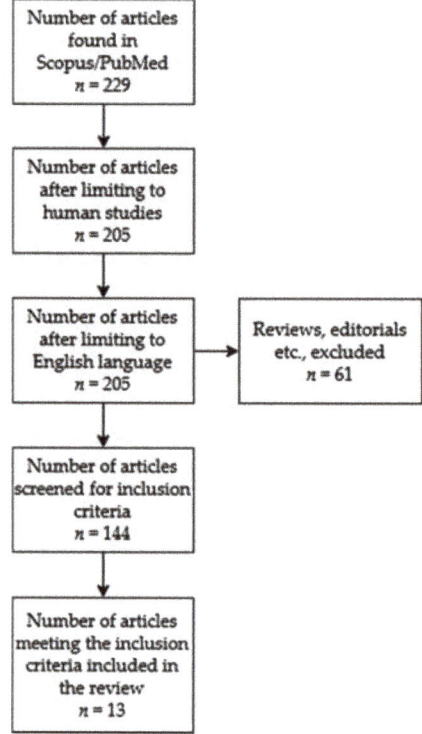

Figure 1. Selection process diagram of articles meeting the eligibility criteria for our review.

2.2. Data Classification

Out of the 13 included studies, we analysed 22 separate DN experimental situations. The experimental situations were classified into five groups according to the mean group VO_{2max} or VO_{2peak} of the participants according to the preliminary testing of each study (Table 1), which allowed us to define their training status as previously published [73,74]. One study did not use the VO_{2max} of participants for training status assessment but used training load instead [75]. Mean percentual change in time-to-completion of given exercise tasks in the experimental DN groups were either included in the article or calculated from the results.

Table 1. Participant training status classification defined by VO_{2max}.

Training Status (Number of Experimental Situations Included)	Sex	VO_{2max} (mL/kg/min)
1—Untrained ($n = 1$)	Males	<45
	Females	<37
2—Recreationally trained ($n = 4$)	Males	45–54.9
	Females	37–48
3—Trained ($n = 4$)	Males	55–64.9
	Females	48–52

Table 1. Cont.

Training Status (Number of Experimental Situations Included)	Sex	VO_{2max} (mL/kg/min)
4—Well-trained (n = 12)	Males	65–71
	Females	52–58
5—Elite (n = 1)	Males	>71
	Females	>58

2.3. Quality Assessment

Risk of bias was assessed using the Physiotherapy Evidence Database (PEDro) scale, which provides a reliable assessment of internal validity [76,77]. Each article was individually assessed by the reviewer (T.H.) using an adjusted 11 item checklist to yield a maximum score of 10.

2.4. Data Extraction

Data were extracted and reviewed by one of the researchers (T.H.). Additionally, the data were independently reviewed by the other researchers (M.K. and P.V.), following a systematic selection list which included the inclusion criteria mentioned in Section 2.1.

2.5. Statistical Analysis

A one-way ANOVA was conducted to determine whether there is a relationship between DN ergogenicity and training status level. Data were classified into three groups according to the training status of participants: untrained + recreationally trained (n = 5), *trained* (n = 4), well-trained + elite (n = 13). There were no outliers as assessed by a boxplot. Data were normally distributed for each group as assessed by the Shapiro–Wilk test ($p > 0.05$), and variances were homogeneous as assessed by Levene's test of homogeneity of variances ($\alpha = 0.05$). A Spearman's rank-order correlation and Pearson correlation coefficient were used to assess the relationship between DN ergogenicity and VO_{2max} after chronic/acute DN intake and between DN ergogenicity and TT test duration. A coefficient of variation (CV) was carried out to assess the frequency distribution of VO_{2max} among the groups of participants and inter-study variability in performance effect. All data analyses were performed using the SPSS statistical package (version 25; SPSS, Chicago, IL, USA) and the GraphPad Prism 8 (GraphPad Software, San Diego, CA, USA). Results are presented as mean ± standard deviation.

3. Results

The reviewed articles included 22 experimental situations presented in Figure 2. The figure shows performance changes in all acute (blue bars) and chronic (red bars) experimental situations reviewed. The effect of DN supplementation is displayed as the percentual mean change in the experimental group. Improvement in performance is interpreted as a negative value as the TT test was finished faster compared to placebo.

The mean changes in performance across the selected experimental situations were −2.63%, −2.83%, −0.49%, −0.27% and −0.31% in untrained (n = 1), recreationally trained (I = 4), trained (n = 4), well-trained (n = 12) and elite (n = 1) groups, respectively.

One-way ANOVA presented a statistically significant difference in performance change among groups with different training status after DN supplementation $F (2, 19) = 11.787$, $p = 0.001$ and $\omega^2 = 0.533$. The positive performance change increased from well-trained + elite (−0.272 ± 0.671%) to trained (−0.490 ± 1.238%) and untrained + recreationally trained (−2.786 ± 1.629%) groups, in that order. Tukey's post-hoc analysis revealed that the increase from well-trained + elite to the untrained + recreationally trained group (2.51, 95% CI (1.12 to 3.91)) was statistically significant ($p = 0.001$), as well as the increase from trained to untrained + recreationally trained (2.30, 95% CI (0.52 to 4.07), $p = 0.010$), but not from well-trained + elite to trained. Statistical analysis was done on a sample of all

22 experimental situations. Therefore, the data were divided according to the training status but not according to the supplementation protocol due to the small sample size for ANOVA analysis.

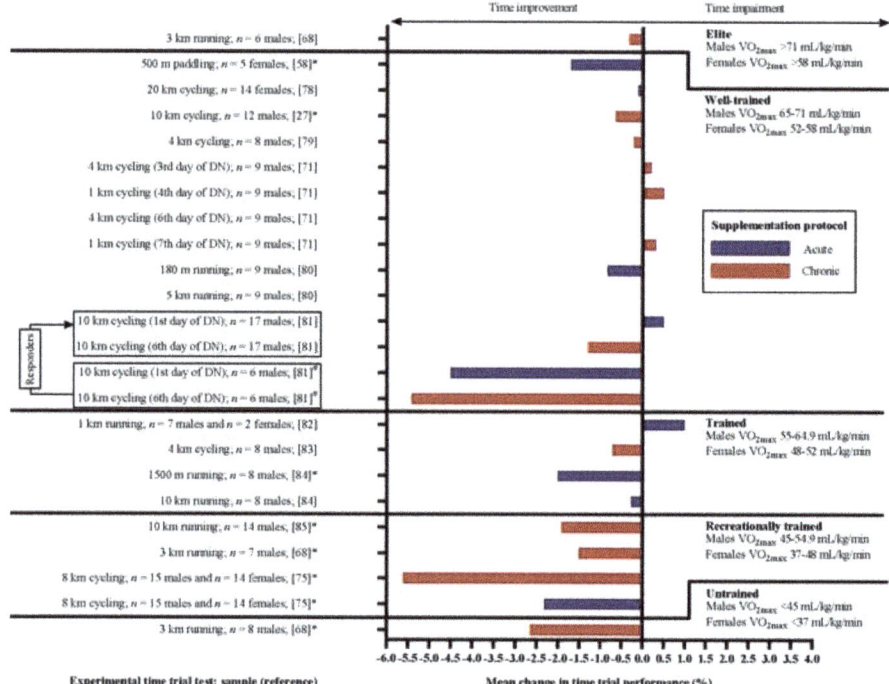

Figure 2. Effects of DN supplementation on TT performance in athletes with different training statuses according to their VO_{2max}. The graph presents the mean percentual changes in time-to-completion of given tasks in the experimental groups. Negative values represent improvement, as the task was finished in less time (bars to the left from y-axis) following acute (blue bars) or chronic (red bars) supplementation. Cited studies are listed in References [27,58,68,71,75,78–85]. * Statistically significant improvement in performance following DN supplementation; # improvement was observed in 6 of 17 participants dividing the group of *well-trained* athletes into "responders" and "non-responders". The two experimental situations are, therefore, divided into four according to the specific reaction to DN supplementation of the participants [81].

A Spearman's rank-order correlation was run to assess the relationship between VO_{2max} and DN ergogenicity in the TT tests after chronic intake of DN. There was a statistically significant, strong positive correlation between VO_{2max} and performance change in TT, i.e., a positive ergogenic effect declines with higher training status ($r_s(9) = 0.810$, $p = 0.003$; Figure 3.). However, Pearson's correlation coefficient showed no significant correlation for acute supplementation ($r(8) = 0.445$, $p = 0.198$; Figure 4). One study did not report VO_{2max} values of participants and, therefore, was excluded from the analysis [75].

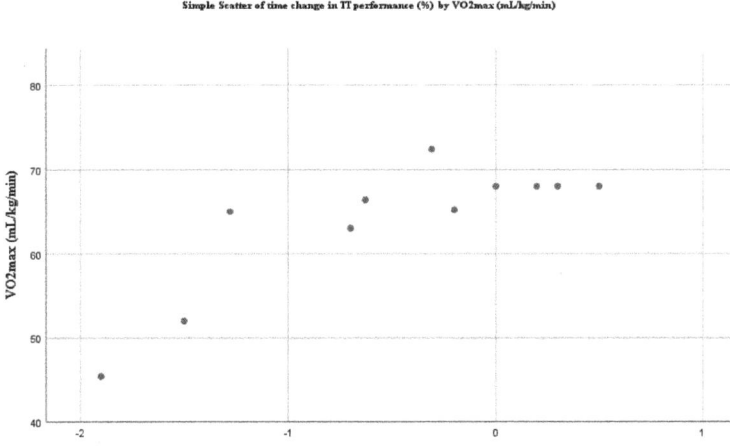

Figure 3. Relationship between VO_{2max} and DN ergogenicity in TT tests: chronic supplementation protocol. Negative values in time change represent improvement as the task was finished in less time.

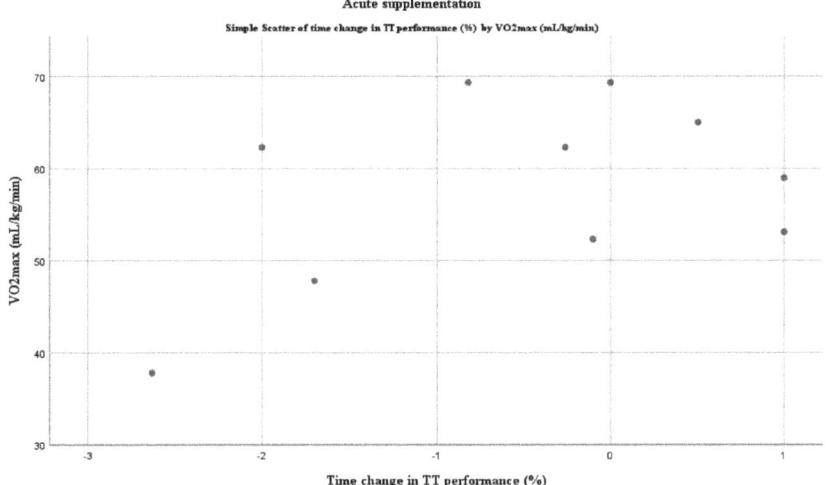

Figure 4. Relationship between VO_{2max} and DN ergogenicity in TT tests: acute supplementation protocol. Negative values in time change represent improvement as the task was finished in less time.

Methodological Quality of Studies

All the reviewed studies that met the eligibility criteria scored 10 out of 10 in PEDro scale as they followed double-blinded crossover placebo-controlled experimental design. Overall, the quality of the reviewed studies was assessed as excellent.

4. Discussion

We reviewed the available research from 2015 to 2019 focused on the relationship between dietary nitrates and TT performance in athletes with different training status according to their VO_{2max}. Statistical analysis of the data collected from 13 articles showed that the higher the training status, the lower the effect on TT performance.

4.1. Dietary Nitrates and Time Trial Performance

Our results demonstrate that DN ergogenicity in TT performance is more likely observed in less-trained individuals than in the highly trained and more consistently after chronic use. These results are in agreement with previously reported data [1]. In contrast, some reviews did not find a statistically significant change in TT performance [86,87]. It was proposed that the $VO_{2max} > 65$ mL/kg/min is not related to ergogenic effects after DN intake [1,10]. However, our results suggest that DN ergogenicity may be lower even in trained athletes, as we did not find a significant difference between the trained and well-trained + elite groups. Significant ergogenic effects were evident in the groups of $VO_{2max} \leq 50$ mL/kg/min and less.

These results suggest there is a strong link between the athlete's training status and DN ergogenicity. The real cause of this phenomenon is still debated. We further provide a discussion on possible causes.

4.2. Dietary Nitrates and Exercise Performance in a High-Altitude Environment

Our results are consistent with other studies suggesting the ergogenicity of DN is diminished in highly-trained endurance athletes, possibly due to the fact of their higher type I MF ratio [1,37,88].

To support the hypothesis of a relationship between ergogenicity and type II MFs, we also reviewed TT studies at simulated high-altitude through normobaric hypoxia ($n = 3$; Figure 5). A high altitude environment with lower pO_2 leads to impairment in O_2 delivery in tissues, and the aerobic energy metabolism pathway is diminished [89]. Therefore, the work efficiency of type I MFs is lowered, and reliance on the anaerobic metabolic pathway and type II MFs is increased [90]. Exercise-induced hypoxemia is amplified in high-altitude hypoxic conditions, and the reliance on type II MFs is expected to be increased [91,92]. Therefore, it has been hypothesised that DN ergogenicity in highly-trained endurance athletes could be augmented due to the increased involvement of type II MFs during TT tests in an environment with lower pO_2 [93–95]. Although performance improvement was observed in highly-trained athletes ($VO_{2max} > 65$ mL/kg/min) after DN intake (−3.2%) [94], yet again, more consistent improvement was more likely observed in less-trained athletes (−3.6 ± 0.4%) [93,94].

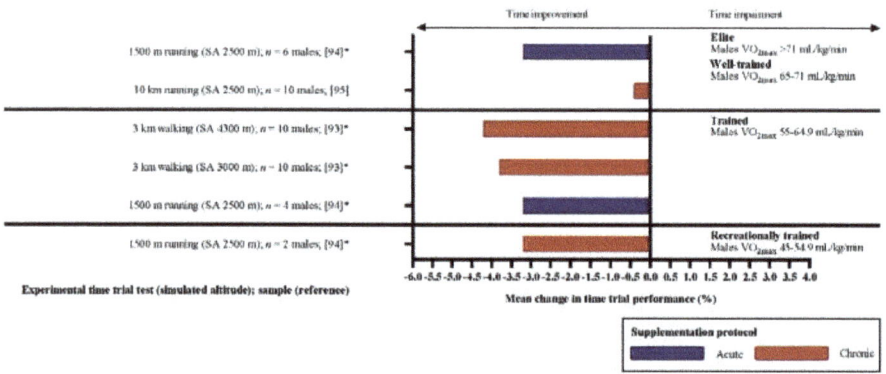

Figure 5. Training status and ergogenicity in simulated high-altitude. Cited studies are listed in References [93–95]. * Statistically significant improvement in performance following DN supplementation.

Additionally, Arnold et al. [95] observed an improvement in the highly trained (−0.4%), but this was not of statistical significance ($p = 0.6$). To this day, data on the ergogenicity of DN at high altitude brings more or less mixed results and, so far, no additional benefits in general [96,97]. Despite the increased pulmonary NO availability and plasma NO_2^- concentrations [98] and lower altitude-induced reduction in endothelial function [99] that have been documented, solid conclusions as to whether a high altitude could augment ergogenicity in highly-trained athletes requires further research.

4.3. Dietary Nitrates Studies Methodology

Nyakayiru et al. [81] observed a statistically significant and positive response in six out of the total of 17 participants during TT performance. Whereas the mean VO_{2max} (65.0 ± 4 mL/kg/min) classified the group as well-trained, the standard deviation suggested that some of the participants were less trained and potentially more likely to be DN responders. In future research, we suggest the grouping of participants to be carefully divided according to training status, because there seems to be a thin line between the high and low ergogenicity of DN and, therefore, statistical evaluation of the results may be affected.

Correctly classifying training status (e.g., VO_{2max} and/or weekly training load) in various athletes may be an essential aspect of increasing the reliability of DN research [73,74]. Table 2 summarises the research characteristics of the reviewed studies, showing that specific TT criteria (distance, test duration) and DN supplementation protocols (acute/chronic, DN dosage) are different across the studies. Notably, groups of participants are somewhat mixed in terms of training status as the diversity of the athlete's VO_{2max} is in some studies quite high (CV = 21.5% in Oskarsson and McGawley [82]).

Twenty-two experimental situations were included in our review with highly variable TT test durations 881 ± 856 s (25–3300 s). No correlation was observed between the TT duration and performance effects ($r_s(20) = -0.237$, $p = 0.288$). There was also no correlation after the TT duration adjustment (i.e., only situations with TT duration > 10 min included; $r_s(10) = 0.064$, $p = 0.843$). However, it may be speculated whether long-duration TT tests (>720 s) could benefit more from DN supplementation as the authors of 10 out of the 12 experimental situations reported ergogenic effects. In contrast, only 5 out of 10 experimental situations (TT test duration < 720 s) reported improvement in exercise performance. It is becoming more evident that DN ergogenicity could be fibre-type specific. Therefore, the duration of the event should be taken into consideration as our results are in contrast with general recommendations for DN use (4–8 min events in Burke et al. [2]).

Inter-study variability in performance effect was high as the coefficient of variation (CV) reached 55%. The lowest and therefore more stable CV was obtained in trained (26%) and well-trained groups (26%) but not in the recreationally trained groups (58%).

Table 2. Relationship between DN supplementation protocol and training status in promoting the ergogenic effects.

Reference	Sex	Training Status	VO$_{2max}$ [a]/VO$_{2peak}$ [b]	CV	A/C	Supplementation Protocol	Test (Test Duration)	Ergogenic *
[75]	M and F	Recreationally trained	-	-	Acute	8.0 mmol (NO$_3^-$) of PN; 2 h before the test	8 km cycling (~20 min)	Yes
[84]	M	Trained	62.3 ± 8.1 mL/kg/min [a]	13.0%		12.8 mmol (NO$_3^-$) of BJC; 3 h before the test	1500 m running (~6 min)	Yes
							10 km running (~45 min)	No
[82]	M	Trained	59.0 ± 2.9 mL/kg/min [a]	4.9%		6.4 mmol (NO$_3^-$) of BJC; 2.5 h before the test	1 km running (~3 min)	No
	F		53.1 ± 11.4 mL/kg/min [a]	21.5%				No
[80]	M	Well-trained	69.3 ± 5.8 mL/kg/min [a]	8.4%		9.9 mmol (NO$_3^-$) of PN; 2.5 h before the test	180 m running (~25 s)	No
							5 km running (~17 min)	No
[81]	M	Well-trained	65.0 ± 4.0 mL/kg/min [b]	6.2%		12.8 mmol (NO$_3^-$) of SN; 3 h before the test	10 km cycling (~17 min)	No [#]
[78]	F	Well-trained	52.3 ± 4.9 mL/kg/min [a]	9.4%		6.4 mmol (NO$_3^-$) of BJC; 2.5 h before the test	20 km cycling (~35 min)	No
[58]	F	Well-trained [†]	47.8 ± 3.7 mL/kg/min [b]	7.7%		12.8 mmol NO$_3^-$ of BJC; 2 h before the test	500 m paddling (~2 min)	Yes
[68]	M	Untrained	37.8 ± 5.8 mL/kg/min [b]	15.3%	Chronic	6-day 5.5 mmol (NO$_3^-$) of SN; 3.5 h before the test	3 km running (~15 min)	Yes
[73]	M and F	Recreationally trained	-	-		15-day 8.0 mmol (NO$_3^-$) of PN; 2 h before the test	8 km cycling (~20 min)	Yes
[68]	M	Recreationally trained	52.0 ± 4.5 mL/kg/min [b]	8.7%		6-day 5.5 mmol (NO$_3^-$) of SN; 3.5 h before the test	3 km running (~12 min)	Yes
[85]	M	Recreationally trained	45.4 ± 5.9 mL/kg/min [b]	13.0%		3-day 8.4 mmol (NO$_3^-$) of BJ; 2 h before the test	10 km running (~55 min)	Yes
[83]	M	Trained	63.0 ± 4.0 mL/kg/min [b]	6.3%		8-day 6.4 mmol (NO$_3^-$) of BJC; 2.5 h before the test	4 km cycling (~6 min)	No
[71]	M	Well-trained	68.0 ± 3.0 mL/kg/min [a]	4.4%		7-day 12.8 mmol (NO$_3^-$) of BJC; 2.5 h before the test	1 km cycling (~80 s)	No
							4 km cycling (<6 min)	No
[79]	M	Well-trained	65.2 ± 4.2 mL/kg/min [a]	6.4%		3-day ~5 mmol (NO$_3^-$) of BC; 1 h before the test	4 km cycling (<6 min)	No
[81]	M	Well-trained	65.0 ± 4.0 mL/kg/min [b]	6.2%		6-day 12.8 mmol (NO$_3^-$) of SN; 3 h before the test	10 km cycling (~17 min)	No [#]
[27]	M	Well-trained	66.4 ± 5.3 mL/kg/min [a]	8.0%		7-day 12.8 mmol (NO$_3^-$) of BJC; 2.75 h before the test	10 km cycling (~15 min)	Yes
[68]	M	Elite	72.4 ± 6.1 mL/kg/min [b]	8.4%		6-day 5.5 mmol (NO$_3^-$) of SN; 3.5 h before the test	3 km running (~10 min)	No

[a] VO$_{2max}$ values; [b] VO$_{2peak}$ values; * Statistically significant change in performance; [#] ergogenic effects in 6 of 17 participants following supplementation [81]; [†] 5 female athletes with VO$_{2peak}$ 47.8 ± 3.7 mL/kg/min (recreationally trained or trained) are presented in the "well-trained" section of this figure because they were described as international-level female kayak athletes and all were 2012 National Squad members with 3/5 athletes competing at the 2012 London Olympic Games [58]. VO$_{2peak}$ could have been lower due to the exercise modality [1]. VO$_{2max}$/VO$_{2peak}$ values are presented as the mean ± SD. Abbreviations: dietary nitrates (DN); male (M); female (F); CV-coefficient of variation; beetroot juice concentrate (BJC); beetroot juice (BJ); potassium nitrate (PN); beetroot crystals (BC); sodium nitrate (SN).

Dosage, time-to-test intake, supplementation protocol and form of DN also differed across the reviewed studies. In eight studies, the dosage exceeded the amount of 8 mmol of NO_3^- (up to 12.8 mmol; $n = 5$) which is the generally recommended amount whether an acute or chronic protocol is chosen [6]. Time-to-test intake is 2–3 h in most studies ($n = 11$). In contrast, in some studies participants were instructed to consume the supplement less close to the test (3.5 h in Porcelli et al. [68]) or closer to the test (1 h in Callahan et al. [79]). A more consistent positive change in performance is likely observed in athletes following a chronic supplementation protocol [1]. Our results showed a strong positive correlation ($r_s(9) = 0.810$, $p = 0.003$) between the VO_{2max} and performance change after chronic DN intake but no correlation in acute intake studies ($r(8) = 0.445$, $p = 0.198$). This suggests that chronic DN intake provides more consistent results for all training status categories and underlines the lower ergogenicity in highly trained athletes. The most common form of DN supplementation is beetroot juice concentrate (BJC) [27,58,71,78,82–84]. Other forms of DN supplementation include raw beetroot juice (BJ) [85], encapsulated potassium nitrate (PN) [75,80] and beetroot crystals (BC) [79] or a water solution containing sodium nitrate (SN) [68,81]. All these variables in the supplementation protocol could potentially interfere with the ergogenic effects. It has been well documented that individual pharmacokinetic responsiveness after DN intake varies [10,28,31].

4.4. The Real Benefit for Elite Athletes?

Significant beneficial effects of DN intake in elite endurance athletes are less likely to be observed. This athletic group demonstrated a high proportion of type I MFs, elite exercise performance close to the athlete's physiological limits or NO_3^--mediated vasodilation in non-prioritized muscles which may lead to reduced O_2 delivery to the essential muscles working very close to their maximal cardiac output [100]. All these factors are now suggested as potential causes of the lower ergogenicity in highly trained athletes.

Although the available laboratory studies do not support DN ergogenicity in well-trained athletes by providing statistically significant outcomes, some might argue whether this is of concern in real sport events. From the perspective of more ecologically valid situations (e.g., sports competitions), even statistically insignificant improvement can change the overall result of TT performance. Therefore, it may be speculated whether the 0.63% change in performance found in our analysis in the well-trained group [27] could change the outcome in a real sports event. Other studies have discussed the same phenomenon. For example, Rokkedal-Lausch et al. [27] concluded: "The improvement in 10-km TT completion time and power output of 0.6% and 1.6%, respectively, in the present study, is of practical relevance for elite and well-trained athletes". Seemingly, the improvement in performance of only 0.6% could make a significant difference when comparing the TT durations of elite cyclists. For example, during the 17 km TT at the 2019 Giro d'Italia (Verona-Verona, winning time 22:07) or during the 31 km TT at the 2019 Tour De France (Saint pée sur Nivelle–Espelette, winning time 40:52) only 0.3% and 0.04%, respectively, separated first and second position [101,102]. Nevertheless, in the laboratory environment, the smallest worthwhile change (SWC) and the typical error of measurement (TEM) should be taken into consideration when interpreting the results [103,104]. According to Hopkins [103], the improvement in an athlete's performance cannot be considered as progressive until it reaches or goes over 0.3% in individual sports, defining this improvement as the SWC. Additionally, the TEMs for TT cycling tests are usually around ~1% depending on the ergometer and time variation for short (~60 s) and long-duration TT (~1 h) in elite athletes, also around ~0.5% and ~1%, respectively, depending on the method and the equipment [105]. Furthermore, if we would focus on a longer duration TT test (several minutes) then the athlete's improvement would have to reach 1.3% (SWC + TEM), so it could be called beneficial [103]. Therefore, even the most considerable TT performance changes observed during cycling ergometry measurements in elite athletes may not be relevant (improvement is lower than SWC + TEM, therefore unclear) in real sports events [103]. Interestingly only 5 of the 13 reviewed studies observed performance improvement after DN supplementation $\geq 1.3\%$ [68,75,81,84,85].

From this point of view, it is evident that translating athlete-specific DN research outcomes into practical interventions requires the determination of their true translational potential. To standardise this, Close et al. [106] recently proposed an excellent 9 step framework, that may assist practitioners in the proper evaluation of performance nutrition research and applying the findings into practice therefore making the dietary choices adopted by their athletes sport-specific and "evidence-based".

4.5. Future Perspectives

Recent results from muscle histology studies show fascinating new insights into the role of NO_3^- in the human body [107–111]. Seemingly NO_3^- can be stored within the muscle tissue cells which could be a very elegant explanation of the crucial role of muscle tissue in NOS production, the NOS-dependent and NO_3^-–NO_2^-–NO pathways [88]. Wylie et al. [66] suggested that there is a relationship between VO_{2max} and NO_3^- substrates within the MFs. In the light of these recent findings, significant improvements in TT performance in athletes with VO_{2max} < 65 mL/kg/min may be explained by lower muscle NO_3^- disposal and NO bioavailability. Therefore, increased DN intake may increase muscle NO_3^- storage capacity and positively affect physical performance [112]. Moreover, it has been hypothesised there could be a potentially positive effect in the treatment of cardiovascular and metabolic diseases as NO_3^- levels are lower in the elderly, untrained and cardiovascular or diabetes patients [111–113]. Therefore, further research in the area of NO_3^- muscle storage and its role not only in physical exercise but also in therapeutic practice is needed.

Based on the above discussion, it remains unclear whether any statistically insignificant changes in highly trained athletes could be affected by MF ratio, non-specific tissue vasodilatation, physiological systems already at their maximal limit of adaption in elite athletes, supplementation protocol, NO_3^- muscle storage or other factors. As such, future research should focus on unifying the study design framework and strict classification of participants according to their training status. Additionally, in the light of recent observations of the fibre-type specific effects of DN, it would be reasonable to focus more on resistance and speed exercise tasks or lactate-anaerobic tasks to compare DN effectiveness among different sports disciplines.

4.6. Limitations of the Study

Our study has limitations which should be noted. Firstly, we only focused on articles published from 2015 and 2019, as we wanted to review the most recent studies and put them in the context of future perspectives as the NO_3^- muscle storage presents a new and fascinating approach in explaining the DN ergogenicity. Secondly, our study did not focus on data related to NO_3^-/NO_2^- blood levels which are the critical substrates for NO production and bioavailability. We managed to associate performance enhancement with chronic use of DN. However, we may speculate whether increased levels of NO_3^-/NO_2^- cause such a performance effect. We had not made the statistical analysis of biochemical data to verify such association (some studies do not provide such data as the authors did not focus on the biochemical analysis). Lastly, we analysed mean percentual changes in the performance of the experimental groups gathered from the selected studies resulting in a certain bias as the results can deviate across the group of participants.

5. Conclusions

In conclusion, reviewed studies from 2015 and 2019 show that ergogenicity of dietary nitrates in time trial performance is more likely to be observed in lesser-trained athletes. Our results suggest that the higher the athlete's training status, the lower the exercise performance improvement. These results are more consistent in chronic dietary nitrates supplementation studies rather than in studies following an acute supplementation protocol. Furthermore, even a minor and statistically insignificant improvement in performance of around 0.31% could make a difference for the elite trained, as the performance differences between the podium athletes are tight. However, research results in elite athletes are inconsistent (e.g., improvement/impairment, statistically significant/insignificant), and research samples are usually small. The smallest worthwhile change and typical error of measurement should be used for critical assessment when evaluating time-trial research results. The performance change should be considered as beneficial only when compared to the sum of the smallest worthwhile change and typical error of measurement for selected training status groups and laboratory tests.

Author Contributions: Conceptualization, T.H. and M.K.; methodology, T.H., M.K. and P.V.; validation, P.V.; formal analysis, T.H. and P.V.; writing—original draft preparation, T.H.; writing—review and editing, T.H., M.K. and P.V.; supervision, M.K.; project administration, T.H.; funding acquisition, T.H. All authors have read and agreed to the published version of the manuscript.

Funding: This article was written at Masaryk University as part of the project "Effect of Dietary Nitrates on Physical Performance" MUNI/A/1201/2018 with the support of the Specific University Research Grant, as provided by the Ministry of Education, Youth and Sports of the Czech Republic.

Acknowledgments: The authors would like to thank our colleague Alexander Floyd for reviewing the grammar and critically reviewing the manuscript.

Conflicts of Interest: The authors declare no conflict of interest.

References

1. Jones, A.M.; Thompson, C.; Wylie, L.J.; Vanhatalo, A. Dietary nitrate and physical performance. *Annu. Rev. Nutr.* **2018**, *38*, 303–328. [CrossRef]
2. Murad, F. Discovery of some of the biological effects of nitric oxide and its role in cell signaling. *Biosci. Rep.* **1999**, *19*, 133–154. [CrossRef] [PubMed]
3. Ignarro, L.J. Nitric oxide: A unique endogenous signaling molecule in vascular biology. *Biosci. Rep.* **1999**, *19*, 51–71. [CrossRef] [PubMed]
4. Furchgott, R.F. Endothelium-derived relaxing factor: Discovery, early studies, and identification as nitric oxide. *Biosci. Rep.* **1999**, *19*, 235–251. [CrossRef] [PubMed]
5. Clifford, T.; Howatson, G.; West, D.J.; Stevenson, E.J. The potential benefits of red beetroot supplementation in health and disease. *Nutrients* **2015**, *7*, 2801–2822. [CrossRef]
6. Burke, L.M. Practical issues in evidence-based use of performance supplements: Supplement interactions, repeated use and individual responses. *Sports Med.* **2017**, *47*, 79–100. [CrossRef]
7. Peeling, P.; Castell, L.M.; Derave, W.; de Hon, O.; Burke, L.M. Sports foods and dietary supplements for optimal function and performance enhancement in track-and-field athletes. *Int. J. Sport Nutr. Exerc. Metab.* **2019**, *29*, 198–209. [CrossRef]
8. Vitale, K.; Getzin, A. Nutrition and supplement update for the endurance athlete: Review and recommendations. *Nutrients* **2019**, *11*, 1289. [CrossRef]
9. Hord, N.G.; Tang, Y.; Bryan, N.S. Food sources of nitrates and nitrites: The physiologic context for potential health benefits. *Am. J. Clin. Nutr.* **2009**, *90*, 1–10. [CrossRef] [PubMed]
10. Jonvik, K.L.; Nyakayiru, J.; van Loon, L.J.C.; Verdijk, L.B. Can elite athletes benefit from dietary nitrate supplementation? *J. Appl. Physiol.* **2015**, *119*, 759–761. [CrossRef]
11. Murad, F. Nitric oxide and cyclic GMP in cell signaling and drug development. *N. Engl. J. Med.* **2006**, *355*, 2003–2011. [CrossRef] [PubMed]
12. Rhodes, P.M.; Leone, A.M.; Francis, P.L.; Struthers, A.D.; Moncada, S. The L-arginine: Nitric oxide pathway is the major source of plasma nitrite in fasted humans. *Biochem. Biophys. Res. Commun.* **1995**, *209*, 590–596. [CrossRef] [PubMed]
13. Lundberg, J.O.; Carlström, M.; Larsen, F.J.; Weitzberg, E. Roles of dietary inorganic nitrate in cardiovascular health and disease. *Cardiovasc. Res.* **2011**, *89*, 525–532. [CrossRef] [PubMed]
14. Kapil, V.; Weitzberg, E.; Lundberg, J.O.; Ahluwalia, A. Clinical evidence demonstrating the utility of inorganic nitrate in cardiovascular health. *Nitric Oxide* **2014**, *38*, 45–57. [CrossRef]
15. Lidder, S.; Webb, A.J. Vascular effects of dietary nitrate (as found in green leafy vegetables and beetroot) via the nitrate-nitrite-nitric oxide pathway. *Br. J. Clin. Pharmacol.* **2013**, *75*, 677–696. [CrossRef]
16. Duncan, C.; Dougall, H.; Johnston, P.; Green, S.; Brogan, R.; Leifert, C.; Smith, L.; Golden, M.; Benjamin, N. Chemical generation of nitric oxide in the mouth from the enterosalivary circulation of dietary nitrate. *Nat. Med.* **1995**, *1*, 546. [CrossRef]

17. Benjamin, N.; O'Driscoll, F.; Dougall, H.; Duncan, C.; Smith, L.; Golden, M.; McKenzie, H. Stomach NO synthesis. *Nature* **1994**, *368*, 502. [CrossRef]
18. James, P.E.; Willis, G.R.; Allen, J.D.; Winyard, P.G.; Jones, A.M. Nitrate pharmacokinetics: Taking note of the difference. *Nitric Oxide* **2015**, *48*, 44–50. [CrossRef]
19. Lundberg, J.O.; Weitzberg, E. NO generation from inorganic nitrate and nitrite: Role in physiology, nutrition and therapeutics. *Arch. Pharm. Res.* **2009**, *32*, 1119–1126. [CrossRef]
20. Domínguez, R.; Maté-Muñoz, J.L.; Cuenca, E.; García-Fernández, P.; Mata-Ordoñez, F.; Lozano-Estevan, M.C.; Veiga-Herreros, P.; da Silva, S.F.; Garnacho-Castaño, M.V. Effects of beetroot juice supplementation on intermittent high-intensity exercise efforts. *J. Int. Soc. Sports Nutr.* **2018**, *15*, 2. [CrossRef]
21. Moncada, S.; Higgs, A. The L-arginine-nitric oxide pathway. *N. Engl. J. Med.* **1993**, *329*, 2002–2012. [CrossRef] [PubMed]
22. Larsen, F.J.; Schiffer, T.A.; Borniquel, S.; Sahlin, K.; Ekblom, B.; Lundberg, J.O.; Weitzberg, E. Dietary inorganic nitrate improves mitochondrial efficiency in humans. *Cell Metab.* **2011**, *13*, 149–159. [CrossRef] [PubMed]
23. Sarti, P.; Forte, E.; Mastronicola, D.; Giuffrè, A.; Arese, M. Cytochrome c oxidase and nitric oxide in action: Molecular mechanisms and pathophysiological implications. *Biochim. Biophys. Acta* **2012**, *1817*, 610–619. [CrossRef] [PubMed]
24. Van Faassen, E.E.; Bahrami, S.; Feelisch, M.; Hogg, N.; Kelm, M.; Kim-Shapiro, D.B.; Kozlov, A.V.; Li, H.; Lundberg, J.O.; Mason, R.; et al. Nitrite as regulator of hypoxic signaling in mammalian physiology. *Med. Res. Rev.* **2009**, *29*, 683–741. [CrossRef]
25. Bailey, S.J.; Fulford, J.; Vanhatalo, A.; Winyard, P.G.; Blackwell, J.R.; DiMenna, F.J.; Wilkerson, D.P.; Benjamin, N.; Jones, A.M. Dietary nitrate supplementation enhances muscle contractile efficiency during knee-extensor exercise in humans. *J. Appl. Physiol.* **2010**, *109*, 135–148. [CrossRef]
26. Coggan, A.R.; Peterson, L.R. Dietary nitrate enhances the contractile properties of human skeletal muscle. *Exerc. Sport Sci. Rev.* **2018**, *46*, 254–261. [CrossRef]
27. Rokkedal-Lausch, T.; Franch, J.; Poulsen, M.K.; Thomsen, L.P.; Weitzberg, E.; Kamavuako, E.N.; Karbing, D.S.; Larsen, R.G. Chronic high-dose beetroot juice supplementation improves time trial performance of well-trained cyclists in normoxia and hypoxia. *Nitric Oxide Biol. Chem.* **2019**, *85*, 44–52. [CrossRef]
28. Wylie, L.J.; Kelly, J.; Bailey, S.J.; Blackwell, J.R.; Skiba, P.F.; Winyard, P.G.; Jeukendrup, A.E.; Vanhatalo, A.; Jones, A.M. Beetroot juice and exercise: Pharmacodynamic and dose-response relationships. *J. Appl. Physiol.* **2013**, *115*, 325–336. [CrossRef]
29. Hoon, M.W.; Jones, A.M.; Johnson, N.A.; Blackwell, J.R.; Broad, E.M.; Lundy, B.; Rice, A.J.; Burke, L.M. The effect of variable doses of inorganic nitrate-rich beetroot juice on simulated 2,000-m rowing performance in trained athletes. *Int. J. Sports Physiol. Perform.* **2014**, *9*, 615–620. [CrossRef]
30. Vanhatalo, A.; Bailey, S.J.; Blackwell, J.R.; DiMenna, F.J.; Pavey, T.G.; Wilkerson, D.P.; Benjamin, N.; Winyard, P.G.; Jones, A.M. Acute and chronic effects of dietary nitrate supplementation on blood pressure and the physiological responses to moderate-intensity and incremental exercise. *Am. J. Physiol. Regul. Integr. Comp. Physiol.* **2010**, *299*, R1121–R1131. [CrossRef]
31. Wylie, L.J.; Ortiz de Zevallos, J.; Isidore, T.; Nyman, L.; Vanhatalo, A.; Bailey, S.J.; Jones, A.M. Dose-dependent effects of dietary nitrate on the oxygen cost of moderate-intensity exercise: Acute vs. chronic supplementation. *Nitric Oxide* **2016**, *57*, 30–39. [CrossRef] [PubMed]
32. Thompson, K.G.; Turner, L.; Prichard, J.; Dodd, F.; Kennedy, D.O.; Haskell, C.; Blackwell, J.R.; Jones, A.M. Influence of dietary nitrate supplementation on physiological and cognitive responses to incremental cycle exercise. *Respir. Physiol. Neurobiol.* **2014**, *193*, 11–20. [CrossRef] [PubMed]
33. Muggeridge, D.J.; Sculthorpe, N.; Grace, F.M.; Willis, G.; Thornhill, L.; Weller, R.B.; James, P.E.; Easton, C. Acute whole body UVA irradiation combined with nitrate ingestion enhances time trial performance in trained cyclists. *Nitric Oxide* **2015**, *48*, 3–9. [CrossRef] [PubMed]
34. Hernández, A.; Schiffer, T.A.; Ivarsson, N.; Cheng, A.J.; Bruton, J.D.; Lundberg, J.O.; Weitzberg, E.; Westerblad, H. Dietary nitrate increases tetanic [Ca2+]i and contractile force in mouse fast-twitch muscle. *J. Physiol.* **2012**, *590*, 3575–3583. [CrossRef] [PubMed]
35. Haider, G.; Folland, J.P. Nitrate supplementation enhances the contractile properties of human skeletal muscle. *Med. Sci. Sports Exerc.* **2014**, *46*, 2234–2243. [CrossRef] [PubMed]

36. Whitfield, J.; Gamu, D.; Heigenhauser, G.J.F.; van Loon, L.J.C.; Spriet, L.L.; Tupling, A.R.; Holloway, G.P. Beetroot juice increases human muscle force without changing Ca2+-handling proteins. *Med. Sci. Sports Exerc.* **2017**, *49*, 2016–2024. [CrossRef]
37. Jones, A.M.; Ferguson, S.K.; Bailey, S.J.; Vanhatalo, A.; Poole, D.C. Fiber Type-Specific Effects of Dietary Nitrate. *Exerc. Sport Sci. Rev.* **2016**, *44*, 53. [CrossRef]
38. Sussman, I.; Erecińska, M.; Wilson, D.F. Regulation of cellular energy metabolism. The Crabtree effect. *Biochim. Biophys. Acta Bioenerg.* **1980**, *591*, 209–223. [CrossRef]
39. Nourry, C.; Fabre, C.; Bart, F.; Grosbois, J.-M.; Berthoin, S.; Mucci, P. Evidence of exercise-induced arterial hypoxemia in prepubescent trained children. *Pediatr. Res.* **2004**, *55*, 674–681. [CrossRef]
40. Lundberg, J.O.; Weitzberg, E. NO-synthase independent NO generation in mammals. *Biochem. Biophys. Res. Commun.* **2010**, *396*, 39–45. [CrossRef]
41. Modin, A.; Björne, H.; Herulf, M.; Alving, K.; Weitzberg, E.; Lundberg, J.O. Nitrite-derived nitric oxide: A possible mediator of "acidic-metabolic" vasodilation. *Acta Physiol. Scand.* **2001**, *171*, 9–16. [CrossRef] [PubMed]
42. Lundberg, J.O.; Weitzberg, E.; Gladwin, M.T. The nitrate-nitrite-nitric oxide pathway in physiology and therapeutics. *Nat. Rev. Drug Discov.* **2008**, *7*, 156–167. [CrossRef] [PubMed]
43. Behnke, B.J.; McDonough, P.; Padilla, D.J.; Musch, T.I.; Poole, D.C. Oxygen exchange profile in rat muscles of contrasting fibre types. *J. Physiol.* **2003**, *549*, 597–605. [CrossRef] [PubMed]
44. McDonough, P.; Behnke, B.J.; Padilla, D.J.; Musch, T.I.; Poole, D.C. Control of microvascular oxygen pressures in rat muscles comprised of different fibre types. *J. Physiol.* **2005**, *563*, 903–913. [CrossRef] [PubMed]
45. Ferreira, L.F.; McDonough, P.; Behnke, B.J.; Musch, T.I.; Poole, D.C. Blood flow and O2 extraction as a function of O2 uptake in muscles composed of different fiber types. *Respir. Physiol. Neurobiol.* **2006**, *153*, 237–249. [CrossRef] [PubMed]
46. Vanin, A.F.; Bevers, L.M.; Slama-Schwok, A.; van Faassen, E.E. Nitric oxide synthase reduces nitrite to NO under anoxia. *Cell. Mol. Life Sci.* **2007**, *64*, 96–103. [CrossRef] [PubMed]
47. Bailey, S.J.; Varnham, R.L.; DiMenna, F.J.; Breese, B.C.; Wylie, L.J.; Jones, A.M. Inorganic nitrate supplementation improves muscle oxygenation, O$_2$ uptake kinetics, and exercise tolerance at high but not low pedal rates. *J. Appl. Physiol.* **2015**, *118*, 1396–1405. [CrossRef] [PubMed]
48. Coggan, A.R.; Leibowitz, J.L.; Kadkhodayan, A.; Thomas, D.P.; Ramamurthy, S.; Spearie, C.A.; Waller, S.; Farmer, M.; Peterson, L.R. Effect of acute dietary nitrate intake on maximal knee extensor speed and power in healthy men and women. *Nitric Oxide* **2015**, *48*, 16–21. [CrossRef]
49. Cermak, N.M.; Res, P.; Stinkens, R.; Lundberg, J.O.; Gibala, M.J.; van Loon, L.J.C. No improvement in endurance performance after a single dose of beetroot juice. *Int. J. Sport Nutr. Exerc. Metab.* **2012**, *22*, 470–478. [CrossRef]
50. Christensen, P.M.; Nyberg, M.; Bangsbo, J. Influence of nitrate supplementation on VO$_2$ kinetics and endurance of elite cyclists. *Scand. J. Med. Sci. Sports* **2013**, *23*, e21–e31. [CrossRef]
51. Mosher, S.L.; Gough, L.A.; Deb, S.; Saunders, B.; Naughton, L.R.M.; Brown, D.R.; Sparks, S.A. High dose Nitrate ingestion does not improve 40 km cycling time trial performance in trained cyclists. *Res. Sports Med.* **2020**, *28*, 138–146. [CrossRef] [PubMed]
52. Boorsma, R.K.; Whitfield, J.; Spriet, L.L. Beetroot juice supplementation does not improve performance of elite 1500-m runners. *Med. Sci. Sports Exerc.* **2014**, *46*, 2326–2334. [CrossRef] [PubMed]
53. Bescós, R.; Ferrer-Roca, V.; Galilea, P.A.; Roig, A.; Drobnic, F.; Sureda, A.; Martorell, M.; Cordova, A.; Tur, J.A.; Pons, A. Sodium nitrate supplementation does not enhance performance of endurance athletes. *Med. Sci. Sports Exerc.* **2012**, *44*, 2400–2409. [CrossRef] [PubMed]
54. Peacock, O.; Tjønna, A.E.; James, P.; Wisløff, U.; Welde, B.; Böhlke, N.; Smith, A.; Stokes, K.; Cook, C.; Sandbakk, Ø. Dietary nitrate does not enhance running performance in elite cross-country skiers. *Med. Sci. Sports Exerc.* **2012**, *44*, 2213–2219. [CrossRef]
55. Coyle, E.F.; Feltner, M.E.; Kautz, S.A.; Hamilton, M.T.; Montain, S.J.; Baylor, A.M.; Abraham, L.D.; Petrek, G.W. Physiological and biomechanical factors associated with elite endurance cycling performance. *Med. Sci. Sports Exerc.* **1991**, *23*, 93–107. [CrossRef]
56. Jeukendrup, A.E.; Craig, N.P.; Hawley, J.A. The bioenergetics of world class cycling. *J. Sci. Med. Sport* **2000**, *3*, 414–433. [CrossRef]

57. Yan, Z.; Okutsu, M.; Akhtar, Y.N.; Lira, V.A. Regulation of exercise-induced fiber type transformation, mitochondrial biogenesis, and angiogenesis in skeletal muscle. *J. Appl. Physiol.* **2010**, *110*, 264–274. [CrossRef]
58. Peeling, P.; Cox, G.R.; Bullock, N.; Burke, L.M. Beetroot juice improves on-water 500 M time-trial performance, and laboratory-based paddling economy in national and international-level kayak athletes. *Int. J. Sport Nutr. Exerc. Metab.* **2015**, *25*, 278–284. [CrossRef]
59. Muggeridge, D.J.; Howe, C.C.F.; Spendiff, O.; Pedlar, C.; James, P.E.; Easton, C. The effects of a single dose of concentrated beetroot juice on performance in trained flatwater kayakers. *Int. J. Sport Nutr. Exerc. Metab.* **2013**, *23*, 498–506. [CrossRef]
60. Johnson, M.A.; Polgar, J.; Weightman, D.; Appleton, D. Data on the distribution of fibre types in thirty-six human muscles. An autopsy study. *J. Neurol. Sci.* **1973**, *18*, 111–129. [CrossRef]
61. Polgar, J.; Johnson, M.A.; Weightman, D.; Appleton, D. Data on fibre size in thirty-six human muscles: An autopsy study. *J. Neurol. Sci.* **1973**, *19*, 307–318. [CrossRef]
62. Jennekens, F.G.I.; Tomlinson, B.E.; Walton, J.N. The sizes of the two main histochemical fibre types in five limb muscles in man: An autopsy study. *J. Neurol. Sci.* **1971**, *13*, 281–292. [CrossRef]
63. Roth, W.; Schwanitz, P.; Pas, P.; Bauer, P. Force-time characteristics of the rowing stroke and corresponding physiological muscle adaptations. *Int. J. Sports Med.* **1993**, *14*, S32–S34. [CrossRef] [PubMed]
64. Shephard, R.J. Science and medicine of canoeing and kayaking. *Sports Med.* **1987**, *4*, 19–33. [CrossRef] [PubMed]
65. Steinacker, J. Physiological aspects of training in rowing. *Int. J. Sports Med.* **1993**, *14* (Suppl. 1), S3.
66. Wylie, L.J.; Park, J.W.; Vanhatalo, A.; Kadach, S.; Black, M.I.; Stoyanov, Z.; Schechter, A.N.; Jones, A.M.; Piknova, B. Human skeletal muscle nitrate store: Influence of dietary nitrate supplementation and exercise. *J. Physiol.* **2019**, *597*, 5565–5576. [CrossRef]
67. Bryan, N.S.; Ivy, J.L. Inorganic nitrite and nitrate: Evidence to support consideration as dietary nutrients. *Nutr. Res.* **2015**, *35*, 643–654. [CrossRef]
68. Porcelli, S.; Ramaglia, M.; Bellistri, G.; Pavei, G.; Pugliese, L.; Montorsi, M.; Rasica, L.; Marzorati, M. Aerobic fitness affects the exercise performance responses to nitrate supplementation. *Med. Sci. Sports Exerc.* **2015**, *47*, 1643–1651. [CrossRef]
69. Tesch, P.A.; Karlsson, J. Muscle fiber types and size in trained and untrained muscles of elite athletes. *J. Appl. Physiol.* **1985**, *59*, 1716–1720. [CrossRef]
70. Proctor, D.N.; Sinning, W.E.; Walro, J.M.; Sieck, G.C.; Lemon, P.W. Oxidative capacity of human muscle fiber types: Effects of age and training status. *J. Appl. Physiol.* **1995**, *78*, 2033–2038. [CrossRef]
71. McQuillan, J.A.; Dulson, D.K.; Laursen, P.B.; Kilding, A.E. Dietary nitrate fails to improve 1 and 4 km cycling performance in highly trained cyclists. *Int. J. Sport Nutr. Exerc. Metab.* **2017**, *27*, 255–263. [CrossRef] [PubMed]
72. Liberati, A.; Altman, D.G.; Tetzlaff, J.; Mulrow, C.; Gøtzsche, P.C.; Ioannidis, J.P.A.; Clarke, M.; Devereaux, P.J.; Kleijnen, J.; Moher, D. The PRISMA statement for reporting systematic reviews and meta-analyses of studies that evaluate health care interventions: Explanation and elaboration. *PLoS Med.* **2009**, *6*, e1000100. [CrossRef] [PubMed]
73. De Pauw, K.; Roelands, B.; Cheung, S.S.; De Geus, B.; Rietjens, G.; Meeusen, R. Guidelines to classify subject groups in sport-science research. *Int. J. Sports Physiol. Perform.* **2013**, *8*, 111–122. [CrossRef] [PubMed]
74. Decroix, L.; Pauw, K.D.; Foster, C.; Meeusen, R. Guidelines to classify female subject groups in sport-science research. *Int. J. Sports Physiol. Perform.* **2016**, *11*, 204–213. [CrossRef] [PubMed]
75. Jo, E.; Fischer, M.; Auslander, A.T.; Beigarten, A.; Daggy, B.; Hansen, K.; Kessler, L.; Osmond, A.; Wang, H.; Wes, R. The effects of multi-day vs. single pre-exercise nitrate supplement dosing on simulated cycling time trial performance and skeletal muscle oxygenation. *J. Strength Cond. Res.* **2019**, *33*, 217–224. [CrossRef] [PubMed]
76. Maher, C.G.; Sherrington, C.; Herbert, R.D.; Moseley, A.M.; Elkins, M. Reliability of the PEDro scale for rating quality of randomized controlled trials. *Phys. Ther.* **2003**, *83*, 713–721. [CrossRef] [PubMed]
77. Verhagen, A.P.; de Vet, H.C.; de Bie, R.A.; Kessels, A.G.; Boers, M.; Bouter, L.M.; Knipschild, P.G. The Delphi list: A criteria list for quality assessment of randomized clinical trials for conducting systematic reviews developed by Delphi consensus. *J. Clin. Epidemiol.* **1998**, *51*, 1235–1241. [CrossRef]

78. Glaister, M.; Pattison, J.R.; Muniz-Pumares, D.; Patterson, S.D.; Foley, P. Effects of dietary nitrate, caffeine, and their combination on 20-km cycling time trial performance. *J. Strength Cond. Res.* **2015**, *29*, 165–174. [CrossRef]
79. Callahan, M.J.; Parr, E.B.; Hawley, J.A.; Burke, L.M. Single and combined effects of beetroot crystals and sodium bicarbonate on 4-km cycling time trial performance. *Int. J. Sport Nutr. Exerc. Metab.* **2017**, *27*, 271–278. [CrossRef]
80. Sandbakk, S.B.; Sandbakk, Ø.; Peacock, O.; James, P.; Welde, B.; Stokes, K.; Böhlke, N.; Tjønna, A.E. Effects of acute supplementation of L-arginine and nitrate on endurance and sprint performance in elite athletes. *Nitric Oxide Biol. Chem.* **2015**, *48*, 10–15. [CrossRef]
81. Nyakayiru, J.M.; Jonvik, K.L.; Pinckaers, P.J.M.; Senden, J.; van Loon, L.J.C.; Verdijk, L.B. No effect of acute and 6-day nitrate supplementation on VO2 and time-trial performance in highly trained cyclists. *Int. J. Sport Nutr. Exerc. Metab.* **2017**, *27*, 11–17. [CrossRef] [PubMed]
82. Oskarsson, J.; McGawley, K. No individual or combined effects of caffeine and beetrootjuice supplementation during submaximal or maximal running. *Appl. Physiol. Nutr. Metab.* **2018**, *43*, 697–703. [CrossRef] [PubMed]
83. McQuillan, J.A.; Dulson, D.K.; Laursen, P.B.; Kilding, A.E. The effect of dietary nitrate supplementation on physiology and performance in trained cyclists. *Int. J. Sports Physiol. Perform.* **2017**, *12*, 684–689. [CrossRef] [PubMed]
84. Shannon, O.M.; Barlow, M.J.; Duckworth, L.; Williams, E.; Wort, G.; Woods, D.; Siervo, M.; O'Hara, J.P. Dietary nitrate supplementation enhances short but not longer duration running time-trial performance. *Eur. J. Appl. Physiol.* **2017**, *117*, 775–785. [CrossRef]
85. de Castro, T.F.; Manoel, F.A.; Figueiredo, D.H.; Figueiredo, D.H.; Machado, F.A. Effect of beetroot juice supplementation on 10-km performance in recreational runners. *Appl. Physiol. Nutr. Metab.* **2019**, *44*, 90–94. [CrossRef]
86. McMahon, N.F.; Leveritt, M.D.; Pavey, T.G. The effect of dietary nitrate supplementation on endurance exercise performance in healthy adults: A systematic review and meta-analysis. *Sports Med.* **2017**, *47*, 735–756. [CrossRef]
87. Hoon, M.W.; Johnson, N.A.; Chapman, P.G.; Burke, L.M. The effect of nitrate supplementation on exercise performance in healthy individuals: A systematic review and meta-analysis. *Int. J. Sport Nutr. Exerc. Metab.* **2013**, *23*, 522–532. [CrossRef]
88. Nyakayiru, J.; van Loon, L.C.; Verdijk, L. Could intramuscular storage of dietary nitrate contribute to its ergogenic effect? A mini-review. *Free Radic. Biol. Med.* **2020**. [CrossRef]
89. Murray, A.J.; Horscroft, J.A. Mitochondrial function at extreme high altitude. *J. Physiol.* **2016**, *594*, 1137–1149. [CrossRef]
90. Murray, A.J. Metabolic adaptation of skeletal muscle to high altitude hypoxia: How new technologies could resolve the controversies. *Genome Med.* **2009**, *1*, 117. [CrossRef]
91. Kelly, J.; Vanhatalo, A.; Bailey, S.J.; Wylie, L.J.; Tucker, C.; List, S.; Winyard, P.G.; Jones, A.M. Dietary nitrate supplementation: Effects on plasma nitrite and pulmonary O2 uptake dynamics during exercise in hypoxia and normoxia. *Am. J. Physiol. Regul. Integr. Comp. Physiol.* **2014**, *307*, R920–R930. [CrossRef] [PubMed]
92. Masschelein, E.; van Thienen, R.; Wang, X.; van Schepdael, A.; Thomis, M.; Hespel, P. Dietary nitrate improves muscle but not cerebral oxygenation status during exercise in hypoxia. *J. Appl. Physiol.* **2012**, *113*, 736–745. [CrossRef] [PubMed]
93. Shannon, O.M.; Duckworth, L.; Barlow, M.J.; Deighton, K.; Matu, J.; Williams, E.L.; Woods, D.; Xie, L.; Stephan, B.C.M.; Siervo, M.; et al. Effects of dietary nitrate supplementation on physiological responses, cognitive function, and exercise performance at moderate and very-high simulated altitude. *Front. Physiol.* **2017**, *8*. [CrossRef] [PubMed]
94. Shannon, O.M.; Duckworth, L.; Barlow, M.J.; Woods, D.; Lara, J.; Siervo, M.; O'Hara, J.P. Dietary nitrate supplementation enhances high-intensity running performance in moderate normobaric hypoxia, independent of aerobic fitness. *Nitric Oxide Biol. Chem.* **2016**, *59*, 63–70. [CrossRef] [PubMed]
95. Arnold, J.T.; Oliver, S.J.; Lewis-Jones, T.M.; Wylie, L.J.; Macdonald, J.H. Beetroot juice does not enhance altitude running performance in well-trained athletes. *Appl. Physiol. Nutr. Metab.* **2015**, *40*, 590–595. [CrossRef]
96. Puype, J.; Ramaekers, M.; van Thienen, R.; Deldicque, L.; Hespel, P. No effect of dietary nitrate supplementation on endurance training in hypoxia. *Scand. J. Med. Sci. Sports* **2015**, *25*, 234–241. [CrossRef]

97. Cumpstey, A.F.; Hennis, P.J.; Gilbert-Kawai, E.T.; Fernandez, B.O.; Grant, D.; Jenner, W.; Poudevigne, M.; Moyses, H.; Levett, D.Z.; Cobb, A.; et al. Effects of dietary nitrate supplementation on microvascular physiology at 4559 m altitude—A randomised controlled trial (Xtreme Alps). *Nitric Oxide* **2020**, *94*, 27–35. [CrossRef]
98. Cumpstey, A.F.; Hennis, P.J.; Gilbert-Kawai, E.T.; Fernandez, B.O.; Poudevigne, M.; Cobb, A.; Meale, P.; Mitchell, K.; Moyses, H.; Pöhnl, H.; et al. Effects of dietary nitrate on respiratory physiology at high altitude—Results from the Xtreme Alps study. *Nitric Oxide* **2017**, *71*, 57–68. [CrossRef]
99. Bakker, E.; Engan, H.; Patrician, A.; Schagatay, E.; Karlsen, T.; Wisløff, U.; Gaustad, S.E. Acute dietary nitrate supplementation improves arterial endothelial function at high altitude: A double-blinded randomized controlled cross over study. *Nitric Oxide* **2015**, *50*, 58–64. [CrossRef]
100. Hultström, M. Commentaries on Viewpoint: Can elite athletes benefit from dietary nitrate supplementation? *J. Appl. Physiol.* **2015**, *119*, 762–769. [CrossRef]
101. Giro d'Italia 2019 | Stage 21 (ITT) | Results. Available online: https://www.procyclingstats.com/race/giro-d-italia/2019/stage-21 (accessed on 10 May 2020).
102. Tour de France 2018 | Stage 20 (ITT) | Results. Available online: https://www.procyclingstats.com/race/tour-de-france/2018/stage-20 (accessed on 10 May 2020).
103. Hopkins, W.G. Measures of reliability in sports medicine and science. *Sports Med.* **2000**, *30*, 1–15. [CrossRef] [PubMed]
104. Atkinson, G.; Nevill, A.M. Statistical methods for assessing measurement error (reliability) in variables relevant to sports medicine. *Sports Med.* **1998**, *26*, 217–238. [CrossRef] [PubMed]
105. Paton, C.D.; Hopkins, W.G. Tests of cycling performance. *Sports Med.* **2001**, *31*, 489–496. [CrossRef] [PubMed]
106. Close, G.L.; Kasper, A.M.; Morton, J.P. From paper to podium: Quantifying the translational potential of performance nutrition research. *Sports Med.* **2019**, *49*, 25–37. [CrossRef] [PubMed]
107. Piknova, B.; Park, J.W.; Swanson, K.M.; Dey, S.; Noguchi, C.T.; Schechter, A.N. Skeletal muscle as an endogenous nitrate reservoir. *Nitric Oxide* **2015**, *47*, 10–16. [CrossRef]
108. Piknova, B.; Park, J.W.; Lam, K.K.; Schechter, A.N. Nitrate as a source of nitrite and nitric oxide during exercise hyperemia in rat skeletal muscle. *Nitric Oxide* **2016**, *55*, 54–61. [CrossRef]
109. Gilliard, C.N.; Lam, J.K.; Cassel, K.S.; Park, J.W.; Schechter, A.N.; Piknova, B. Effect of dietary nitrate levels on nitrate fluxes in rat skeletal muscle and liver. *Nitric Oxide* **2018**, *75*, 1–7. [CrossRef]
110. Srihirun, S.; Park, J.W.; Teng, R.; Sawaengdee, W.; Piknova, B.; Schechter, A.N. Nitrate uptake and metabolism in human skeletal muscle cell cultures. *Nitric Oxide* **2020**, *94*, 1–8. [CrossRef]
111. Kapur, S.; Bédard, S.; Marcotte, B.; Côté, C.H.; Marette, A. Expression of nitric oxide synthase in skeletal muscle: A novel role for nitric oxide as a modulator of insulin action. *Diabetes* **1997**, *46*, 1691–1700. [CrossRef]
112. Nyakayiru, J.; Kouw, I.W.K.; Cermak, N.M.; Senden, J.M.; van Loon, L.J.C.; Verdijk, L.B. Sodium nitrate ingestion increases skeletal muscle nitrate content in humans. *J. Appl. Physiol.* **2017**, *123*, 637–644. [CrossRef]
113. McDonagh, S.T.J.; Wylie, L.J.; Webster, J.M.A.; Vanhatalo, A.; Jones, A.M. Influence of dietary nitrate food forms on nitrate metabolism and blood pressure in healthy normotensive adults. *Nitric Oxide* **2018**, *72*, 66–74. [CrossRef] [PubMed]

© 2020 by the authors. Licensee MDPI, Basel, Switzerland. This article is an open access article distributed under the terms and conditions of the Creative Commons Attribution (CC BY) license (http://creativecommons.org/licenses/by/4.0/).

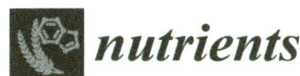

Article

The Influence of Cyclical Ketogenic Reduction Diet vs. Nutritionally Balanced Reduction Diet on Body Composition, Strength, and Endurance Performance in Healthy Young Males: A Randomized Controlled Trial

Pavel Kysel [1], Denisa Haluzíková [1], Radka Petráková Doležalová [1], Ivana Laňková [2,3], Zdeňka Lacinová [2,4], Barbora Judita Kasperová [3], Jaroslava Trnovská [2], Viktorie Hrádková [3], Miloš Mráz [3], Zdeněk Vilikus [1,*] and Martin Haluzík [3,4,*]

- [1] Department of Sports Medicine, First Faculty of Medicine and General University Hospital, 12000 Prague, Czech Republic; kysel@palestra.cz (P.K.); dhalu@lf1.cuni.cz (D.H.); radka.petrakovadolezalova@vfn.cz (R.P.D.)
- [2] Centre for Experimental Medicine, Institute for Clinical and Experimental Medicine, 12000 Prague, Czech Republic; laki@ikem.cz (I.L.); lacz@ikem.cz (Z.L.); troj@ikem.cz (J.T.)
- [3] Diabetes Centre, Institute for Clinical and Experimental Medicine, 12000 Prague, Czech Republic; kapb@ikem.cz (B.J.K.); hrav@ikem.cz (V.H.); mrzm@ikem.cz (M.M.)
- [4] Institute of Medical Biochemistry and Laboratory Diagnostics, First Faculty of Medicine, Charles University and General University Hospital, 12000 Prague, Czech Republic
- * Correspondence: zvili@lf1.cuni.cz (Z.V.); halm@ikem.cz (M.H.)

Received: 31 August 2020; Accepted: 15 September 2020; Published: 16 September 2020

Abstract: (1) Background: The influence of ketogenic diet on physical fitness remains controversial. We performed a randomized controlled trial to compare the effect of cyclical ketogenic reduction diet (CKD) vs. nutritionally balanced reduction diet (RD) on body composition, muscle strength, and endurance performance. (2) Methods: 25 healthy young males undergoing regular resistance training combined with aerobic training were randomized to CKD ($n = 13$) or RD ($n = 12$). Body composition, muscle strength and spiroergometric parameters were measured at baseline and after eight weeks of intervention. (3) Results: Both CKD and RD decreased body weight, body fat, and BMI. Lean body mass and body water decreased in CKD and did not significantly change in RD group. Muscle strength parameters were not affected in CKD while in RD group lat pull-down and leg press values increased. Similarly, endurance performance was not changed in CKD group while in RD group peak workload and peak oxygen uptake increased. (4) Conclusions: Our data show that in healthy young males undergoing resistance and aerobic training comparable weight reduction were achieved by CKD and RD. In RD group; improved muscle strength and endurance performance was noted relative to neutral effect of CKD that also slightly reduced lean body mass.

Keywords: body composition; ketogenic diet; strength parameters; endurance; training

1. Introduction

The last decade has been characterized by the search for alternative dietary ways to achieve optimal body composition while maintaining or improving physical fitness and sports performance to promote healthy lifestyle and prevent chronic diseases [1,2]. Current trends in sports nutrition are increasingly reaching for the minimization of the carbohydrate component with ketogenic diet becoming a very popular approach, in particular in endurance athletes [3,4].

According to current definitions, carbohydrate intake within the range of 50–150 g per day can be described as non-ketogenic low-carbohydrate regimens [5]. Ketogenic diet is most commonly defined by a daily carbohydrate intake below 50 g per day or energy provision from carbohydrates for up to 10% of total energy intake [6]. Out of the frequently used approaches, targeted ketogenic diet allows carbohydrates to be consumed immediately around exercise to sustain performance without affecting ketosis [7]. The cyclical ketogenic diet (CKD) alternates periods of ketogenic dieting with periods of high-carbohydrate consumption [8]. The period of high-carbohydrate eating is supposed to refill muscle glycogen to sustain exercise performance [9].

The influence of ketogenic diets on sports performance is still the topic of an ongoing debate [10,11] with often conflicting results [12]. The overreaching mainstream nutrition philosophy for endurance athletes emphasizes a carbohydrate-dominant, low fat paradigm. Under these dietary conditions, carbohydrates are utilized as predominant fuel source to cover high volumes of aerobic exercise [13]. The appeal of low carbohydrate high fat diet for endurance athletes is likely due to the shift in fuel utilization, from a carbohydrate-centric model with limited glycogen sources to predominant fat utilization with much bigger and longer-lasting fat stores [14]. This metabolic shift, seen after a period of dietary alteration, is often referred to as being "fat-adapted", which has been well-documented in studies since the 1980s [15]. Substantial reduction in carbohydrate intake promotes utilization of ketones and, according to some studies, it may enhance physical performance due to minimizing the reliance of body metabolism on carbohydrates [16,17] and reduce lactate deposition leading to enhanced recovery [18]. Importantly, ketogenic diets are, in particular in the short-term run, a very efficacious way to reduce body weight not only in physically active subjects but also in patients with obesity, type 2 diabetes and other chronic lifestyle diseases [19–21]. Nevertheless, it has to be noted that long-term compliance and efficacy of ketogenic diet is not optimal and most of the studies had rather limited duration [19,22].

Here we performed a randomized controlled trial to compare the effect of the cyclical ketogenic reduction diet (CKD) vs. nutritionally balanced reduction diet (RD) on body composition, muscle strength, and endurance performance in healthy young males undergoing regular resistance training three times/week combined with aerobic training three times/week. We hypothesized that CKD will be more efficacious in inducing fat loss as compared to RD while maintaining aerobic performance. To this end, we explored the effect of eight weeks of CKD vs. RD combined with regular exercise on body composition, and measures of strength and aerobic performance.

2. Materials and Methods

Twenty-five males of various fitness levels with minimum of one-year experience in resistance training recruited from colleges of physical education and through a website with readers interested in fitness and diets. Inclusion criteria were as follows: age between 18 and 30 years and a minimum one-year experience with resistance and aerobic training. Subject recruitment began in April 2019 and lasted until January 2020. Persons interested in participating were screened to ascertain they meet the minimum criteria for the enrollment into the study.

Exclusion criteria were current injuries or health conditions that might have affected sports performance or put them at risk for further injuries including the presence of cardiovascular diseases, diabetes mellitus, arterial hypertension, or any other diseases that required pharmacological treatment. Additionally, subjects taking any performance enhancing supplements (i.e., creatine, β-hydroxy β-methyl butyrate, caffeine, protein powder, weight gainer, thermogenics, etc.), were required to discontinue consumption at least one week prior to baseline testing and continue abstaining from their use for the remainder of the study. The study was approved (ethic approval code 764/18 S-IV)by the Human Ethics Review Board, First Faculty of Medicine and General University Hospital, Prague, Czech Republic and was performed in agreement with the principles of the Declaration of Helsinki as revised in 2008. Prior to randomization, all subjects were required to sign an informed consent.

Using electronic randomization system, subjects were randomly assigned to follow either a CKD or RD (both with total caloric intake reduction by 500 kcal/day) while participating in three strength workouts and three aerobic workouts per week (30 min run, heart rate around 130–140 beats/min.) for 8 weeks. Total caloric intake reduction by 500 kcal/day is counted from balanced hypocaloric diet with a reduction of energy intake by 500 to 1000 kcal from the usual caloric intake. The U.S. Food and Drug Administration (FDA) recommends such diets as the "standard treatment" for clinical trials (FDA, 1996)

Subject randomization and follow-up during the study is depicted in CONSORT diagram in Figure 1.

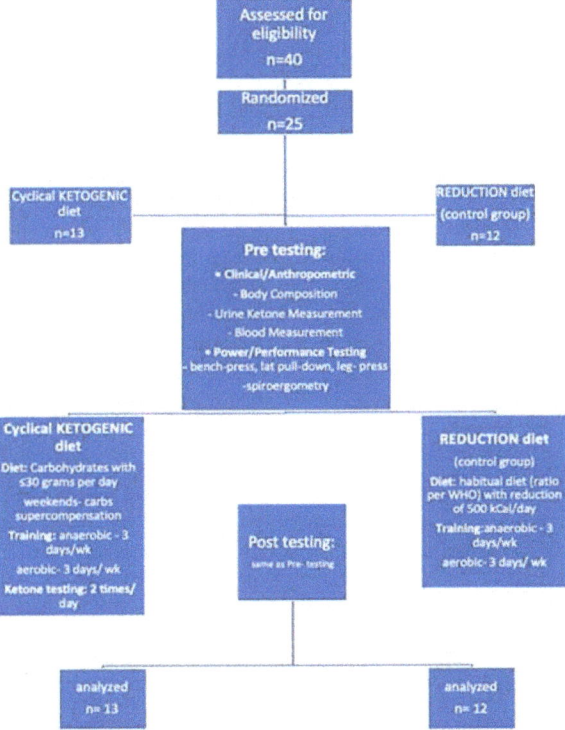

Figure 1. CONSORT diagram of subjects participating in an 8-week program while consuming a cyclical ketogenic reduction diet (CKD) or nutritionally balanced reduction diet (RD).

2.1. Baseline and Postinterventional Testing

Data collection during baseline and post-intervention testing included medical history, anthropometric examination, power performance test, bicycle spiroergometry, and blood drawings to obtain laboratory data. BMI was calculated by the scale, using the height measurement. Accurate height was measured using a basic stadiometer (Seca 222, Seca Co., London, UK).

2.1.1. Biochemical and Anthropometric Examination

At baseline, all subjects were weighted, and their BMI was calculated. Body composition was measured using InBody Body Composition Analyzers (InBody230, InBody Co., Ltd., Seoul, Korea). Body weight and other body composition measurements (lean body mass, body fat mass, BMI, water content, and percentage of body fat) were taken with minimal clothes, no shoes, and measured to the nearest 0.5 kg.

Blood samples for biochemical measurements were taken prior to initiation of study and at the end of the study after 8 weeks of diet. Serum was obtained by centrifugation and samples were subsequently stored in aliquots at −80 °C until further analysis. The maximal storage time was 8 months.

Biochemical parameters liver test, urea, creatinine, and circulating lipids were measured to exclude liver, kidney, or lipid disorder. Creatine kinase and lactate dehydrogenase were measured to explore a possible influence of the diets on muscle regeneration. β-hydroxy-butyrate was measured to confirm a compliance to ketogenic diet.

β-hydroxy-butyrate was measured using TECOM Analytical Systems (TECOM Analytical Systems CS spol. s r.o., Prague, Czech Republic). Other biochemical parameters were measured by spectrophotometric methods using ARCHITECT c Systems device (Abbott Park, IL, USA.) in the Department of Biochemistry of the Institute for Clinical and Experimental Medicine in Prague.

2.1.2. Strength and Aerobic Performance Testing

Power and performance testing were conducted over a 5-day period. Subjects signed for an hour block to participate in each test. Each block had a maximum of 5 subjects in a gym and the spiroergometry was reserved for each of them for an hour. Subjects were instructed to arrive at the gym 30 min prior to testing times and not to train for at least 24 h before testing. A strength performance testing for power output in the three exercises—bench-press, lat pull-down, and leg-press was performed as follows: The subjects underwent an adequate warm up. After resting for two to four minutes the subjects than performed a one-repetition maximum attempt of each exercise with proper technique. If the lift/press was successful, after resting for another two to four minutes the load was increased by 5–10% and another lift/press was attempted. If the subject failed to perform the lift/press, after resting for two to four minutes they attempted the lift/press with weight reduced by 2.5–5%.

2.1.3. Methodology of Strength Testing

Upon arrival, the primary researcher explained the testing procedures and protocols and demonstrated each test. Subjects were instructed to warm up. Power and aerobic performance test administrators and personal researchers were blinded to the randomized group allocations. Each proband participated in bench press, lat pull-down, and leg-press to assess the maximum power performance.

2.1.4. Aerobic Performance Testing

Aerobic performance testing was carried out by bicycle spiroergometry using analyzer of respiratory gases (Quark CPET, 1850 Bates Ave, Concord, CA 94520, Cosmed, USA). This metabolic cart measures expired airflow by means of a pneumotach connected to the mouthpiece. A sample line is connected to the pneumotach from which air is continuously pumped to O_2 and CO_2 gas analyzers. Prior to testing, the pneumotach was calibrated with six samples from a 3 L calibration syringe. The gas analyzers were also calibrated before each test to room air and calibration gases (15.21% O_2 and 5.52% CO_2, respectively). Heart rate (HR) was continuously recorded during exercise by electrocardiography (Fukuda Denshi FX-8322 Cardimax ECG, 17725 N. E. 65th Street Bldg. C, Redmond, WA. 98052 USA).

Prior to exercise, the subjects were instructed to maintain a pedal cadence between 70 and 90 rpm during exercise and to exercise to volitional fatigue. We used a modified exercise step protocol 0.33 W.min^{-1} as described by Gordon et al. [23]. The test was terminated when the subject was unable to maintain a pedaling cadence of 40 rpm.

Maximal oxygen consumption was assessed by the attainment of the following criteria: (1) a plateau ($\Delta VO_2 \leq 50$ mL/min at VO_2 peak and the closest neighboring data point) in VO_2 with increases in external work, (2) maximal respiratory exchange ratio (RER) ≥ 1.10, and (3) maximal HR within 10 b/min of the age-predicted maximum (220-age). All subjects met the first two criteria.

Breath-by-breath gas exchange data from all tests were transferred to a spreadsheet program (MS Excel 365) for further analysis. In addition, data from the VO$_2$max tests were time-averaged using 10 s intervals to examine the incidence of an oxygen plateau.

2.2. Diet Protocol

Subjects were randomly assigned by electronic randomization system to either CKD or RD group for 8 weeks. Subjects had a mandatory dietary session with a nutritionist prior to the beginning of the study which provided detailed instructions on accurately keeping dietary food intake records. All food record data were entered and analyzed using the DietSystem application (DietSystem App, DietSystem App, s.r.o., Czech Republic).

2.2.1. Cyclical Ketogenic Reduction Diet

Total intake of energy was assigned to each participant based on lifestyle (individually calculated according to somatotype, physical activity, type of work, etc.) and was reduced by 500 kcal per day. Five days of low-carbohydrate phase, nutrient ratio (carbohydrates up to 30 g; proteins 1.6 g/kg; fats: calculation of energy intake instead of carbohydrates) in order to induce and maintain ketosis. Following with 2 days of carbohydrate phase (weekends): nutrient ratio (carbohydrates 8–10 g/1 kg of non-fat tissue, 70% intake; proteins 15%; and fat 15%).

2.2.2. Reduction Diet

Principles of healthy nutrition, nutrient ratio (carbohydrates 55%, fat 30%, proteins 15% of total energy intake). The overall caloric intake (individually calculated according to somatotype, physical activity, type of work, etc.) was reduced by 500 kcal per day.

Both groups were given detailed instructions on acceptable foods for both types of diets. In addition, subjects were given an 8-week low-carbohydrate meal plan or reduction diet meal plan as per randomization.

2.3. Training Protocol

2.3.1. Development of Strength Skills

The plan was designed to develop maximum strength in the tested exercise and the muscles involved. 3 differently focused trainings per week were performed:

- Focused on chest—bench press.
- Focused on the muscles of the lower limbs—leg press.
- Focused on the back muscles—lat pull-down.

One training unit lasted approximately 60 min. For each training unit, the full focus was on the technique of execution and time under tension. Each training unit was performed with the maximum possible effort to achieve the maximum results. The prescribed intensity in the form of load was individualized and based on the entry measurements. The technical design, time under tension and maximum effort must were similar for all subjects (maximum effort = maximum possible intensity in compliance with technical parameters and number of repetitions) under tension and maximum effort were similar for all subjects (maximum effort = maximum possible intensity in compliance with technical parameters and number of repetitions)

2.3.2. Development of Endurance Skills

The plan consisted of a 30-min run at constant heart rate (at approximately 70% max TF or around 130–140 heart beats/minute).

2.3.3. Supervision of Adherence to Training and Diet Protocols

Overall adherence to diet was checked once weekly by a nutritionist. Furthermore, adherence to CKD was evaluated through urinary ketone measurements performed twice daily and by measurement of blood β-hydroxybutyrate at the end of the study.

Training compliance was monitored through mandatory check-in procedures in a gym, and also by a sport tester for aerobic performance (TomTom Runner Cardio, TomTom, The Netherlands).

2.4. Post-Intervention Testing

Data collection procedures were the same as baseline testing procedures. To ensure reliability, power measures and performance testing were completed by the same researcher as at baseline for each subject. In addition, subjects conducted their testing at the same time and with the same personal researcher as pre-testing. Results from all tests were compared to the individual's baseline values and provided to the subjects after data analysis.

2.5. Statistical Analysis

Statistical analysis was performed using Sigma Stat software (SPSS Inc., Chicago, IL, USA). Graphs were drawn using SigmaPlot 13.0 software (SPSS Inc., Chicago, IL, USA). The results are expressed as mean ± standard deviation (SD). Differences of body composition (body fat %, weight, BMI, lean body mass, and fat mass), biochemical, and strength or aerobic performance parameters between CKD and RD were evaluated using one-way ANOVA followed by Holm-Sidak test. Paired t-test was used for the assessment of intra group differences as appropriate. Statistical significance was assigned to $p < 0.05$.

3. Results

3.1. The Influence of Cyclical Ketogenic Reduction Diet vs. Nutritionally Balanced Reduction Diet on Anthropometric and Biochemical Parameters

Both CKD and RD decreased body weight (Figure 2), body fat mass and body mass index with comparable effects of both approaches (Table 1). Lean body mass and body water content was significantly reduced by CKD (Figures 3 and 4 and Table 1) while it was not influenced by RD.

Table 1. Anthropometric and biochemical parameters of subjects on cyclical ketogenic reduction diet or nutritionally balanced reduction diet at baseline and after 8 weeks of diet.

	Cyclical Ketogenic Diet (CKD)		Reduction Diet (RD)		ANOVA
	V1-before	V2-after	V1-before	V2-after	
Number (*n*)	13	13	12	12	
Age (year)	23 ± 5	NA	24 ± 4	NA	NS
Height (cm)	181 ± 6	NA	186 ± 10	NA	NS
BMI (kg/m^2)	26.1 ± 3.7	24.6 ± 3.3 *	26.9 ± 4.3	25.5 ± 4.2 *	NS
WEIGHT (kg)	85.6 ± 13.4	81.0 ± 12.0 *	93.0 ± 17.5	88.5 ± 17.4 *	NS
MUSCLES (kg)	41.8 ± 4.5	40.0 ± 4.6 *	43.5 ± 5.3	43.1 ± 5.3	NS
FAT (kg)	12.9 ± 6.9	11.0 ± 5.8 *	17.6 ± 9.8	13.6 ± 9.0 *	NS
% FAT	14.5 ± 5.5	13.0 ± 5.1 *	17.9 ± 6.9	14.2 ± 6.9 *	NS
WATER (kg)	53.2 ± 5.6	51.0 ± 5.6 *	55.1 ± 6.4	54.8 ± 6.5	NS
CK (ukat/L)	4.40 ± 2.81	2.81 ± 1.21	3.80 ± 2.03	3.03 ± 2.03	NS
LDH (ukat/L)	2.68 ± 0.60	2.47 ± 0.42	2.74 ± 0.44	2.55 ± 0.33	NS
β-OH-butyrate (mmol/L)	0.2 ± 0.07	0.38 ± 0.25 *	0.24 ± 0.12	0.12 ± 0.04	NS

Data are mean ± SD. Statistical significance is from One-way ANOVA and paired *t*-test (V1—baseline testing vs. V2—testing after 8 weeks of diet). * $p < 0.05$ vs. V1. BMI: Body mass index; CK: Creatine kinase; LDH: Lactate dehydrogenase; β-OH-butyrate—β-hydroxy-butyrate. NS: Not significant. NA : not avalible.

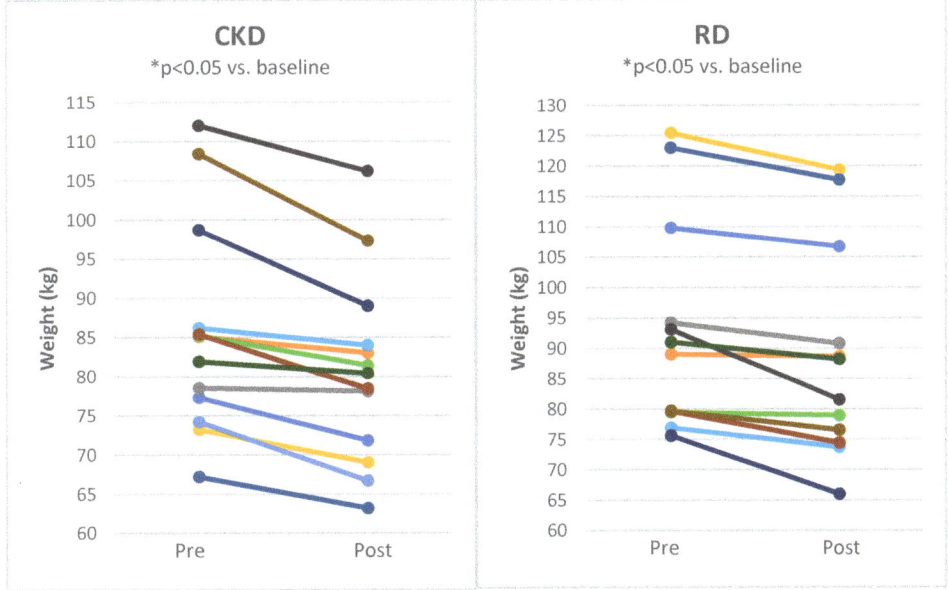

Figure 2. Individual responses of body weight for subjects before and after 8 weeks of cyclical ketogenic reduction diet (CKD) and nutritionally balanced reduction diet (RD). Statistical significance is from paired t-test * $p < 0.05$ vs. baseline.

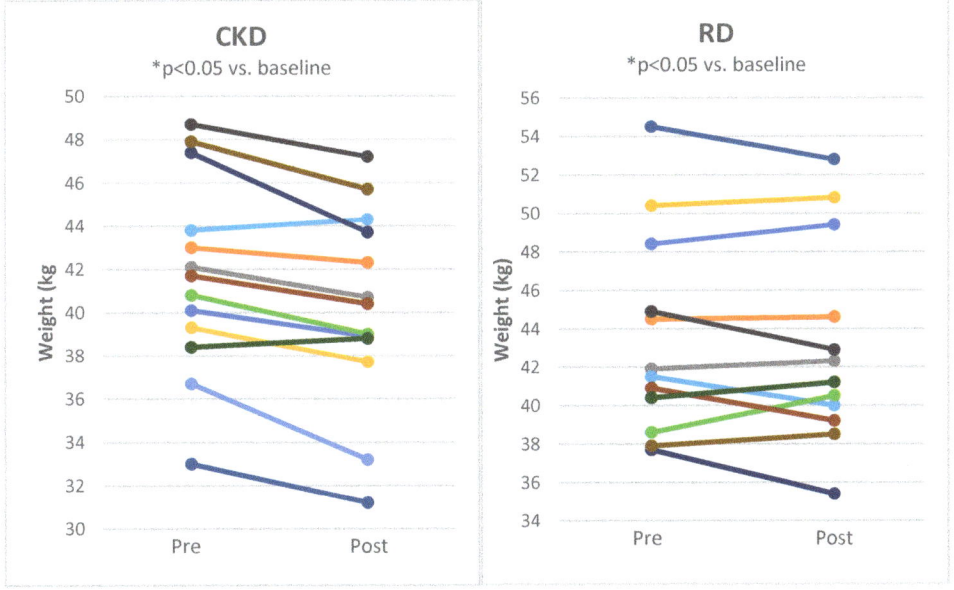

Figure 3. Individual responses of lean body mass for subjects before and after 8 weeks of cyclical ketogenic reduction diet (CKD) and nutritionally balanced reduction diet (RD). Statistical significance is from paired t-test * $p < 0.05$ vs. baseline.

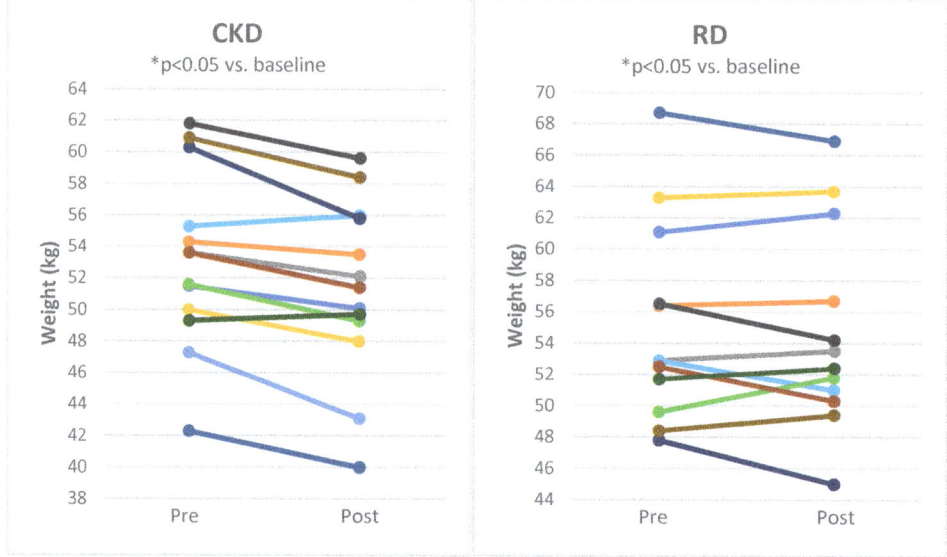

Figure 4. Individual responses of body water weight for subjects before and after 8 weeks of cyclical ketogenic reduction diet (CKD) and nutritionally balanced reduction diet (RD). Statistical significance is from paired t-test * $p < 0.05$ vs. baseline.

None of the diets significantly affected serum concentration of creatine kinase or lactate dehydrogenase (Table 1), liver tests, urea, creatinine, or circulating lipids (data not shown). β-hydroxy-butyrate significantly increased in CKD group while it was unaffected in subjects on reduction diet (Table 1).

3.2. The Influence of Cyclical Ketogenic Reduction Diet vs. Nutritionally Balanced Reduction Diet on Muscle Strength Parameters

The muscle strength parameters were assessed as maximum weight lifted during bench press, lat pull-down, and leg press. CKD did not affect any of these parameters (Table 2). On the contrary, in subjects on RD lat pull-down and leg press values significantly increased (Table 2).

Table 2. The effect of cyclical ketogenic reduction diet and nutritionally balanced reduction diet on strength parameters.

	Cyclical Ketogenic Diet (CKD)		Reduction Diet (RD)		ANOVA
	V1-before	V2-after	V1-before	V2-after	
Bench press (BP)	90.0 ± 24.2	90.0 ± 23.7	84.2 ± 21.8	87.7 ± 20.1	NS
Lat pull-down (LPD)	74.2 ± 15.7	76.0 ± 15.0	70.4 ± 14.8	75.2 ± 17.1 *	NS
Leg press (LP)	138.0 ± 21.1	142.0 ± 16.3	127.8 ± 22.0	140 ± 22.8 *	NS

Data are mean ± SD. Statistical significance is from One-way ANOVA and paired *t*-test (V1—baseline testing vs. V2—testing after 8 weeks of diet). * $p < 0.05$ vs. V1. NS: Not significant. NA : not avalible.

3.3. The Influence of Cyclical Ketogenic Reduction Diet vs. Nutritionally Balanced Reduction Diet on Spiroergometric Parameters

Spiroergometric parameters are shown in Table 3. Respiratory exchange ratio decreased in subjects on CKD while it did not change in subjects on RD. None of other spiroergometric parameters were significantly affected in CKD group.

Table 3. The effect of cyclical ketogenic reduction diet and nutritionally balanced reduction diet on aerobic performance parameters.

	Cyclical Ketogenic Diet (CKD)		Reduction Diet (RD)		ANOVA
	V1-before	V2-after	V1-before	V2-after	
TFmax	180.9 ± 10.2	178.0 ± 11.3	178.9 ± 11.8	179.0 ± 10.2	NS
Rmax	1.27 ± 0.08	1.2 ± 0.12 *	1.21 ± 0.04	1.16 ± 0.10	0.04
Wmax	297.0 ± 48.5	298.0 ± 54.3	282.1 ± 34.3	296.0 ± 35.9 *	NS
VEmax	121.0 ± 28.5	136.0 ± 30.0	113.2 ± 20.3	124.0 ± 21.3	NS
VO_2max/kg	40.2 ± 4.1	43.0 ± 5.4	35.2 ± 6.0	38.2 ± 6.3 *	0.007
VO_2max/TF	19.0 ± 3.3	20.0 ± 3.4	18.0 ± 1.9	18.9 ± 1.6	NS
Wmax/kg	3.53 ± 0.42	3.6 ± 0.39	3.13 ± 0.52	3.36 ± 0.59 *	NS
W170max/kg	3.27 ± 0.65	3.4 ± 0.37	2.8 ± 0.74	3.06 ± 0.83 *	NS

Data are mean ± SD. Statistical significance is from One-way ANOVA and paired *t*-test (V1—baseline testing vs. V2—testing after 8 weeks of diet). * $p < 0.05$ vs. V1 TFmax—maximal heart rate; Rmax—respiratory exchange ratio; Wmax—peak workload; VEmax—maximal pulmonary ventilation; VO_2 max/kg—peak oxygen uptake; VO_2max/TF—peak pulse oxygen; Wmax.kg peak workload/kg; W170 max/kg—physical working capacity (at a heart rate of 170/min). NS: Not significant. NA : not avalible.

In contrast, in RD group peak workload, peak oxygen uptake/kg, peak workload/kg, and physical working capacity at a heart rate of 170/min increased after 8 weeks of intervention.

4. Discussion

The most important finding of this study is that eight weeks of regular aerobic exercise combined with exercise training complemented by two different dietary approaches—cyclical ketogenic reduction diet or nutritionally balanced reduction diet—significantly decreased body weight and body fat in healthy young men to a similar degree while having differential influence on body composition, strength parameters, and aerobic performance.

Despite comparable influence of both diets on body weight, we detected distinctions in their effects on body composition. In CKD group, the drop of body weight was due to a combination of decreased body fat, body water, and a slight, but significant, decline in lean body mass. On the contrary, in RD patients neither body water nor lean body mass were significantly affected and the weight reduction was predominantly due to body fat loss. The influence of ketogenic diet combined with different forms of exercise on body composition has been studied both in athletes and in patients with obesity and other comorbidities on numerous occasions. In some of the trials, isocaloric [24] or hypocaloric ketogenic diet [25] did not significantly change lean body mass while reducing body fat. On the contrary and in agreement with our current data, Perissious and colleagues found a reduction in lean body mass in patients with obesity undergoing exercise program while being on low carbohydrate diet [26]. Differential effect of ketogenic vs. nutritionally balanced diet under hyperenergetic conditions has also been described in a study in healthy men undergoing an eight-week resistance training program. Under these conditions, lean body mass increased only in control diet while it was unaffected in the ketogenic diet group [27]. Finally, ad libitum low carbohydrate ketogenic diet reduced body mass and lean body mass without compromising performance in powerlifting and Olympic weightlifting athletes [28]. In our study, a slight decrease in lean body mass did not impair strength parameters as compared to baseline values. Nevertheless, we have noted that in RD patients both lat pull-down and leg-press significantly increased after eight weeks of intervention as compared to no change in subjects on CKD.

While neutral effect of CKD on strength parameters in our study could have been expected based on the previously published data [29,30], we hypothesized that ketogenic diet could be more efficacious in improving endurance parameters as compared to nutritionally-balanced reduction diet as suggested by some previous trials [31]. The increasing popularity of ketogenic diets in endurance athletes is based on the hypothesis that predominant fat utilization over the use of carbohydrates may improve energy availability during endurance exercise along with accelerated recovery [10]. Bailey and Hennesy recently reviewed available data on the influence of ketogenic diet on endurance in athletes. They included seven studies into their analysis and concluded that limited and heterogenous findings prohibit definitive conclusions [16]. In our study, we found decreased respiratory exchange ratio in CKD groups after eight weeks of intervention as compared with no effect of RD suggesting a shift towards lipid oxidation, which is in agreement with the mode of action of ketogenic diet and previously published data [32]. However, none of the endurance parameters as measured by spiroergometry have been affected in CKD group. On the contrary, in RD group peak oxygen uptake and peak workload significantly increased after eight weeks of intervention. Our data suggesting lack of improvement of endurance performance by ketogenic diet go in similar direction with results published by Burke and colleagues in 2017 [33] and reproduced by the same group in 2020 [34] where they found decreased endurance parameters in elite race walkers after ketogenic diet. By contrast, in one of the early studies, low carbohydrate diet improved endurance times during moderate exercise in moderately obese patients along with significant reductions in body weight and body fat mass [35]. Nevertheless, despite more pronounced fat loss the improvement on endurance performance with low carbohydrate diet was comparable to that of high carbohydrate diet group.

When interpreted the results of our study within the context of currently published data it is important to consider its strengths and limitations. The randomized design and the good compliance of the subjects to dietary and treatment regimens can be consider strong points of our trial. On the other hand, the limitations include relatively short duration, low number of subjects and inclusion of only male participants.

Taken together our data are in general agreement with most of the previously published studies [36] showing little or no benefit of ketogenic diet on endurance capacity. However, it should be noted that contribution of fatty acids to metabolic response may differ with respect to duration and intensity of exercise [37,38], exact type of training and numerous other characteristics. The utilization of fatty acids increases with prolonged bouts of exercise of moderate intensity suggesting that ketogenic diet might be useful especially with longer duration of aerobic exercise.

5. Conclusions

In summary, our data show that in healthy young males undergoing resistance and aerobic training comparable weight reduction can be achieved with ketogenic and nutritionally balanced reduction diet. In RD group, improved muscle strength and endurance performance was noted relative to neutral effect of CKD on these parameters. Furthermore, CKD also slightly reduced lean body mass. Our study thus demonstrates that the cyclical ketogenic reduction diet effectively reduces body weight but is not an effective strategy to increase anaerobic or strength performance in healthy young men. All in all, further randomized studies of longer duration are still needed to explore whether the response to different diets is affected by long-term adaptation responses and whether it differs in males and females or subjects with various types and levels of fitness.

Author Contributions: Conceptualization, P.K., D.H., R.P.D., M.H., and Z.V.; methodology, P.K., I.L., Z.L., B.J.K., J.T., V.H., M.M., D.H., Z.V., and R.P.D.; writing—original draft preparation, P.K., M.H., and Z.V.; and writing—review and editing, all authors. All authors have read and agreed to the published version of the manuscript.

Funding: This research was funded by Funded by CZ-RO ("Institute for Clinical and Experimental Medicine—IKEM, IN 00023001") and RVO VFN 64165 to M.H.

Conflicts of Interest: The authors declare no conflict of interest.

References

1. Mozaffarian, D. Dietary and Policy Priorities for Cardiovascular Disease, Diabetes, and Obesity: A Comprehensive Review. *Circulation* **2016**, *133*, 187–225. [CrossRef]
2. Burke, L.M.; Kiens, B.; Ivy, J.L. Carbohydrates and fat for training and recovery. *J. Sports Sci.* **2004**, *22*, 15–30. [CrossRef] [PubMed]

3. Kaspar, M.B.; Austin, K.; Huecker, M.; Sarav, M. Ketogenic Diet: From the Historical Records to Use in Elite Athletes. *Curr. Nutr. Rep.* **2019**, *8*, 340–346. [CrossRef]
4. Hawley, J.A.; Brouns, F.; Jeukendrup, A. Strategies to enhance fat utilisation during exercise. *Sports Med.* **1998**, *25*, 241–257. [CrossRef] [PubMed]
5. Pilis, K.; Pilis, A.; Stec, K.; Pilis, W.; Langfort, J.; Letkiewicz, S.; Michalski, C.; Czuba, M.; Zych, M.; Chalimoniuk, M. Three-Year Chronic Consumption of Low-Carbohydrate Diet Impairs Exercise Performance and Has a Small Unfavorable Effect on Lipid Profile in Middle-Aged Men. *Nutrients* **2018**, *10*, 1914. [CrossRef]
6. Westman, E.C.; Feinman, R.D.; Mavropoulos, J.C.; Vernon, M.C.; Volek, J.S.; Wortman, J.A.; Yancy, W.S.; Phinney, S.D. Low-carbohydrate nutrition and metabolism. *Am. J. Clin. Nutr.* **2007**, *86*, 276–284. [CrossRef]
7. Webster, C.C.; Swart, J.; Noakes, T.D.; Smith, J.A. A Carbohydrate Ingestion Intervention in an Elite Athlete Who Follows a Low-Carbohydrate High-Fat Diet. *Int. J. Sports Physiol. Perform.* **2018**, *13*, 957–960. [CrossRef]
8. Noakes, T.D.; Windt, J. Evidence that supports the prescription of low-carbohydrate high-fat diets: A narrative review. *Br. J. Sports Med.* **2017**, *51*, 133–139. [CrossRef] [PubMed]
9. Miller, S.L.; Wolfe, R.R. Physical exercise as a modulator of adaptation to low and high carbohydrate and low and high fat intakes. *Eur. J. Clin. Nutr.* **1999**, *53* (Suppl. 1), S112–S119. [CrossRef]
10. Pinckaers, P.J.; Churchward-Venne, T.A.; Bailey, D.; van Loon, L.J. Ketone Bodies and Exercise Performance: The Next Magic Bullet or Merely Hype? *Sports Med.* **2017**, *47*, 383–391. [CrossRef]
11. McSwiney, F.T.; Doyle, L.; Plews, D.J.; Zinn, C. Impact of Ketogenic Diet on Athletes: Current Insights. *Open Access J. Sports Med.* **2019**, *10*, 171–183. [CrossRef] [PubMed]
12. Heatherly, A.J.; Killen, L.G.; Smith, A.F.; Waldman, H.S.; Seltmann, C.L.; Hollingsworth, A.; O'Neal, E.K. Effects of Ad libitum Low-Carbohydrate High-Fat Dieting in Middle-Age Male Runners. *Med. Sci. Sports Exerc.* **2018**, *50*, 570–579. [CrossRef] [PubMed]
13. Burke, L.M. Re-Examining High-Fat Diets for Sports Performance: Did We Call the "Nail in the Coffin" Too Soon? *Sports Med.* **2015**, *45* (Suppl. 1), S33–S49. [CrossRef]
14. Yeo, W.K.; Carey, A.L.; Burke, L.; Spriet, L.L.; Hawley, J.A. Fat adaptation in well-trained athletes: Effects on cell metabolism. *Appl. Physiol. Nutr. Metab.* **2011**, *36*, 12–22. [CrossRef] [PubMed]
15. Phinney, S.D.; Bistrian, B.R.; Evans, W.J.; Gervino, E.; Blackburn, G.L. The human metabolic response to chronic ketosis without caloric restriction: Preservation of submaximal exercise capability with reduced carbohydrate oxidation. *Metabolism* **1983**, *32*, 769–776. [CrossRef]
16. Bailey, C.P.; Hennessy, E. A review of the ketogenic diet for endurance athletes: Performance enhancer or placebo effect? *J. Int. Soc. Sports Nutr.* **2020**, *17*, 33. [CrossRef]
17. Hawley, J.A.; Burke, L.M.; Phillips, S.M.; Spriet, L.L. Nutritional modulation of training-induced skeletal muscle adaptations. *J. Appl. Physiol.* **2011**, *110*, 834–845. [CrossRef]
18. Ma, S.; Huang, Q.; Tominaga, T.; Liu, C.; Suzuki, K. An 8-Week Ketogenic Diet Alternated Interleukin-6, Ketolytic and Lipolytic Gene Expression, and Enhanced Exercise Capacity in Mice. *Nutrients* **2018**, *10*, 1696. [CrossRef]
19. Bolla, A.M.; Caretto, A.; Laurenzi, A.; Scavini, M.; Piemonti, L. Low-Carb and Ketogenic Diets in Type 1 and Type 2 Diabetes. *Nutrients* **2019**, *11*, 962. [CrossRef]
20. Bazzano, L.A.; Hu, T.; Reynolds, K.; Yao, L.; Bunol, C.; Liu, Y.; Chen, C.S.; Klag, M.J.; Whelton, P.K.; He, J. Effects of low-carbohydrate and low-fat diets: A randomized trial. *Ann. Intern. Med.* **2014**, *161*, 309–318. [CrossRef]
21. Kelly, T.; Unwin, D.; Finucane, F. Low-Carbohydrate Diets in the Management of Obesity and Type 2 Diabetes: A Review from Clinicians Using the Approach in Practice. *Int. J. Environ. Res. Public Health* **2020**, *17*, 2557. [CrossRef]
22. Brouns, F. Overweight and diabetes prevention: Is a low-carbohydrate-high-fat diet recommendable? *Eur. J. Nutr.* **2018**, *57*, 1301–1312. [CrossRef] [PubMed]
23. Gordon, D.; Schaitel, K.; Pennefather, A.; Gernigon, M.; Keiller, D.; Barnes, R. The incidence of plateau at VO(2max) is affected by a bout of prior-priming exercise. *Clin. Physiol. Funct. Imaging* **2012**, *32*, 39–44. [CrossRef] [PubMed]
24. Merra, G.; Miranda, R.; Barrucco, S.; Gualtieri, P.; Mazza, M.; Moriconi, E.; Marchetti, M.; Chang, T.F.; De Lorenzo, A.; Di Renzo, L. Very-low-calorie ketogenic diet with aminoacid supplement versus very low restricted-calorie diet for preserving muscle mass during weight loss: A pilot double-blind study. *Eur. Rev. Med. Pharmacol Sci.* **2016**, *20*, 2613–2621. [PubMed]

25. Moreno, B.; Bellido, D.; Sajoux, I.; Goday, A.; Saavedra, D.; Crujeiras, A.B.; Casanueva, F.F. Comparison of a very low-calorie-ketogenic diet with a standard low-calorie diet in the treatment of obesity. *Endocrine* **2014**, *47*, 793–805. [CrossRef]
26. Perissiou, M.; Borkoles, E.; Kobayashi, K.; Polman, R. The Effect of an 8 Week Prescribed Exercise and Low-Carbohydrate Diet on Cardiorespiratory Fitness, Body Composition and Cardiometabolic Risk Factors in Obese Individuals: A Randomised Controlled Trial. *Nutrients* **2020**, *12*, 482. [CrossRef]
27. Vargas, S.; Romance, R.; Petro, J.L.; Bonilla, D.A.; Galancho, I.; Espinar, S.; Kreider, R.B.; Benitez-Porres, J. Efficacy of ketogenic diet on body composition during resistance training in trained men: A randomized controlled trial. *J. Int. Soc. Sports Nutr.* **2018**, *15*, 31. [CrossRef]
28. Greene, D.A.; Varley, B.J.; Hartwig, T.B.; Chapman, P.; Rigney, M. A Low-Carbohydrate Ketogenic Diet Reduces Body Mass Without Compromising Performance in Powerlifting and Olympic Weightlifting Athletes. *J. Strength Cond Res.* **2018**, *32*, 3373–3382. [CrossRef]
29. Wilson, J.M.; Lowery, R.P.; Roberts, M.D.; Sharp, M.H.; Joy, J.M.; Shields, K.A.; Partl, J.; Volek, J.S.; D'Agostino, D. The Effects of Ketogenic Dieting on Body Composition, Strength, Power, and Hormonal Profiles in Resistance Training Males. *J. Strength Cond Res.* **2017**. [CrossRef]
30. Kephart, W.C.; Pledge, C.D.; Roberson, P.A.; Mumford, P.W.; Romero, M.A.; Mobley, C.B.; Martin, J.S.; Young, K.C.; Lowery, R.P.; Wilson, J.M.; et al. The Three-Month Effects of a Ketogenic Diet on Body Composition, Blood Parameters, and Performance Metrics in CrossFit Trainees: A Pilot Study. *Sports* **2018**, *6*, 1. [CrossRef]
31. McSwiney, F.T.; Wardrop, B.; Hyde, P.N.; Lafountain, R.A.; Volek, J.S.; Doyle, L. Keto-adaptation enhances exercise performance and body composition responses to training in endurance athletes. *Metabolism* **2018**, *81*, 25–34. [CrossRef]
32. Rubini, A.; Bosco, G.; Lodi, A.; Cenci, L.; Parmagnani, A.; Grimaldi, K.; Zhongjin, Y.; Paoli, A. Effects of Twenty Days of the Ketogenic Diet on Metabolic and Respiratory Parameters in Healthy Subjects. *Lung* **2015**, *193*, 939–945. [CrossRef] [PubMed]
33. Burke, L.M.; Ross, M.L.; Garvican-Lewis, L.A.; Welvaert, M.; Heikura, I.A.; Forbes, S.G.; Mirtschin, J.G.; Cato, L.E.; Strobel, N.; Sharma, A.P.; et al. Low carbohydrate, high fat diet impairs exercise economy and negates the performance benefit from intensified training in elite race walkers. *J. Physiol.* **2017**, *595*, 2785–2807. [CrossRef]
34. Burke, L.M.; Sharma, A.P.; Heikura, I.A.; Forbes, S.F.; Holloway, M.; McKay, A.K.A.; Bone, J.L.; Leckey, J.J.; Welvaert, M.; Ross, M.L. Crisis of confidence averted: Impairment of exercise economy and performance in elite race walkers by ketogenic low carbohydrate, high fat (LCHF) diet is reproducible. *PLoS ONE* **2020**, *15*, e0234027. [CrossRef]
35. Phinney, S.D.; Horton, E.S.; Sims, E.A.; Hanson, J.S.; Danforth, E., Jr.; LaGrange, B.M. Capacity for moderate exercise in obese subjects after adaptation to a hypocaloric, ketogenic diet. *J. Clin. Invest.* **1980**, *66*, 1152–1161. [CrossRef]
36. Harvey, K.L.; Holcomb, L.E.; Kolwicz, S.C., Jr. Ketogenic Diets and Exercise Performance. *Nutrients* **2019**, *11*, 2296. [CrossRef]
37. Egan, B.; Zierath, J.R. Exercise metabolism and the molecular regulation of skeletal muscle adaptation. *Cell Metab.* **2013**, *17*, 162–184. [CrossRef]
38. Evans, M.; Cogan, K.E.; Egan, B. Metabolism of ketone bodies during exercise and training: Physiological basis for exogenous supplementation. *J. Physiol.* **2017**, *595*, 2857–2871. [CrossRef]

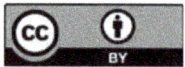

© 2020 by the authors. Licensee MDPI, Basel, Switzerland. This article is an open access article distributed under the terms and conditions of the Creative Commons Attribution (CC BY) license (http://creativecommons.org/licenses/by/4.0/).

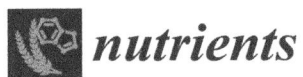

Review

Nutritional Ergogenic Aids in Racquet Sports: A Systematic Review

Néstor Vicente-Salar [1,2,*,†], Guillermo Santos-Sánchez [3,†,‡] and Enrique Roche [1,2,4]

1. Biochemistry and Cell Therapy Unit, Institute of Bioengineering, University Miguel Hernandez, 03201 Elche, Spain; eroche@umh.es
2. Department of Applied Biology-Nutrition, Alicante Institute for Health and Biomedical Research (ISABIAL-FISABIO Foundation), University Miguel Hernandez, 03201 Elche, Spain
3. Departamento de Tecnología de la Alimentación y Nutrición, Universidad Católica de Murcia, 30107 Murcia, Spain; gsantos-ibis@us.es
4. CIBER Fisiopatología de la Obesidad y Nutrición (CIBEROBN), Instituto de Salud Carlos III (ISCIII), 28029 Madrid, Spain
* Correspondence: nvicente@umh.es
† To be considered as equal first author.
‡ Present Address: Departamento de Bioquímica Médica y Biología Molecular e Inmunología, Universidad de Sevilla, 41009 Seville, Spain.

Received: 27 August 2020; Accepted: 15 September 2020; Published: 17 September 2020

Abstract: A nutritional ergogenic aid (NEA) can help athletes optimize performance, but an evidence-based analysis is required in order to support training outcomes or competition performance in specific events. Racquet sports players are regularly exposed to a high-intensity workload throughout the tournament season. The activity during a match is characterized by variable durations (2–4 h) of repeated high-intensity bouts interspersed with standardized rest periods. Medline/PubMed, Scopus, and EBSCO were searched from their inception until February 2020 for randomized controlled trials (RCTs). Two independent reviewers extracted data, after which they assessed the risk of bias and the quality of trials. Out of 439 articles found, 21 met the predefined criteria: tennis (15 trials), badminton (three trials), paddle (one trial), and squash (two trials). Among all the studied NEAs, acute dosages of caffeine (3–6 mg/kg) 30–60 min before a match have been proven to improve specific skills and accuracy but may not contribute to improve perceived exertion. Currently, creatine, sodium bicarbonate, sodium citrate, beetroot juice, citrulline, and glycerol need more studies to strengthen the evidence regarding improved performance in racquet sports.

Keywords: racquet sports; ergogenic aid; performance; sport supplement

1. Introduction

Racquet sports are included in the family of ball sports and more specifically, among those using an implement. They are characterized by the use of a manual racquet to propel an implement (a ball, shuttlecock, etc.) between two or four players with the objective of placing it in a position with no return possibilities for the opponent. There are two different game formats: (a) passing the implement over a net in a divided field (tennis, badminton, paddle and table tennis) or (b) hitting the implement onto a wall in a shared field (squash and racquetball) [1].

Racquet sports are acyclic disciplines with very intense workload cycles, which are interrupted by small pauses that allow for an incomplete recovery. Therefore, metabolic demands in racquet sports alternate between both anaerobic and aerobic energy sources. Anaerobic energy comes from intramuscular ATP and phosphocreatine (PC), as well as from anaerobic glycolysis, the three of which are used during high intensity, short duration points, changes of direction, and hits. On the other hand, the aerobic system is involved during long points of moderate intensity, playing a primary role in delaying fatigue, and indirectly, favoring concentration, technical skills, and maintaining workload during a match [2–5].

As a result of this fact, the average heart rate (HR) during a match reaches up to 60–80% of HR maximum (HRmax), increasing to 90% of HRmax in high-intensity situations [6–8]. Nonetheless, HRmax does not provide clear information regarding real energy demands or the metabolic pathways involved, since this parameter is affected by dehydration, heat stress, age, and playing techniques [9]. Measuring blood lactate concentration during a match could report more accurately the energetic pathways used by racquet sports players. Ranges vary from 1.0–4.0 mmol/L to 8.0–12.0 mmol/L during prolonged high-intensity matches [2,10–12], supporting the key role of glycolytic pathways during the match.

An ergogenic aid is any training method, mechanical device, nutritional or pharmacological approach, or psychological technique that can improve exercise performance capacity and/or improve training adaptations [13]. Therefore, a nutritional ergogenic aid (NEA) is defined as those nutritional supplements taken orally containing a nutritional ingredient that intends to complement diet. The objective of these supplements is to improve sports performance without exerting harmful effects on the individual [14].

The consumption of NEAs has been increasing in recent years around the world, which has led to a great variety of research with the aim of estimating their intake and use. In fact, sales of dietary supplements grew 6.1% in 2017, achieving an income of 39.8 billion dollars in the US [15]. A meta-analysis published in 2015 concluded that elite athletes used many more dietary supplements than non-elite athletes, and the prevalence of use was similar in men and women [16]. The NEAs most frequently used by high-level tennis players tend to be creatine and caffeine [17] while among international rank squash players, sodium bicarbonate is also frequently consumed in addition to the two aforementioned NEAs [18]. Normally, NEA recommendations in high-level racquet sports players are directed by personal trainers, coaches, or sports dietitian–nutritionists. However, proper counseling based on current scientific evidence is required.

In this line, several organizations such as the Australian Institute of Sport (AIS) or the World Anti-Doping Agency (WADA) propose classifications of sports supplements grouped into different categories according to effectiveness, legality, and safety. Nevertheless, there are not policies regarding the regulation of alleged benefits and safety claims [19,20]. Thus, athletes find themselves under the influence of companies' advertising, which claims improved performance and recovery through the consumption of a wide range of products without scientific evidence regarding their effect, dosage, or instructions for use.

The main aim of this systematic review was to evaluate the scientific evidence concerning NEAs in the improvement of performance of racquet sports athletes specifically through published RCTs.

2. Materials and Methods

The conduct and reporting of the current systematic review conform to the Preferred Reporting Items for Systematic Reviews and Meta-Analyses (PRISMA) [21]. Five racquet sports were analyzed regarding the effectiveness of certain nutritional ergogenic aids: tennis, badminton, squash, table tennis, and paddle.

2.1. Systematic Search

Relevant articles were identified by title and abstract in the electronic databases Medline, Scopus, and EBSCO (since inception to 20 February 2020) using the search strategy in Table 1. The electronic search was supplemented by a manual review of reference lists from relevant publications and reviews to find additional publications on the subject.

Table 1. Combined terms used in the search for studies in the database. [1] Mesh terms were used in the search; [2] Term not included in the Mesh search; [3] nutritional ergogenic aid (NEAs) filed in the A group of the Australian Institute of Sport (AIS).

Pubmed [1]			Scopus and EBSCO		
NEA		Sport	NEA [3]		Sport
Dietary supplements		Racquet Sports	Dietary supplements		Racquet Sports
Caffeine		Tennis	Ergogenic aid		Tennis
Creatine			Caffeine		Badminton
Beta-alanine	AND		Creatine	AND	Table tennis
Sodium Bicarbonate			Beta-alanine		Squash and sport
Ergogenic aid [2]			Sodium Bicarbonate		Paddle
			Nitrate		
			Beetroot juice		
			Glycerol		

2.2. Data Extraction

Two reviewers (N.V.-S. and G.S.-S.) independently extracted the following data from each study using a predefined Microsoft Excel data extraction form including the number of participants within each group, participant characteristics, racquet sport discipline, and supplementation intervention characteristics, end points, measurement methods, and results in order to produce an overview table of all eligible studies.

2.3. Study Selection

Studies were eligible for inclusion if they met each of the following criteria: (a) not using any doping substances established by the World Anti-Doping Agency (WADA), (b) using a randomized controlled trial (RCT) design that included one group taking supplementation and 1+ groups receiving a placebo or not taking supplementation, (c) not including any ergogenic aids classified within group A by the Australian Sports Commission (AIS) because of their high evidence grade [22], (d) not presenting supplementation as a source of nutrients, such as bars, gels, or drinks rich in carbohydrates and electrolytes, and (e) not being gray literature (abstracts, conference proceedings, or editorials) or reviews.

2.4. Quality Assessment and Publication Bias

Characteristics of the retrieved RCTs were evaluated using the 'risk-of-bias' assessment tool following the recommendations by the Cochrane Handbook for Systematic Reviews of Interventions [23,24]. This evaluation was carried out by two reviewers (N.V.S. and G.S.S.) working independently in order to present bias comprehensively. The following criteria were analyzed: randomized treatment order and carry-over effect (selection bias), blinding of participants and research staff to group allocation (performance bias), blinding of outcome assessor (detection bias), incomplete outcome data (attrition bias), selective reporting (reporting bias), and other bias (it was assessed if there was controlled diet, exercise use of supplements or drugs, and sport stratification when a mixture of disciplines was analyzed). Then, the retrieved RCTs were classified as being of "high", "unclear", or "low" risk of bias. Effect size was calculated using Cohen´s d test.

3. Results

3.1. Included Studies

A total of 438 studies were screened by title and abstract, and 377 were assessed for eligibility criteria (full-text screening). From the retrieved articles, twenty-one met all the inclusion criteria and were included in the systematic review (Figure 1, Tables 2 and 3). Thirteen RTCs were found in the Medline database (eleven for tennis and two for badminton), seven were found in the Scopus database (three for tennis, one for badminton, two for squash, and one for paddle) where one article was not available despite requesting it from its main author; and none were retrieved from the EBSCO database (because all those found there were repeated). Additionally, one article that was not found through the initial search but was found in a review published in the Medline database was added for full-text analysis. The PRISMA flowchart was applied to illustrate the step-by-step exclusion of unrelated/duplicate retrieved records, leading to the final selection of twenty-one RCTs that met the predefined inclusion criteria (Figure 1).

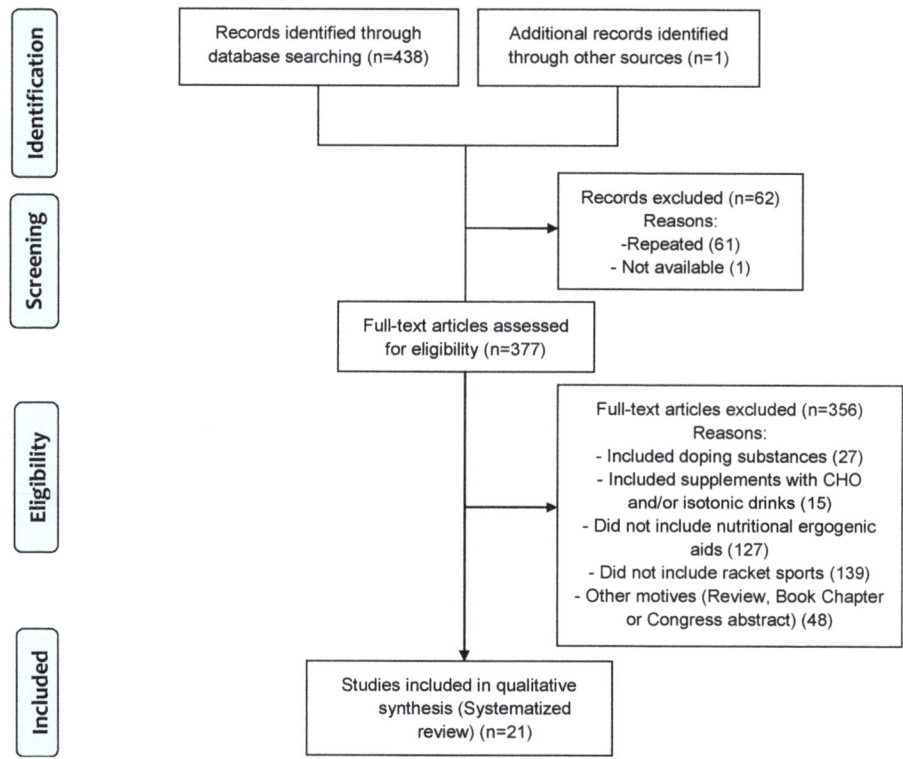

Figure 1. Preferred Reporting Items for Systematic Reviews and Meta-Analyses (PRISMA) flow chart [21] of the study selection process.

Table 2. Included studies on nutritional ergogenic aids in tennis. BCAAs: Branched-chain amino acids; FFA: Blood free fatty acids; Gly: Blood glycerol; HR: Heart rate; Lac: Blood lactate; LTPT: Leuven Tennis Performance Test; LTST: Loughborough Tennis Skill Test; NO: Nitric oxide; Pl: Placebo; RSA: repeated-sprint ability shuttle test; STPT: Skill Tennis Performance Test; Trp/BCAAs: Blood tryptophan/branched-chain amino acids ratio; u-EPI: Urine epinephrine; u-NE: Urine norepinephrine. ↑: Significant increase compared to placebo/control group; ↓: Significant decrease compared to placebo/control group; ↔: without changes compared to placebo/control group.

Study	NEA	Dosage/Time	Participants	Age (yrs)	Level	Blinded/Double Blinded	Duration	Exercise Protocol	Measurements	Main Outcomes
[25]	Caffeine	-0.2 (women)-0.25 (men) mg/kg/0 min before match and every 15 min during a match	16 (8 men/ 8 women)	25.4 ± 1.9/ 20.4 ± 2.8	National ranking (Germany)	DB	1 day	3 matches (2 of 75 min/match and 1 of 90 min/match with only rest between match 2 and 3 of 30 min) + Accuracy and sprint test	- Lac - Glu - Gly - FFA - u-EPI - u-NE - Sprints - Accuracy hit - Perceived exertion	↔ Lac ↔ Glu ↔ Gly ↔ FFA ↑ u-EPI ↔ u-NE ↔ Sprints ↔ Accuracy hit ↔ Perceptual training intensity
[26]	Caffeine	-5 mg/kg/60 min before pre-test. -0.75 mg/kg/Each 1 h after start pre-test and during protocol	13 men	20.4 ± 0.9	National ranking (Belgium)	DB	1 day	LTPT + Sprint test + Court session (120 min) + LTPT	- Sprints - Serve quality - Backhand stroke quality - Volley errors and fatigue - HR - Perceived exertion	↔ Sprints ↔ Serve quality ↑ Backhand stroke ↑ Volley errors and fatigue ↔ HR ↔ Perceptual training intensity
[27]	Caffeine	-3 mg/kg/30 min before match	12 men	18.3 ± 3.0	National ranking (Australia)	B	1 day	1 match of 160 min/match	- Lac - Glu - CK - Prolactin - Fluid loss - Serve and stroke velocity - Serve kinematics - Perceptual skills - HR - Perceived exertion	↔ Lac ↔ Glu ↔ CK ↔ Prolactin ↔ Fluid loss ↑ Serve velocity in 4th set ↔ Serve kinematics ↔ Perceptual skills ↔ HR ↔ Perceptual training intensity

Table 2. Cont.

Study	NEA	Dosage/Time	Participants	Age (yrs)	Level	Blinded/Double Blinded	Duration	Exercise Protocol	Measurements	Main Outcomes
[28]	Caffeine	- 6 mg/kg/60 min before test	16 (8 men/8 women)	20.7 ± 1.7	National ranking (USA)	DB	1 day	Intermittent treadmill exercise (45 min) + Tennis skills test	- Successful shots - HR - Perceived exertion	↑ Total shot successes ↔ HR ↔ Perceptual training intensity
[29]	Caffeine	- 80 mg/30 min before test	12 (6 men/6 women)	18–22	University players (UK)	DB	1 day	3 days of sleep restriction follow a day of accuracy serve test	- Accuracy serve	↔ Accuracy serve
[30]	Caffeine	- 3 mg/kg/60 min before test	14 (10 men/4 women)	16.4 ± 1.2	Elite-level Junior players (Spain)	DB	1 day	Tennis specific test + Simulated Match of best-of-3-sets system	- Handgrip force - Serve velocity - Running speed - Number of sprints - Distance - HR - Sweat rate	↑ Handgrip force ↔ Serve velocity ↑ Only in high intensity ↑ Number of sprints ↔ Distance ↔ HR ↑ Sweat rate
[31]	Caffeine	- 6 mg/kg/60 min before test	10 (5 men/5 women)	19.9 ± 1.8	National ranking (USA)	DB	1 day	Tennis serve trial + Shuttle run sprint + Tennis serve trial	- Accuracy serve - Shuttle run time - Likert scale	↑ Accuracy serve (depending of conditions of time and distance ↔ Shuttle run time ↔ Feelings
[32]	Creatine	- 20 g/day (4 × 5g/day)/ During 5 days before test	8 men	20.4 ± 0.9	National ranking (Belgium)	DB	5 days	LTPT + Shuttle run sprint	- Quality of 1st and 2nd service - Stroke quality - Sprint power - Lac	↔ Service quality ↔ Stroke quality ↔ Sprint power ↔ Lac
[33]	Creatine	- 0.3 g/kg in loading phase (6 days) - 0.03 g/day in maintenance phase (28 days)	36 men	22.5 ± 4.9–28.8 ± 4.8	ITN 3	DB	5 weeks	- Service test + Ball machine ground stroke drill + Intermittent sprint test + Strength test	- Serving velocity - Stroke velocity - Sprinting velocity - Strength - HR - Perceived exertion	↔ Serving velocity ↔ Stroke velocity ↔ Sprinting velocity ↔ Strength ↔ HR ↔ Perceptual training intensity

142

Table 2. Cont.

Study	NEA	Dosage/Time	Participants	Age (yrs)	Level	Blinded/Double Blinded	Duration	Exercise Protocol	Measurements	Main Outcomes
[34]	Sodium Bicarbonate	- 0.3 g/kg/70 min before test - 0.1 g/kg/During test	9 men	21.8 ± 2.4	College Tennis players (Taiwan)	DB	1 day	- LIST + Simulated match (50 min) + LIST	- Lac - pH - Serve consistency - Stroke consistency - Serve Accuracy - Stroke Accuracy - HR - Perceived exertion	↑ Lac ↔ pH Keeps serve consistency while PI ↓ Keeps stroke consistency while PI ↓ ↔ Serve Accuracy ↔ Stroke Accuracy ↔ HR ↔ Perceptual training intensity
[35]	Sodium Citrate	- 0.5 g/kg/120 min before test	10 men	17.0 ± 1.0	Junior National Ranking (Brazil)	DB	1 day	STPT + RSA + Simulated match (60 min) + STPT + RSA	- Lac - pH - Stroke consistency - Stroke accuracy - Number strokes - Time of sprints - Perceived exertion	↑ Lac ↑ pH ↑ Stroke consistency ↔ Stroke accuracy ↔ Number strokes ↔ Time of sprints ↔ Perceptual training intensity
[36]	Beetroot juice	- 70 mL (6.4 mmol of NO$_3^-$)/3 h before test	13 men	25.4 ± 5.1	ATP and National ranking (Spain)	DB	1 day	- Serve velocity test + Counter movement jump + Isometric handgrip strength + Agility and sprint test	- Serve velocity - Jump height - Handgrip force - Agility - Sprint velocity - Perceived exertion	↔ Serve velocity ↔ Jump height ↔ Handgrip force ↔ Agility ↔ Sprint velocity ↔ Perceptual training intensity
[37]	Citrulline-malate	- 8 g/60 min before test	17 women	51.0 ± 9.0	Masters ranking in USTA (USA)	DB	1 day	- Isometric handgrip strength + Counter movement jump + Wingate cycling test	- Handgrip force - Peak vertical power - Anaerobic capacity - Relative peak power - Explosive power - Sustained power	↑ Handgrip strength ↔ Jump power ↔ Anaerobic capacity ↑ Relative peak power ↑ Explosive power ↔ Sustained power

Table 2. Cont.

Study	NEA	Dosage/Time	Participants	Age (yrs)	Level	Blinded/Double Blinded	Duration	Exercise Protocol	Measurements	Main Outcomes
[38]	BCAAs + Arginine + Citrulline	- 0.17 g/kg BCAAs (Leu-Ile-Val = 10:7:3) + 0.05 g/kg Arginine + 0.05 g/kg Citrulline/80 min before test	9 men	25.6 ± 0.7	National Ranking (Taiwan)	B	1 day	Perceptual-motor performance test (LIST modified) + Simulated match (120 min) + Perceptual-motor performance test (LIST modified)	- Lac	↔ Lac
									- Gly	↔ Gly
									- Glu	↔ Glu
									- FFA	↔ FFA
									- NO	↑ NO
									- Trp/BCAAs	↓ Trp/BCAAs
									- HR	↓ HR
									- Stroke Accuracy	Prevents a high decrease in stroke accuracy compared with PI
									- Stroke consistency	Keeps stroke consistency while PI ↓
									- Stroke velocity	Keeps stroke velocity while PI ↓
									- Perceived exertion	↓ Perceptual training intensity
									- Change in body Weight	↑ Body weight vs. PI
[39]	Glycerol	- 1 g/kg/150 min before test - 0.5 g/kg/15 min after test	11 men	27.0 ± 2.0	Ranking 4-5 in USTA (USA)	DB	1 day	Tennis specific test + Simulated match (75 min) + Tennis specific test	- Plasma osmolality	↑ Plasma osmolality vs. PI (only pre- and post-exercise)
									- Change in plasma volume	↑ Plasma volume vs. PI (only pre- and post-exercise)
									- Electrolytes	↔ Electrolytes
									- Urine volume	↓ Urine volume
									- Sprint velocity	↔ Sprint velocity
									- Agility	↔ Agility
									- Stroke accuracy	↔ Stroke accuracy
									- Serve accuracy	↔ Serve accuracy

Table 3. Included studies on nutritional ergogenic aids in badminton, squash, and paddle. Glu: Blood glucose; HR: Heart rate; Lac: Blood lactate. ↑: Significant increase compared to placebo/control group; ↓: Significant decrease compared to placebo/control group; ↔: without changes compared to placebo/control group.

Badminton

Study	NEA	Dosage/Time	Participants	Age (yrs)	Level	Blinded/Double Blinded	Duration	Exercise Protocol	Measurements	Main Outcomes
[40]	Caffeine	- 3 mg/kg/60 min before test	16 men	25.4 ± 7.3	National ranking (Spain)	DB	1 day	Handgrip force + Jump tests + Agility Test + Simulated match (45 min)	- Handgrip maximal force	↔ Handgrip force
									- Smash jump	↔ Smash jump
									- Squat jump	↑ Squat jump height/power
									- Countermovement Jump (CJ)	↑ CJ height/power
									- Agility	↔ Agility
									- Number of impacts	↑ Number of impacts
									- HR	↔ HR
									- Perceived exertion	↔ Perceptual training intensity
									- Lac	↔ Lac
									- Glu	↔ Glu
[41]	Caffeine	- 4 mg/kg/60 min before exercise - 4 mg/kg /during 2nd Badminton specific test	12 men	28 ± 9	National ranking (United Kingdom)	DB	1 day	Badminton specific test + Fatigue protocol (33 min) + Badminton specific test	- Errors in anticipation	↓ Errors in anticipation
									- Accuracy serve	↔ Accuracy serve
									- Reaction time	↓ Reaction time
									- Time sprints	↓ Time sprints
									- HR	↔ HR
									- Perceived exertion	↓ Perceptual training intensity
[42]	Sodium bicarbonate	- 300 mg/kg/90 min before test	30 men	21	Student players (Indonesia)	?	1 day	Treadmill testing to exhaustion	- pH	↑ pH
									- Lac	↑ Lac
									- Time to exhaustion	↑ Time to Exhaustion
[42]	Sodium citrate	- 300 mg/kg/90 min before test	30 men	21	Student players (Indonesia)	?	1 day	Treadmill testing to exhaustion	- pH	↓ pH
									- Lac	↑ Lac
									- Time to exhaustion	↑ Time to Exhaustion

Table 3. Cont.

Study	NEA	Dosage/Time	Participants	Age (yrs)	Level	Blinded/Double Blinded	Duration	Exercise Protocol	Measurements	Main Outcomes
Squash										
[43]	Creatine	- 0.3 g/kg/day (4 × 0.075 g /kg/day)/during 5 days before test	9 (8 men/1 woman)	21.3 ± 0.3	National ranking (UK)	DB	5 days	Court set sprint test	- Lac - Sprint time - Likert scale - HR	↔Lact ↓ Sprint time ↔ Feelings ↔HR
[44]	Creatine + Guarana	- 1000 mg creatine + 1500 mg guarana + 133 mg Caffeine/Half dosage at 30 min and rest at 0 min before test.	8	18.2 ± 3.7	National ranking (France)	?	1 day	Cognitive tests + Cycle ergometer sprint test + Cognitive tests + Submaximal test with cognitive test	- Peak Power - Fatigue - Reaction time - Reaction time under pressure - Visual response reaction time - Ocular motility response time	↑ Peak power ↓ Fatigue ↔Reaction time ↓ Reaction time under time pressure ↓ Visual response reaction time ↓ Ocular motility response time
Paddle										
[45]	Caffeine	6 mg/Kg/30 min before test	12 men	27.7 ± 3.7	Amateur (Brazil)	B	1 day	Specific paddle training (45 min) + Handgrip strength and Volley test	- Isometric handgrip strength - Volley precision - HR - Perceived exertion	↔ Handgrip strength ↑ % Correct hits ↓ % Errors ↔ HR ↔ Perceptual training intensity

3.2. Risk of Bias and Quality Assessment of Studies

The risk of bias of the included studies is illustrated in Table 4. The RCTs of Pluim; 2006 [33] and Hartono; 2017 [42] were parallel group trials, so the criteria of random sequence generation and allocation concealment were used instead of randomized treatment order and carry-over effect respectively. Most of the trials assessed showed an unclear level in the criteria of selection bias, both in the randomized treatment order and in the evaluation of the carry-over effect. Only the trials by Vergauwen; 1998, [26] Lopez-Samanes; 2020 [36] and Abian; 2015 [40] suitably described the tools used for randomization treatment, while trials by Wu; 2010 [34], Yang; 2017 [38], Abian; 2015 [40] and Muller; 2019 [45] used tests to check if the washout time between conditions was suitable. Moreover, most of the studies also showed a high risk of detection bias except for trials by Gallo-Salazar; 2015 [30] and Abian; 2015 [40], which specifically indicated that blinding was kept until the statistical analysis was performed. Five studies [27,38,42,44,45] were at a high risk of performance bias due to incomplete blinding or a lack of blinding.

Table 4. Quality assessment of the included studies. Cross-over studies where A = Randomized treatment order; B = Carry-over effect; C = Performance bias; D = Detection bias; E = Attrition bias; F = Reporting bias; G = Other bias. * Parallel studies where A = Random sequence generation and B = Allocation concealment.

Study	A	B	C	D	E	F	G
[25]	−	?	+	−	?	+	?
[26]	+	?	+	−	+	+	?
[27]	−	?	−	−	+	+	+
[28]	−	?	+	−	+	+	?
[29]	?	?	?	−	+	+	?
[30]	?	?	+	+	+	+	+
[31]	?	?	+	−	+	+	?
[32]	?	?	+	−	+	+	+
[33] *	?	?	+	−	+	+	?
[36]	+	?	+	−	+	+	?
[37]	?	−	+	−	+	+	?
[39]	?	?	?	−	+	+	?
[34]	?	+	+	−	+	+	+
[35]	?	?	+	−	+	+	?
[38]	?	+	−	−	+	+	+
[40]	+	+	+	+	+	+	+

Table 4. Cont.

Study	A	B	C	D	E	F	G
[41]	?	?	+	−	+	+	+
[42] *	?	?	−	−	+	+	−
[43]	?	?	?	−	+	+	+
[44]	?	?	−	−	+	+	−
[45]	?	+	−	−	+	+	?

+ Low Risk of bias
− High Risk of bias
? Unclear

3.3. Participants

Age in all the examined studies ranged from 16.4 to 51.0 years old, so that included from junior to master players. Level ranged from university to professional level in both sexes, with a majority of players being males ($n = 266$) as compared to females ($n = 27$). Tennis was the racquet sport about which more studies on NEAs were checked ($n = 15$), followed by badminton ($n = 3$), squash ($n = 2$), and paddle ($n = 1$), but no study was found for table tennis. In the case of NEAs, caffeine was the most evaluated supplement ($n = 10$) followed by creatine monohydrate ($n = 4$), plasma buffers ($n = 3$), nitric oxide (NO) precursors ($n = 3$), and hydration agents ($n = 1$).

3.4. Nutritional Ergogenic Aids and Intervention Characteristics in Tennis

Caffeine was the most tested NEA with seven studies (Table 2). All trials had a duration of 1 day with variations in concentrations and timing. Most studies selected used a caffeine dosage of 3–6 mg/kg 30–60 min before the tests [26–28,30,31], with improvements in specific tennis skills such as accuracy serve, backhand stroke, serve velocity in last sets, total number of successful shots, handgrip force, and number of sprints compared with control groups. Other protocols with continued administration during tests but a smaller dosage (0.2–0.25 mg/kg) [25] or the same quantity of caffeine given to each player (80 mg) [29] only show an increase in urine epinephrine or no changes compared with control groups respectively.

Regarding creatine monohydrate, only two studies evaluated its efficiency. Neither a high dosage for five days (20 g/day) [32] nor a load period of six days (0.3 g/kg) followed by a maintenance period (0.03 g/kg) until completing five weeks [33] offered advantages compared to control groups.

NEAs related to plasma buffer function were evaluated by two one-day duration studies. A load of 0.3 g/kg sodium bicarbonate 70 min before test and continuous intake of 0.1 g/kg during test showed maintenance of serve and stroke consistency (number of balls landed within the singles court on the designated side) compared to the control group [34], while 0.5 g/kg sodium citrate 120 min before test increased stroke consistency [35]. Both NEAs increased plasma lactate significantly, but only sodium citrate was accompanied by an increase in blood pH.

Three studies about NO precursors were found. The intake of 70 mL beetroot juice 3 h before the test did not show differences compared to control [36]. On the other hand, only citrulline malate supplementation (80 g 60 min before the trial) [37] or together with arginine and BCAAs (0.05 g/kg 80 min before test) [38] showed improvements compared with control. Citrulline malate improved handgrip strength and relative peak power, and citrulline + arginine + BCAAs avoided the decrease of stroke accuracy and kept stroke consistency and stroke velocity.

Lastly, regarding hydration agents, glycerol was the only NEA found in just one study [39]. The consumption of 1 g/kg glycerol 150 min before the trial and 0.5 g/kg 15 min after it increased body weight, plasma osmolality, and plasma volume, and decreased urine volume.

3.5. Nutritional Ergogenic Aids and Intervention Characteristics in Badminton, Squash, and Paddle

Caffeine was tested in badminton male players 60 min before exercise protocol with a dosage ranging from 3 to 4 mg/kg [40,41]. It showed improvements in jumps and the number of impacts accompanied with a decrease in errors in anticipation, reaction time, and time of sprints (Table 3). In addition, in paddle, caffeine showed ergogenic effects. The intake of 6 mg/kg caffeine 30 min before the exercise protocol in twelve amateur male players increased the percentage of correct hits, diminishing errors [45].

Different plasma buffers were evaluated by one study in badminton male players [42]. A load of 0.3 g/kg sodium bicarbonate or 0.3 g/kg sodium citrate 90 min before the test showed an increase in time to exhaustion with both supplements (51.3 and 44.4% respectively). Both NEAs increased plasma lactate, but only sodium bicarbonate showed an increase in plasma pH.

Finally, the effect of creatine was evaluated in squash players by two studies, one of them with a load of 0.3 g/kg/day for 5 days before test [43], and the other with acute supplementation of a mixed product composed by 1 g creatine + 1.5 g guarana + 133 mg caffeine [44]. The creatine loading protocol showed a decrease in sprint time, while acute supplementation with guarana and caffeine increased peak power and decreased fatigue, reaction time under pressure, and time visual response.

4. Discussion

4.1. Effects of Caffeine in Racquet Sports

Caffeine has shown to be an effective ergogenic aid for aerobic and anaerobic exercise with improvements in performance and the perceptions of exertion and muscle pain with dosage ranging from 2.35 to 5 mg/kg [46,47]. A similar dosage range was used in most of the racquet sports studies that showed positive effects and a low risk of bias [26,30,40,41] with the exception of Hornery; 2007 [27] due to its methodology of randomization and blinding. Even using higher doses (6 mg/kg), the positive effects are verified [28,31,45] but with a moderate risk of bias due to aspects of randomization or blinding.

In tennis, caffeine improved power skills such as backhand stroke, serve velocity, handgrip force, and the number and velocity of sprints, as well as mental aspects such as the accuracy serve or total number of successful shots. Lower dosages such as 0.2–0.25 mg/kg before and during a tennis match or approximately 1 mg/kg 30 min before a serve test only increased epinephrine levels in urine but they have not shown any performance improvements [25,29]. Moreover, both studies have a moderate risk of bias since the control of randomization, the carry-over effect, the differences in caffeine dosage between sexes, and the lack of certain control groups could be affecting the results. In another study [26], it was shown that the use of a carbohydrate drink with or without caffeine showed improvements in sprints and serve quality compared with the placebo group. As there were no differences between both conditions, it is not possible to evaluate the real effect of caffeine in this study. Furthermore, although an increase in sweat rate has been observed with low caffeine dosages (3 mg/kg) in junior tennis players [30], several studies have disproved a dehydration risk [14].

On the other hand, handgrip force was not affected in badminton and paddle [40,45], but squat and counter jump height or power were significantly better than in the placebo group in badminton [40], offering a specific advantage in this discipline due to the net height in this sport.

In short resistance training, positive results have been observed regarding caffeine consumption in the reduction of perceived exercise exertion [47]. However, no changes were observed in racquet sports (long duration intermittent sports) with the only exception of using two intakes of 4 mg/kg caffeine before and after the first half of a badminton specific test and combining them with carbohydrates [41]. Despite these null effects, the number of total successful shots (with medium effect size (d = 0.57)) and volley precision (high effect size (d = 0.86)) were improved in tennis and paddle respectively using a high caffeine dosage (6 mg/kg) [28,45].

Therefore, the use of an acute ergogenic dosage of caffeine (3–6 mg/kg) 30–60 min before a match is better than the intake of smaller concentrations, despite its continuous use during the match. Due to the large seasons with accumulative long duration matches such as tennis, caffeine consumption could be a useful aid for all competitive levels, since it may maintain physical and mental conditions. More studies with a high caffeine dosage during long periods of intermittent exercise and in combination with carbohydrates are needed in order to prove caffeine capacity to elicit high accuracy and synergetic effects.

4.2. Effects of Creatine Monohydrate in Racquet Sports

Commonly, creatine monohydrate supplementation has been used as a strategy to increase muscle mass and strength during training, but it has been also reported to improve power and anaerobic capacity [48–50]. Thus, the use of creatine in intermittent sports such as racquet sports is of high interest since about 75% of top 100 rank tennis players take it [17]. However, up to the present, there is no evidence for recommendation.

Neither specific tennis skills, such serve or stroke, nor general physical aptitudes, such as sprints or strength (typical short-duration high-intensity movements), were improved with different protocols involving only a creatine load (20 g/day for 5 days) or load and maintenance (0.3 g/day for 6 days and 0.03 g/kg for 28 days) [32,33]. Both creatine protocols were used in two studies that had a low to moderate risk of bias.

On the contrary, in one study on squash, the intake of 0.3 g/kg creatine for 5 days was capable of improving the sprint time in a specific test on court [43]. Due to the heterogeneity of sprint protocols, it is not possible to reach a solid conclusion regarding its effect and the effect of moderate bias due to lack of information about the randomization method, carry-over effect and missing information about placebo composition. Moreover, the combination of 1 g of creatine + 1.5 g of guarana + 133 mg of caffeine in an acute dosage improved several physical and alertness aptitudes in squash players, but it has not been ruled out that the stimulant effect of guarana and caffeine were behind them [44]. Therefore, this fact—together with the lack of blinded groups—led to a high risk of bias.

Further studies should evaluate the sprint capacity or service and stroke skills with a high dosage (16 g/day or 0.3 g/kg/day) for a longer period (at least 14 days), as has been shown in previous works [49,50]. Further studies should also consider protocols that emulate long games. In addition, despite not showing any clear improvements in specific tennis skills, creatine consumption during the pre-season could be beneficial for the maintenance or increase of lean mass [50].

4.3. Effects of Buffering Supplements in Racquet Sports

High-intensity intermittent exercise tends to accumulate acid (H^+) and carbon dioxide (CO_2) in the muscle and blood. Bicarbonate coming from CO_2 acts as the primary mechanism to counteract plasma acidification. The efficiency of acute sodium bicarbonate supplementation is influenced by exercise duration. Specifically, extended duration (>4 min) sports have shown diverse results, with sodium bicarbonate improving performance in running and cycling, but not in rowing, rugby, water polo, or basketball [51].

An acute dosage (0.3 g/kg) and a continuous intake for a >4 min specific tennis test (0.1 g/kg) did not improve accuracy or perceptual exercise exertion but kept serve (small effect size (d = 0.42)) and stroke consistency (small effect size (d = 0.09)), which decreased in placebo condition [34] with a low risk of bias. On the other hand, in badminton players, only an acute dosage of 0.3 g/kg increased time to exhaustion in a treadmill test, but not in a specific test in a high risk of bias study, since the randomized method, allocation concealment, blinding method and control of diet, other supplementation consumption, and exercise load were poorly controlled [42]. Although the blood lactate level was higher than in the placebo groups in both studies, this could be due to the carboxylate co-transporter, which extracts lactate and H^+ from working muscle cell to circulation after an increase in extracellular pH [52] and an increase of glycolytic activity. Despite no changes observed in extracellular pH between placebo and sodium bicarbonate before and after tests in tennis players [34], changes between pre- and post-tests with supplementation may be enough to activate lactate extrusion due to an enhance of glycolytic metabolism.

Other buffer supplements such as sodium citrate, used for causing less gastrointestinal distress than other supplements, also showed significant high values of blood lactate compared to placebo after an acute dosage (0.3–0.5 g/kg) 90–120 min before exercise [35,42]. Nevertheless, an increase in extracellular pH was observed in tennis players, [35] which decreased in badminton players [42], but there are contradictions about it, since the text of the study indicates otherwise. On the other hand, sodium citrate was able to increase stroke consistency (high effect size (d = 1.41)) in junior tennis players, just as sodium bicarbonate did, but it did not present effects in accuracy and perceptual exercise exertion in protocols of >4 min duration [35]. With a non-specific badminton test, sodium citrate was able to improve the time to exhaustion in a treadmill test [42]. Both studies have a moderate to high risk of bias due mainly to the blinding methodology and the control of the intake of other supplementation.

More studies with a higher number of subjects would be needed with the aim of achieving strong evidence about improvements in tennis skills as well as evidencing possible synergies between different buffers (for example, beta-alanine) and other NEAs.

4.4. Effects of Nitric Oxide (NO) Precursors in Racquet Sports

It is well known that NO plays a relevant role as a second messenger. Its production is also related to an increase in blood flow, which enhances nutrient and hormone delivery. NO also has a favorable impact on resistance and endurance training adaptations [53,54]. Recent systematic reviews and meta-analysis about NO synthase-independent pathway supplements showed that potassium nitrate and sodium nitrate were less effective than beetroot juice on endurance exercise. The use of beetroot juice supplementation containing 12–6 mmol nitrate displayed significant improvements in time to exhaustion in a cycling race of 5–30 min duration but slightly non-significant improvements in time trial or graded-exercise performance [55,56].

In intermittent sports such as tennis, beetroot juice containing 6.4 mmol nitrate did not show any improvements in either explosive movements (serve velocity, jump, sprint, handgrip force) or perceptual exertion in high-level tennis players [36] with a low risk of bias. These results are similar to the ones found in recent studies in which short and high-intensity movements (such as countermovement jump, isometric strength, or muscular movement concentric velocity) were evaluated after the consumption of beetroot juice containing 6.4–17.7 mmol nitrate [57–59]. It seems that the effect of beetroot juice could be beneficial in endurance performance due to nitrate conversion to NO, affecting improvement in aerobic adenosine triphosphate (ATP) synthesis due to a reduction of VO_2. In intermittent and short-term exercise, where the anaerobic alactic system is the main source of energy, the effects are less clear. Only one-third of the studies evaluated in a recent systematic review of intermittent exercise protocols [60] showed significant results in different variables of power compared with the placebo group during repeated-sprint tests.

On the other hand, NO synthase-dependent pathway supplements, such as arginine or citrulline, have shown different results. While arginine supplementation has demonstrated improvements in both aerobic and anaerobic performance with acute (0.15 g/kg) or chronic (1.5–2.0 g/day for 4–7 weeks or 10–12 g/day for 8 weeks) protocols [61], acute protocols of citrulline supplementation (3–6 g) showed a small effect size (0.2) on high-intensity strength and power performance in resistance exercise [62]. In master female tennis players (51.0 ± 9.0 years), acute protocol with 8 g of citrulline improved handgrip strength and power peak in a specific anaerobic test, but not the capacity of sustained power or jump power [37]. Due to the lack of a washing time between conditions and control of the consumption of other stimulant substances, the risk of bias is moderate. Further studies are necessary to analyze the role of citrulline supplementation in the performance of younger racquet sports players.

Yang et al. (2017) [38] showed improvements regarding the prevention of a decrease in stroke accuracy and keeping stroke consistency and velocity (as opposed to a worsening in the placebo group) using 0.05/kg citrulline +0.05 g/kg arginine +0.17 g/kg branched-chain amino acids (BCAAs). The study presented a low risk of bias. Additionally, perceived exertion after the test decreased significantly. These results appear to be due to a lower plasma tryptophan/BCAAs ratio than placebo, since theoretically, BCAAs compete for the same tryptophan transporter across the blood–brain barrier, avoiding serotonin formation and, consequently, central fatigue instauration [63]. It is common to use a mixture of several NEAs in one product with the objective to obtain a synergic effect, but further studies are necessary in order to verify the true effects of citrulline or arginine by themselves, without the presence of the BCAAs being able to distort them.

4.5. Effects of Glycerol Supplementation in Racquet Sports

Finally, glycerol is a naturally occurring metabolite that acts as a plasma expander and could help athletes prevent dehydration and improve thermoregulatory and cardiovascular changes [14]. Until 2018, the World Anti-Doping Agency (WADA) considered glycerol a banned substance, since it was hypothesized that it may alter athlete biological passport [64]. In any case, the results of its supplementation are mixed both in endurance and anaerobic disciplines [14]. In intermittent sports such as tennis, 1.0 g/kg glycerol before followed by 0.5 g/kg after 75 min of simulated match, in environmental conditions in the range of 29–38 °C and 50–90% relative humidity (emulating conditions of important tennis tournaments such as The Australian Open Grand Slam or Miami ATP Masters 1000), was not capable of improving accuracy in serves or strokes, sprint velocity, or agility, in spite of its effect increasing pre- and post-exercise plasma volume and osmolality [39]. This study has a moderate risk of bias, since its randomized method, carry-over effect, blinding method and control of diet, and other supplementation and drug consumption were poorly controlled. More research is needed to determine glycerol's supposed potential efficacy in racquet sports during more time-prolonged matches or during several matches on the same day or on consecutive days in hot conditions.

5. Conclusions

Caffeine is the NEA showing clearer evidence of benefits for racquet sport players. Acute dosages (3–6 mg/kg) 30–60 min before a match may improve specific skills and accuracy but may not contribute to improve perceived exertion. Even though some evidence concludes that other NEAs, such as creatine, sodium bicarbonate, sodium citrate, beetroot juice, citrulline and glycerol, could play an interesting role in improving performance, more studies are needed to strengthen the evidence (Table 5).

Table 5. NEA recommendations from current evidence. Green: High level of recommendation due to the high number and quality of studies and the effects produced; Orange: Low level of recommendation due to the low number and/or quality of studies and the effects produced; Red: Not recommended due to the low number and quality of studies and contradictory or low effects.

NEA	Effects	Posology
Caffeine	- Improves specific racquet sports skills - Improves sprints and jumps - Improves mental performance and maybe accuracy	3–6 mg/kg 30–60 min before competition
Creatine	- May improve sprints	0.3 g/kg for 5 days
Sodium Bicarbonate	- May improve specific racquet sports skills - May hold up time to exhaustion	0.3 g /kg 70–90 min before competition
Sodium Citrate	- May improve specific racquet sports skills - May hold up time to exhaustion	0.3–0.5 g/kg 90–120 min before competition
Beetroot juice	- No effects	6.4 mmol 3 h before competition
Citrulline-malate	- May improve handgrip strength - May improve peak power	8 g 60 min before competition
Glycerol	- No effects	1 g/kg 150 min before competition and 0.5 g/kg 15 min after it.

Author Contributions: Conceptualization, N.V.-S. and G.S.-S.; methodology, N.V.-S. and G.S.-S.; protocol drafting, N.V.-S. and G.S.-S.; risk of bias, N.V.-S. and G.S.-S.; quality assessment, N.V.-S. and G.S.-S.; data extraction, N.V.-S. and G.S.-S.; literature search, N.V.-S. and G.S.-S.; search flowchart, N.V.-S.; writing—original draft preparation, N.V.-S. and E.R.; writing—review and editing, N.V.-S., G.S.-S. and E.R. All authors have read and agreed to the published version of the manuscript.

Funding: This study was supported by the official funding agency for biomedical research of the Spanish government, Institute of Health Carlos III (ISCIII) through CIBEROBN CB12/03/30038), which is co-funded by the European Regional Development Fund.

Acknowledgments: CIBEROBN is an initiative of Instituto de Salud Carlos III, Spain.

Conflicts of Interest: The authors declare no conflict of interest.

References

1. Lees, A. Science and the major racket sports: A review. *J. Sports Sci.* **2003**, *21*, 707–732. [CrossRef] [PubMed]
2. Martínez, B.S.A. Estudio de las características fisiológicas del tenis. *Coach. Sport Sci. Rev.* **2014**, *64*, 2–3.
3. Manrique, D.C.; Gonzalez-Badillo, J.J. Analysis of the characteristics of competitive badminton. *Br. J. Sports Med.* **2003**, *37*, 62–66. [CrossRef] [PubMed]
4. Kondrič, M.; Zagatto, A.M.; Sekulić, D. The physiological demands of table tennis: A review. *J. Sports Sci. Med.* **2013**, *12*, 362.
5. Majumdar, P.; Yadav, D. The effectiveness of training routine with reference to the physiological demand of squash match play. *Int. J. Appl. Sport. Sci.* **2009**, *21*, 28–44.
6. Vicén, P.A. *Análisis de la Estructura del Juego y Parámetros Morfológicos y Fisiológicos en Bádminton*; Facultad de Ciencias de la Actividad Física y del Deporte (INEF): Madrid, Spain, 2015.
7. Zagatto, A.M.; Morel, E.A.; Gobatto, C.A. Physiological responses and characteristics of table tennis matches determined in official tournaments. *J. Strength Cond. Res.* **2010**, *24*, 942–949. [CrossRef]
8. Wilkinson, M.; Leedale-Brown, D.; Winter, E.M. Reproducibility of physiological and performance measures from a squash-specific fitness test. *Int. J. Sports Physiol. Perform.* **2009**, *4*, 41–53. [CrossRef]
9. Fernández, J.F.; Villanueva, A.M.; Pluim, B.M.; Cepeda, N.T. Aspectos físicos y fisiológicos del tenis de competición (II). *Arch Med. Deport.* **2007**, *24*, 37–43.
10. Bergeron, M.F.; Maresh, C.; Kraemer, W.; Abraham, A.; Conroy, B.; Gabaree, C. Tennis: A physiological profile during match play. *Int. J. Sports Med.* **1991**, *12*, 474–479. [CrossRef]
11. Phomsoupha, M.; Laffaye, G. The science of badminton: Game characteristics, anthropometry, physiology, visual fitness and biomechanics. *Sport Med.* **2015**, *45*, 473–495. [CrossRef]

12. Kingsley, M.; James, N.; Kilduff, L.P.; Dietzig, R.E.; Dietzig, B. An exercise protocol that simulates the activity patterns of elite junior squash. *J. Sports Sci.* **2006**, *24*, 1291–1296. [CrossRef] [PubMed]
13. Porrini, M.; Del Bo', C. Ergogenic aids and supplements. In *Sport Endocrinol*; Karger Publishers: Basel, Switzerland, 2016; pp. 128–152.
14. Kerksick, C.M.; Wilborn, C.D.; Roberts, M.D.; Smith-Ryan, A.; Kleiner, S.M.; Jäger, R.; Collins, R.; Cooke, M.; Davis, J.N.; Galvan, E.; et al. ISSN exercise & sports nutrition review update: Research & recommendations. *J. Int. Soc. Sports Nutr.* **2018**, *15*, 38. [CrossRef] [PubMed]
15. 2018 Sports Nutrition and Weight Management Report. Available online: https://www.newhope.com/market-data-and-analysis/top-takeaways-2018-sports-nutrition-and-weight-management-report (accessed on 5 September 2020).
16. Knapik, J.J.; Steelman, R.A.; Hoedebecke, S.S.; Austin, K.G.; Farina, E.K.; Lieberman, H.R. Prevalence of dietary supplement use by athletes: Systematic review and meta-analysis. *Sport Med.* **2016**, *46*, 103–123. [CrossRef] [PubMed]
17. López-Samanes, Á.; Moreno-Pérez, V.; Kovacs, M.S.; Pallarés, J.G.; Mora-Rodríguez, R.; Ortega, J.F. Use of nutritional supplements and ergogenic aids in professional tennis players. *Nutr. Hosp.* **2017**, *34*, 1463–1468. [CrossRef]
18. Ventura Comes, A.; Sánchez-Oliver, A.J.; Martínez-Sanz, J.M.; Domínguez, R. Analysis of nutritional supplements consumption by squash players. *Nutrients* **2018**, *10*, 1341. [CrossRef]
19. Maughan, R.; Greenhaff, P.L.; Hespel, P. Dietary supplements for athletes: Emerging trends and recurring themes. *J. Sports Sci.* **2011**, *29*, S57–S66. [CrossRef]
20. Martínez-Sanz, J.M.; Sospedra, I.; Ortiz, C.M.; Baladía, E.; Gil-Izquierdo, A.; Ortiz-Moncada, R. Intended or unintended doping? A review of the presence of doping substances in dietary supplements used in sports. *Nutrients* **2017**, *9*, 1093. [CrossRef]
21. Moher, D.; Liberati, A.; Tetzlaff, J.; Altman, D.G.; Group, P. Preferred reporting items for systematic reviews and meta-analyses: The PRISMA statement. *PLoS Med.* **2009**, *6*, e1000097. [CrossRef]
22. AIS Sports Supplements Evidence Map. Available online: https://www.ais.gov.au/nutrition/supplements/evidence_map (accessed on 5 September 2020).
23. Higgins, J.P.; Altman, D.G.; Gøtzsche, P.C.; Jüni, P.; Moher, D.; Oxman, A.; Savovic, J.; Schulz, K.F.; Weeks, L.; Sterne, J.A.; et al. The Cochrane Collaboration's Tool for Assessing Risk of Bias in Randomised Trials. *BMJ* **2011**, *343*, d5928. [CrossRef]
24. Ding, H.; Hu, G.L.; Zheng, X.Y.; Chen, Q.; Threapleton, D.E.; Zhou, Z.H. The method quality of cross-over studies involved in Cochrane Systematic Reviews. *PLoS ONE* **2015**, *10*, e0120519. [CrossRef]
25. Ferrauti, A.; Weber, H.; Struder, K. Metabolic and ergogenic effects of carbohydrate and caffeine beverages in tennis. *J. Sports Med. Phys. Fit.* **1997**, *31*, 258–266. [CrossRef]
26. Vergauwen, L.; Brouns, F.; Hespel, P. Carbohydrate supplementation improves stroke performance in tennis. *Med. Sci. Sports Exerc.* **1998**, *30*, 1289–1295. [CrossRef] [PubMed]
27. Hornery, D.J.; Farrow, D.; Mujika, I.; Young, W.B. Caffeine, carbohydrate, and cooling use during prolonged simulated tennis. *Int. J. Sports Physiol. Perform.* **2007**, *2*, 423–438. [CrossRef] [PubMed]
28. Klein, C.S.; Clawson, A.; Martin, M.; Saunders, M.J.; Flohr, J.A.; Bechtel, M.K.; Dunham, W.; Hancock, M.; Womack, C.J. The effect of caffeine on performance in collegiate tennis players. *J. Caffeine Res.* **2012**, *2*, 111–116. [CrossRef]
29. Reyner, L.A.; Horne, J.A. Sleep restriction and serving accuracy in performance tennis players, and effects of caffeine. *Physiol. Behav.* **2013**, *120*, 93–96. [CrossRef]
30. Gallo-Salazar, C.; Areces, F.; Abián-Vicén, J.; Lara, B.; Salinero, J.J.; Gonzalez-Millán, C.; Portillo, J.; Muñoz, V.; Juarez, D.; Del Coso, J.; et al. Enhancing physical performance in elite junior tennis players with a caffeinated energy drink. *Int. J. Sports Physiol. Perform.* **2015**, *10*, 305–310. [CrossRef]
31. Poire, B.; Killen, L.G.; Green, J.M.; Neal, E.K.O.; Renfroe, L.G. Effects of Caffeine on Tennis Serve Accuracy. *Int. J. Exerc. Sci.* **2019**, *12*, 1290.
32. Op't Eijnde, B.; Vergauwen, L.; Hespel, P. Creatine loading does not impact on stroke performance in tennis. *Int. J. Sports Med.* **2001**, *22*, 76–80. [CrossRef]
33. Pluim, B.; Ferrauti, A.; Broekhof, F.; Deutekom, M.; Gotzmann, A.; Kuipers, H.; Weber, K. The effects of creatine supplementation on selected factors of tennis specific training. *Br. J. Sports Med.* **2006**, *40*, 507–512. [CrossRef]

34. Wu, C.-L.; Shih, M.-C.; Yang, C.-C.; Huang, M.-H.; Chang, C.-K. Sodium bicarbonate supplementation prevents skilled tennis performance decline after a simulated match. *J. Int. Soc. Sports Nutr.* **2010**, *7*, 33. [CrossRef]
35. Cunha, V.C.; Aoki, M.S.; Zourdos, M.C.; Gomes, R.V.; Barbosa, W.P.; Massa, M.; Moreira, A.; Capitani, C.D. Sodium citrate supplementation enhances tennis skill performance: A crossover, placebo-controlled, double blind study. *J. Int. Soc. Sports Nutr.* **2019**, *16*, 32. [CrossRef]
36. López-Samanes, Á.; Pérez-López, A.; Moreno-Pérez, V.; Nakamura, F.Y.; Acebes-Sánchez, J.; Quintana-Milla, I.; Sánchez-Oliver, A.J.; Moreno-Pérez, D.; Fernández-Elías, V.E.; Domínguez, R. Effects of Beetroot Juice Ingestion on Physical Performance in Highly Competitive Tennis Players. *Nutrients* **2020**, *12*, 584. [CrossRef]
37. Glenn, J.M.; Gray, M.; Jensen, A.; Stone, M.S.; Vincenzo, J.L. Acute citrulline-malate supplementation improves maximal strength and anaerobic power in female, masters athletes tennis players. *Eur. J. Sport Sci.* **2016**, *16*, 1095–1103. [CrossRef] [PubMed]
38. Yang, C.C.; Wu, C.L.; Chen, I.F.; Chang, C.K. Prevention of perceptual-motor decline by branched-chain amino acids, arginine, citrulline after tennis match. *Scand. J. Med. Sci. Sports* **2017**, *27*, 935–944. [CrossRef] [PubMed]
39. Magal, M.; Webster, M.J.; Sistrunk, L.E.; Whitehead, M.T.; Evans, R.K.; Boyd, J.C. Comparison of glycerol and water hydration regimens on tennis-related performance. *Med. Sci. Sports Exerc.* **2003**, *35*, 150–156. [CrossRef] [PubMed]
40. Abian, P.; Del Coso, J.; Salinero, J.J.; Gallo-Salazar, C.; Areces, F.; Ruiz-Vicente, D.; Lara, B.; Soriano, L.; Muñoz, V.; Abian-Vicen, J.; et al. The ingestion of a caffeinated energy drink improves jump performance and activity patterns in elite badminton players. *J. Sports Sci.* **2015**, *33*, 1042–1050. [CrossRef]
41. Clarke, N.D.; Duncan, M.J. Effect of carbohydrate and caffeine ingestion on badminton performance. *Int. J. Sports Physiol. Perform.* **2016**, *11*, 108–115. [CrossRef]
42. Hartono, S. The effects of sodium bicarbonate and sodium citrate on blood pH, HCO3-, lactate metabolism and time to exhaustion. *Sport Mont.* **2017**, *15*, 13–16.
43. Romer, L.; Barrington, J.; Jeukendrup, A. Effects of oral creatine supplementation on high intensity, intermittent exercise performance in competitive squash players. *Int. J. Sports Med.* **2001**, *22*, 546–552. [CrossRef]
44. Pomportes, L.; Davranche, K.; Hays, A.; Brisswalter, J. Effet d'un complexe créatine–guarana sur la puissance musculaire et la performance cognitive chez des sportifs de haut niveau de performance. *Sci. Sports* **2015**, *30*, 188–195. [CrossRef]
45. Müller, C.B.; Goulart, C.; Vecchio, F.B.D. Acute effects of caffeine consumption on performance in specific test paddle. *Rev. Bras. Cienc. Esporte* **2019**, *41*, 26–33. [CrossRef]
46. Ivy, J.L.; Kammer, L.; Ding, Z.; Wang, B.; Bernard, J.R.; Liao, Y.-H.; Hwang, J. Improved cycling time-trial performance after ingestion of a caffeine energy drink. *Int. J. Sport Nutr. Exerc. Metab.* **2009**, *19*, 61–78. [CrossRef] [PubMed]
47. Duncan, M.J.; Stanley, M.; Parkhouse, N.; Cook, K.; Smith, M. Acute caffeine ingestion enhances strength performance and reduces perceived exertion and muscle pain perception during resistance exercise. *Eur. J. Sport Sci.* **2013**, *13*, 392–399. [CrossRef] [PubMed]
48. Nemezio, K.M.D.A.; Bertuzzi, R.; Correia-Oliveira, C.R.; Gualano, B.; Bishop, D.J.; Lima-Silva, A.E. Effect of creatine loading on oxygen uptake during a 1-km cycling time trial. *Med. Sci. Sports Exerc.* **2015**, *47*, 2660–2668. [CrossRef]
49. Yáñez-Silva, A.; Buzzachera, C.F.; Piçarro, I.D.C.; Januario, R.S.; Ferreira, L.H.; McAnulty, S.R.; Utter, A.C.; Souza-Junior, T.P. Effect of low dose, short-term creatine supplementation on muscle power output in elite youth soccer players. *J. Int. Soc. Sports Nutr.* **2017**, *14*, 5. [CrossRef]
50. Kreider, R.B.; Ferreira, M.; Wilson, M.; Grindstaff, P.; Plisk, S.; Reinardy, J.; Cantler, E.; Almada, A.L. Effects of creatine supplementation on body composition, strength, and sprint performance. *Med. Sci. Sports Exerc.* **1998**, *30*, 73–82. [CrossRef]
51. Hadzic, M.; Eckstein, M.L.; Schugardt, M. The impact of sodium bicarbonate on performance in response to exercise duration in athletes: A systematic review. *J. Sports Sci. Med.* **2019**, *18*, 271.
52. Hollidge-Horvat, M.; Parolin, M.; Wong, D.; Jones, N.; Heigenhauser, G. Effect of induced metabolic alkalosis on human skeletal muscle metabolism during exercise. *Am. J. Physiol. Endocrinol. Metab.* **2000**, *278*, E316–E329. [CrossRef]

53. Besco, R.; Sureda, A.; Tur, J.A.; Pons, A. The effect of nitric-oxide-related supplements on human performance. *Sports Med.* **2012**, *42*, 99–117. [CrossRef]
54. Rothschild, J.A.; Bishop, D.J. Effects of dietary supplements on adaptations to endurance training. *Sports Med.* **2020**, *50*, 25–53. [CrossRef]
55. McMahon, N.F.; Leveritt, M.D.; Pavey, T.G. The effect of dietary nitrate supplementation on endurance exercise performance in healthy adults: A systematic review and meta-analysis. *Sports Med.* **2017**, *47*, 735–756. [CrossRef] [PubMed]
56. Lorenzo Calvo, J.; Alorda-Capo, F.; Pareja-Galeano, H.; Jiménez, S.L. Influence of nitrate supplementation on endurance cyclic sports performance: A systematic review. *Nutrients* **2020**, *12*, 1796. [CrossRef] [PubMed]
57. Jonvik, K.L.; Hoogervorst, D.; Peelen, H.B.; de Niet, M.; Verdijk, L.B.; van Loon, L.J.; van Dijk, J.W. The impact of beetroot juice supplementation on muscular endurance, maximal strength and countermovement jump performance. *Eur. J. Sport Sci.* **2020**, 1–8. [CrossRef] [PubMed]
58. Ranchal-Sanchez, A.; Diaz-Bernier, V.M.; La Florida-Villagran, D.; Alonso, C.; Llorente-Cantarero, F.J.; Campos-Perez, J. Acute Effects of Beetroot Juice Supplements on Resistance Training: A Randomized Double-Blind Crossover. *Nutrients* **2020**, *12*, 1912. [CrossRef]
59. Cuenca, E.; Jodra, P.; Pérez-López, A.; González-Rodríguez, L.G.; Fernandes da Silva, S.; Veiga-Herreros, P.; Domínguez, R. Effects of beetroot juice supplementation on performance and fatigue in a 30-s all-out sprint exercise: A randomized, double-blind cross-over study. *Nutrients* **2018**, *10*, 1222. [CrossRef]
60. Rojas-Valverde, D.; Montoya-Rodríguez, J.; Azofeifa-Mora, C.; Sanchez-Urena, B. Effectiveness of beetroot juice derived nitrates supplementation on fatigue resistance during repeated-sprints: A systematic review. *Crit Rev. Food Sci. Nutr.* **2020**, 1–12. [CrossRef]
61. Viribay, A.; Burgos, J.; Fernández-Landa, J.; Seco-Calvo, J.; Mielgo-Ayuso, J. Effects of Arginine Supplementation on Athletic Performance Based on Energy Metabolism: A Systematic Review and Meta-Analysis. *Nutrients* **2020**, *12*, 1300. [CrossRef]
62. Trexler, E.T.; Persky, A.M.; Ryan, E.D.; Schwartz, T.A.; Stoner, L.; Smith-Ryan, A.E. Acute effects of citrulline supplementation on high-intensity strength and power performance: A systematic review and meta-analysis. *Sports Med.* **2019**, *49*, 707–718. [CrossRef]
63. Blomstrand, E.; Hassmén, P.; Ek, S.; Ekblom, B.; Newsholme, E. Influence of ingesting a solution of branched-chain amino acids on perceived exertion during exercise. *Acta Physiol. Scand.* **1997**, *159*, 41–49. [CrossRef]
64. WADA-AMA. Available online: https://www.wada-ama.org/en/questions-answers/prohibited-list-qa (accessed on 7 August 2020).

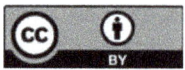

© 2020 by the authors. Licensee MDPI, Basel, Switzerland. This article is an open access article distributed under the terms and conditions of the Creative Commons Attribution (CC BY) license (http://creativecommons.org/licenses/by/4.0/).

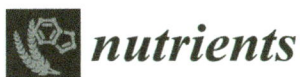

Article

Pre-Sleep Low Glycemic Index Modified Starch Does Not Improve Next-Morning Fuel Selection or Running Performance in Male and Female Endurance Athletes

Monique D. Dudar [1], Emilie D. Bode [1], Karly R. Fishkin [1], Rochelle A. Brown [1], Madeleine M. Carre [1], Noa R. Mills [1], Michael J. Ormsbee [2,3] and Stephen J. Ives [1,*]

1. Health and Human Physiological Sciences, Skidmore College, Saratoga Springs, NY 12866, USA; mdudar@skidmore.edu (M.D.D.); ebode@skidmore.edu (E.D.B.); kfishkin@skidmore.edu (K.R.F.); rbrown@skidmore.edu (R.A.B.); mcarre@skidmore.edu (M.M.C.); nmills@skidmore.edu (N.R.M.)
2. Department of Nutrition, Food, and Exercise Sciences, Institute of Sport Sciences and Medicine, Florida State University, Tallahassee, FL 32306, USA; mormsbee@fsu.edu
3. Department of Biokinetics, Exercise and Leisure Sciences, School of Health Sciences, University of KwaZulu-Natal, Durban 4041, South Africa
* Correspondence: sives@skidmore.edu; Tel.: +1-518-580-8366

Received: 30 August 2020; Accepted: 17 September 2020; Published: 22 September 2020

Abstract: To determine the effects of pre-sleep supplementation with a novel low glycemic index (LGI) carbohydrate (CHO) on next-morning substrate utilization, gastrointestinal distress (GID), and endurance running performance (5-km time-trial, TT). Using a double-blind, randomized, placebo (PLA) controlled, crossover design, trained participants ($n = 14$; 28 ± 9 years, 8/6 male/female, 55 ± 7 mL/kg/min) consumed a LGI, high glycemic index (HGI), or 0 kcal PLA supplement ≥ 2 h after their last meal and <30 min prior to sleep. Upon arrival, resting energy expenditure (REE), substrate utilization, blood glucose, satiety, and GID were assessed. An incremental exercise test (IET) was performed at 55, 65, and 75% peak volume of oxygen consumption (VO_{2peak}) with GID, rating of perceived exertion (RPE) and substrate utilization recorded each stage. Finally, participants completed the 5-km TT. There were no differences in any baseline measure. During IET, CHO utilization tended to be greater with LGI (PLA, 56 ± 11; HGI, 60 ± 14; LGI, 63 ± 14%, $p = 0.16$, $\eta^2 = 0.14$). GID was unaffected by supplementation at any point ($p > 0.05$). Performance was also unaffected by supplement (PLA, 21.6 ± 9.5; HGI, 23.0 ± 7.8; LGI, 24.1 ± 4.5 min, $p = 0.94$, $\eta^2 = 0.01$). Pre-sleep CHO supplementation did not affect next-morning resting metabolism, BG, GID, or 5-km TT performance. The trend towards higher CHO utilization during IET after pre-sleep LGI, suggests that such supplementation increases morning CHO availability.

Keywords: exercise; carbohydrates; time trial; substrate utilization; fat oxidation; fatigue; gastrointestinal distress; satiety

1. Introduction

The importance of pre-exercise nutrition for exercise performance has been well documented [1–6]. However, given that many competitive endurance activities (training and/or competition) are scheduled early in the morning, there exists a major limitation: inadequate time in the morning prior to the event to properly fuel for sport. In addition, endurance athletes seldom consume much, if anything, before training or competitions of 75–90 min in duration [7–11]. Unfortunately, this behavior may result in sub-optimal physiological conditions such as carbohydrate depletion, dehydration, and fatigue [12], which will adversely impact training quality and performance. This issue highlights the need to develop strategies to provide adequate nutrition from foods, beverages, and/or supplements that athletes can consume pre-sleep without inducing gastrointestinal distress (GID) or disrupting normal sleep patterns [6,8]. As an intervention, the incorporation of a pre-sleep meal may provide an added "window of opportunity" for optimizing next-morning pre-race carbohydrate (CHO) availability and exercise performance.

Glucose is the body's preferred energy substrate during endurance exercise. Currently, high glycemic index (HGI) CHOs are utilized by most athletes for pre- and/or intra-exercise nutrition due to their rapid breakdown which drastically increases blood glucose availability. However, complications such as GID, may arise with the consumption of HGI CHO sources prior to or during exercise due to the gastrointestinal sensitivity to nutrient intake [13]. Consequently, this raises the question as to the role of low glycemic index (LGI) CHO for exercise performance and nutrient timing. Contrary to a HGI, a LGI slowly digests carbohydrates, thus providing more stable and long-lasting glucose release, which may lower GID, both of which may better support endurance exercise performance [14].

Previous literature agrees that consuming LGI CHO prior to exercise results in enhanced fat oxidation [15–18], and likely improved exercise performance [14,19]. However, not all studies agree [20–23]. Stevenson and colleagues [22,23] investigated the effects of a low vs. high glycemic index evening meal, approximately 16 h prior (at 19:00 p.m.), on next-morning metabolic responses at rest and during exercise in males [23] and females [22]. Though in these studies [22,23] participants were fed a standard HGI breakfast (at 08:00 a.m.) three hours prior to a 60-min run at 65% VO_{2max}. Although the breakfast elicited immediate post-prandial effects (lower glycemic and insulinemic responses), there was no significant effect of the previous evening's dinner glycemic index on substrate utilization at rest or during running [22,23]. Though, given that meals were consumed 16 h prior to testing, and participants were given a standardized HGI breakfast in the morning, it is not surprising that any residual metabolic effects could not be detected. Given these limitations, it remains unknown if pre-sleep CHO supplementation can optimize next-morning endurance athlete fuel selection and performance, and whether low or high glycemic index would be preferential.

Though a LGI is touted as an efficacious source of CHO, a novel hydrothermally modified LGI starch supplement was developed to manage glucose levels by providing a slow and steady release of glucose to the body and brain for up to ten hours at a time [24]. In fact, data indicate a lower peak and less rapid rate of decline in blood glucose than conventional cornstarch, which is already considered a LGI CHO [25,26]. Currently, only a few studies have included the use of this novel LGI CHO supplement [15,17,21,27] all of which included supplement ingestion either before, during, or after exercise. No studies have investigated the effects of pre-sleep ingestion of a modified CHO on next-morning exercise metabolism and performance. However, there is a plethora of data investigating protein pre-sleep. The only study, to date, that investigated pre-sleep CHO-type beverage was conducted by Ormsbee et al. (2016) [28]. The authors investigated the effect of pre-sleep chocolate milk (HGI and protein) on endurance performance and found that chocolate milk resulted in increased carbohydrate oxidation in the morning, but effects did not translate to 10-km running performance improvements in females [28]. Given these data, we want to explore the effects of pre-sleep LGI CHO since it has the potential to have a positive impact based on the slow/long-lasting release of glucose, the lasting satiety, and if a HGI increases CHO oxidation, it is reasonable to suspect that LGI CHO would have the opposite effect, as noted in acute day of studies.

Accordingly, the purpose of this study was to determine the effects of nighttime pre-sleep supplementation with a novel LGI CHO on the next morning: (1) resting metabolism and GID; (2) metabolic and GID responses to incremental exercise; and (3) 5-km time trial running performance in trained male and female endurance athletes. It was hypothesized that the nighttime pre-sleep consumption of LGI CHO would, in the next morning, enhance fat utilization during exercise, decrease GID, and improve 5-km running time compared to a HGI CHO and a placebo (PLA) control.

2. Materials and Methods

2.1. Subjects

Trained male ($n = 8$) and female ($n = 6$) endurance runners between the ages of 18 and 45 years were recruited to participate in this study from local running clubs, triathlon teams, by word of mouth, flyers, and through an email distribution around the Skidmore College campus. Participants were included if they met the peak volume of oxygen consumption (VO_{2peak}) qualifications (women: $VO_{2peak} \geq 40$ mL·kg^{-1}·min^{-1} and men: $VO_{2peak} \geq 45$ mL·kg^{-1}·min^{-1}). Menstrual cycle status was recorded for all female participants, though they were scheduled independently of the menstrual cycle phase; notably, 3 out of 6 female participants did not have a menstrual cycle due to hormonal or contraceptive therapy. Participants were excluded if they smoked, had uncontrolled thyroid conditions, had been diagnosed with cardiac or metabolic disorders, regularly consumed anti-inflammatory drugs or any dietary supplements intended to improve performance, or had musculoskeletal injury that limited performance. All experimental procedures and risks of participation were explained verbally and in writing prior to participants providing written informed consent. Approval for this study was granted by the Human Subjects Institutional Review Board (IRB# 1901-786) of Skidmore College and is in accordance with the most recent revisions of the Declaration of Helsinki.

2.2. General Procedures

This was a double-blinded randomized placebo-controlled study included four total trials: one familiarization trial and three experimental trials. For the experimental trials, participants were randomly assigned to consume either (1) LGI, (2) HGI, or (3) PLA at least 2 h after their last meal and within 30 min prior to sleep on the evening before returning to the laboratory. Participants then arrived to the lab in the morning after an overnight fast (~7–9 h after supplement consumption) for an incremental exercise test (IET) and 5-km time trial (TT) (See Figure 1). Prior to the first experimental trial, participants were required to complete a one-day dietary food and exercise log. Participants were asked to replicate this diet and exercise, as closely as possible, prior to subsequent exercise trials. Participants abstained from the use of non-steroidal anti-inflammatory drugs, caffeine, alcohol, and/or vigorous activity at least 24 h prior to each experimental trial.

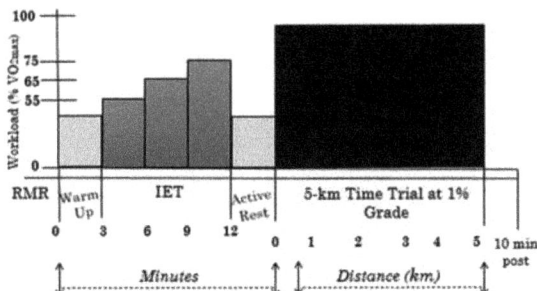

Figure 1. Experimental Overview; RMR = resting metabolic rate; IET: incremental exercise test.

2.3. Supplementation

Over the span of the study, all participants were randomized to the order in which they received each of the following three supplements: (1) 532 mL of water mixed with 75 g of a HMS (LGI; Orange Flavor, SuperStarch®, The UCAN Co., Woodbridge, CT, USA) (270 kcal; 0 g PRO; 66 g CHO; 0 g FAT), (2) 532 mL of water mixed with 75 g of a HGI glucose-based supplement (Orange flavor, Gatorade®, PepsiCo, Inc., Purchase, NY, USA) (270 kcal; 0 g PRO; 67 g CHO; 0 g FAT), and (3) 532 mL of water mixed with a color and flavor-matched, non-nutritive PLA (PLA; Orange CRUSH flavor packet and Benefiber), with a volume of the powder visually similar to the other experimental conditions. Beverages were of similar taste, appearance, and consistency. The supplements were pre-packaged in inconspicuously labeled/coded opaque containers by a researcher not otherwise involved in the study.

2.4. Familiarization Protocol

Participants filled out a physical activity readiness questionnaire (PAR-Q), ACSM health preparticipation screening questionnaire, and a menstrual cycle history form (females only). Height was measured using a stadiometer (Seca 213, portable stadiometer, Chino, CA, USA), while body composition and weight were measured using air displacement plethysmography (BOD POD; COSMED, Chicago, IL, USA) [29].

Peak volume of oxygen consumption (VO_{2peak}) testing was performed to assess baseline cardiorespiratory fitness and inclusion in the study. Gas exchange and ventilatory parameters were measured with a metabolic cart system (TrueOne 2400 Parvomedics, Salt Lake City, UT, USA) [30]. For each individual trial, the metabolic system was calibrated by a flow-calibration with a 3-L calibration syringe and gas analyzer calibration with gas mixture of known concentrations of oxygen (O_2) and carbon dioxide (CO_2) (16% O_2; 4% CO_2) according to manufacturer specifications, in addition to environmental data for standardization purposes. Participants were fitted with a nose clip, two-way non-rebreathe valve, and mouthpiece which was supported by a headpiece in order to collect expiratory gases for analysis by the metabolic cart. The VO_{2peak} protocol was performed on a treadmill (Woodway PPS Med, Waukesha, WI) and the protocol required a self-selected constant pace that was "comfortable but challenging." Once the appropriate speed was determined, grade was increased at a rate of 2% every two minutes until the participant reached volitional fatigue [28]. During the last 15 s of each stage, HR was measured using a chest worn HR monitor (H7, Polar USA, Lake Success, NY, USA) and RPE was measured on a 1–10 categorical ratio scale.

2.5. Experimental Protocol

A recovery period of >72 h was required after the familiarization trial and between each testing day for all participants. On average, the time between trials was 192 ± 168 h. As sleep may have influenced exercise performance we asked participants to self-report their sleep duration prior to each visit. Participants then returned to the laboratory the following morning in a fasted, but well-hydrated, state between 05:30 and 08:30 a.m. Upon arrival, participants were asked to provide a urine sample to measure urine specific gravity using a hand-held refractometer to confirm hydration status [8]. Participants were provided with 250 mL of water to consume at their leisure before exercise and an additional 250 mL of water if their urine specific gravity indicated dehydration (>1.020). Thereafter, baseline measurements for height, weight, body composition, resting HR, satiety, GID, resting energy expenditure (REE), and capillary blood glucose (BG) were collected. GID and satiety were measured via a 100-mm visual analog scale (VAS) during baseline and one-minute post 5-km TT for each of the three experimental trials [31–33]. Each VAS scale was marked with "0 mm" (no GID; extreme hunger) and "100 mm" (extreme GID; extremely full) and participants were asked to draw a vertical line indicating their perceived GID and satiety accordingly. Both VAS and categorical scale have been documented in the literature as reliable perceptual measures of pain or discomfort [31–33].

REE was collected while participants rested quietly in a seated position with the headpiece and mask on for 15 min in a climate-controlled room with the metabolic cart system described above. Respiratory exchange ratio (RER) was recorded and relative substrate utilization (%FAT and %CHO) was estimated [34]. The last ten minutes were used for data analysis. Resting HR was then measured followed by blood sampling via finger stick. Capillary BG concentrations were measured using a commercially available glucometer (OneTouch Ultra 2 LifeScan, Milpitas, CA, USA) [35].

2.6. Incremental Exercise Test and 5-km Time Trial

Fifteen minutes following completion of baseline measurements, participants completed a three-minute warm up at a self-selected pace on the treadmill. Following the warm up, participants completed an incremental exercise test (IET) comprising of three stages of three minutes each at exercise intensities of 55, 65, and 75% of VO_{2peak} [34]. HR, RPE, and GID were recorded during the last 15 s of each three minute each stage. GID and RPE were measured during exercise using a categorical scale [31–33]. Upon completion of the IET, participants were given a five-minute active rest period where they were instructed to walk on the treadmill at a comfortable pace to allow their HR to return closer to baseline. Participants were allowed to use the restroom quickly as long as a researcher monitored them for safety. Following the active rest period, participants completed a 5-km TT. The TT was conducted rather than time-to-exhaustion to better mimic competition and pacing demands [36] and due to greater reliability in the repeatability of the results [37]. Participants were instructed to treat each TT as a competitive event and accordingly provide maximal effort. Participants could only see their distance during the TT and the time and speed were blinded. Additionally, participants ran both the IET and 5-km TT at 1% grade to best simulate the oxygen cost of outdoor running [38]. HR, RPE, and GID measurements were taken every 1 km. BG and HR were measured immediately post exercise and 10 min post exercise. HR, GID (VAS), and satiety (VAS) were also recorded one minute post 5-km TT.

2.7. Statistical Analysis

A sample size estimation was conducted (G*power, sample size estimator v.3.1.9.4; Kiel, Germany) for F-test family in a repeated measures design, using the following parameters: average effect size of night time supplementation of 0.39 on CHO oxidation [28], alpha level of 0.05, and minimal power of 0.8, which revealed a minimum sample size of 13 participants. Enrollment was targeted beyond this minimum in the possible event of dropout. All statistical analyses were performed using commercially available software (SPSS v.25, IBM, Armonk, NY, USA). A one-way repeated measures ANOVA was used to determine if differences existed at baseline across conditions (PLA, HGI, LGI). A two-way repeated measures ANOVA was used to analyze the potential impact of condition (PLA, HGI, LGI), exercise intensity (55, 65, 75% VO_{2peak}), and their potential interaction on HR, RPE, GID, RER, % FAT and % CHO utilization. Two-way repeated measures ANOVA models were used to compare condition (PLA, HGI, LGI), distance (each km), and their potential interaction on RPE, HR, and GID during the 5-km TT. Lastly, a two-way ANOVA was used to determine potential differences across condition (PLA, HGI, LGI), time (baseline, one and ten minutes post 5-km TT), and their potential interaction on BG. Tests of normality were performed and Greenhouse–Geisser corrections were utilized if sphericity was violated. As men and women were recruited for this study, exploratory multi-variate ANOVA measures were conducted including sex as an independent covariate in the model for the above analyses. Significant main effects were followed up using Tukey's Honestly Significant Difference, and p values were complemented by effect size, which in this model we used partial eta squared (η^2). Alpha was set at 0.05. Data are presented as means ± standard deviation.

3. Results

3.1. Participants

Fourteen healthy endurance trained males ($n = 8$) and females ($n = 6$) completed all visits for this study. An overview of subject characteristics is presented in Table 1. There were no differences in self-reported sleep duration between visits ($p = 0.56$, $\eta^2 = 0.05$, Table 1).

Table 1. Subject Characteristics.

Characteristic	Combined	Male	Female
Sex (n, M/F)	14	8	6
Age (years)	28 ± 9	29 ± 9	27 ± 10
Height (cm)	169.3 ± 10.4	176.0 ± 7.1	160.4 ± 6.8 *
Weight (kg)	64.3 ± 9.8	70.1 ± 7.8	56.5 ± 6.2 *

Table 1. Cont.

Characteristic	Combined	Male	Female
Body fat (%)	18.9 ± 5.6	14.7 ± 3.5	23.9 ± 2.5 *
VO_{2peak} (mL·kg^{-1}·min^{-1})	55.4 ± 6.9	59.5 ± 5.5	49.9 ± 4.3 *

Note: Data expressed as means ± SD. VO_{2peak}, peak oxygen uptake. * $p < 0.05$ male vs. female.

3.2. Effects of Supplement on Baseline Measures

Resting metabolic data are displayed in Table 2. There was no significant effect of supplement on baseline REE (PLA, 1689 ± 278; HGI, 1701 ± 308; LGI, 1732 ± 287 kcal·day^{-1}, $p = 0.72$, $\eta^2 = 0.03$; Table 2). There was a significant interaction of supplement and sex for baseline RER, and thus relative substrate utilization where males displayed a higher %FAT (PLA, 47.6 ± 5.4; HGI, 51.3 ± 11.5; LGI, 48.9 ± 11.8%, $p = 0.02$, $\eta^2 = 0.28$) utilization compared to females (PLA, 46.9 ± 13.9; HGI, 28.3 ± 13.7; LGI, 34.5 ± 22.2%, $p = 0.02$, $\eta^2 = 0.28$) at rest for HGI and LGI. However, all other baseline measures were unaffected by the supplement at baseline (all $p > 0.05$, Table 2).

Table 2. Baseline Measurements.

	Supplement			
Variable	PLA	HGI	LGI	p Value
Visual Analogue Scale (VAS) (mm)				
Gastrointestinal Distress (GID)	22.4 ± 25.8	20.6 ± 22.5	26.2 ± 26.0	0.59
Satiety	55.3 ± 13.3	53.6 ± 23.0	50.3 ± 27.2	0.73
Substrate Oxidation				
FAT (%)	47.3 ± 9.5	41.4 ± 16.8	42.7 ± 17.8	0.16
Carbohydrate (CHO) (%)	53.2 ± 9.6	59.1 ± 16.9	57.8 ± 18.0	0.16
VO_2 (mL/kg/min)	3.9 ± 0.4	3.8 ± 0.4	3.8 ± 0.4	0.84
Resting Energy Expenditure (REE) (kcal·day^{-1})	1689 ± 278	1701 ± 308	1732 ± 287	0.72
HR (bpm)	57.7 ± 8.8	57.3 ± 10.6	59.9 ± 10.0	0.06
Blood Glucose (BG) (mg·dL^{-1})	97.7 ± 8.1	99.4 ± 8.8	98.4 ± 9.3	0.85
Urine Specific Gravity (USG) (a.u.)	1.02 ± 0.01	1.02 ± 0.01	1.02 ± 0.01	0.91
Sleep (h)	7.2 ± 0.8	7.2 ± 0.9	6.9 ± 1.2	0.68

Note: Data are means ± SD. PLA: placebo; HGI: high glycemic index; LGI: low glycemic index; VAS: visual analogue scale; GID: gastrointestinal distress; REE: resting energy expenditure; BG: blood glucose; USG: urine specific gravity. Data expressed as means ± SD.

3.3. Effects of Supplement on the Response to the Incremental Exercise Test (IET)

On average, during the IET, the LGI supplement tended to utilize less FAT (PLA, 44.1 ± 10.5; HGI, 39.7 ± 13.0; LGI, 37.5 ± 13.7%, $p = 0.17$, $\eta^2 = 0.14$) and more CHO (PLA, 56.4 ± 10.6; HGI, 60.1 ± 14.3; LGI, 63.1 ± 13.9%, $p = 0.17$, $\eta^2 = 0.14$; Figure 2) than the other two supplements, though this did not reach statistical significance. During the IET, there was no significant effect of supplement on VO_2 ($p = 0.23$, $\eta^2 = 0.11$, Figure 2C) or RER ($p = 0.17$, $\eta^2 = 0.14$, Figure 2D). There was a tendency for an interaction of supplement with intensity for VO_2 where values tended to be lower with the PLA during the lower intensity but equalized in the latter stages ($p = 0.08$, $\eta^2 = 0.18$, Figure 2D). Expectedly, all metabolic parameters were significantly affected by exercise intensity (all $p < 0.001$, all $\eta^2 > 0.90$, Figure 2A–D). The IET elicited an increase in GID ($p = 0.04$, $\eta^2 = 0.23$, Figure 3) and RPE ($p = 0.00$, $\eta^2 = 1.00$, data not shown). Supplementation had no effect on GID ($p = 0.28$, $\eta^2 = 0.10$, Figure 3) or RPE ($p = 0.55$, $\eta^2 = 0.05$, data not shown).

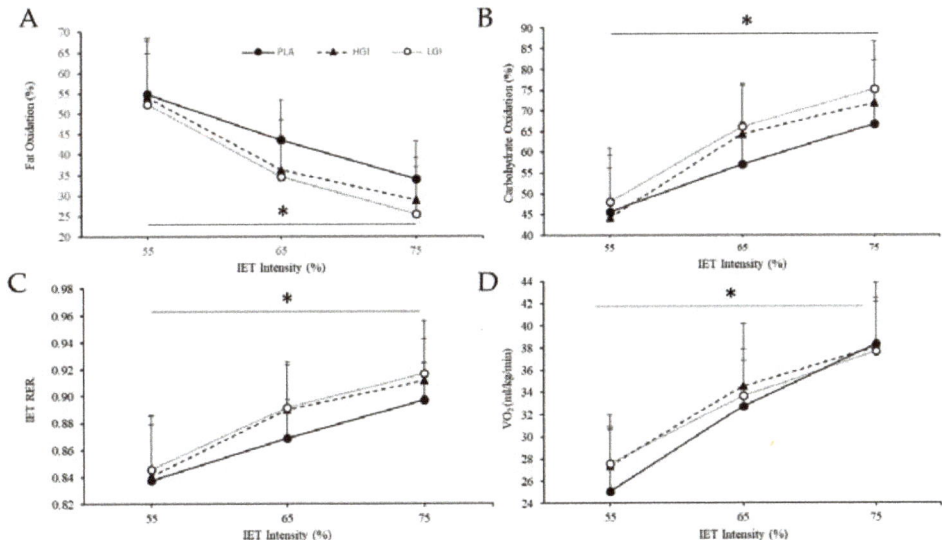

Figure 2. Metabolic Response to incremental exercise test (IET) at 55, 65, and 75% of VO_{2peak} between placebo (PLA), high glycemic index (HGI), and low glycemic index (LGI) supplements ($n = 14$). (**A**) Relative fat utilization (%FAT), (**B**) relative carbohydrate utilization (%CHO), (**C**) respiratory exchange ratio, and (**D**) VO_2. Data expressed as means ± SD. * effect of intensity, $p < 0.001$.

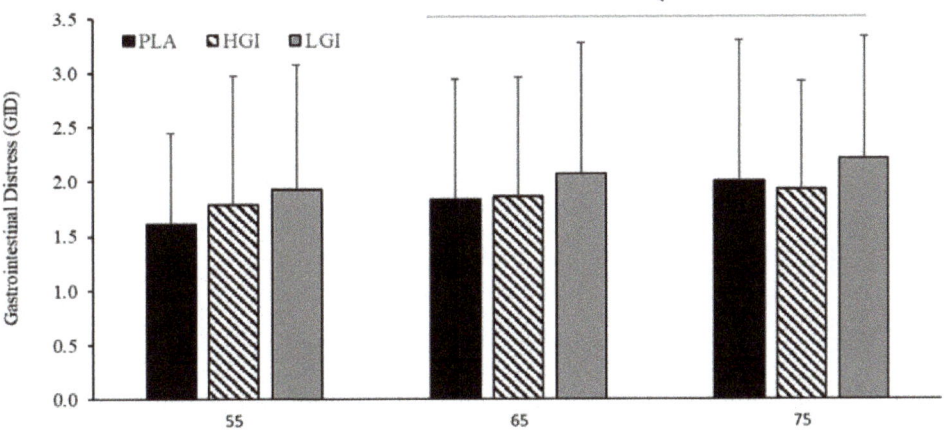

Figure 3. Gastrointestinal distress (GID; categorical scale) during incremental exercise trial (IET) at 55, 65, and 75% of VO_{2peak} ($n = 14$) between placebo (PLA), high glycemic index (HGI), and low glycemic index (LGI) supplements. Data expressed as means ± SD. * effect of intensity, $p = 0.04$.

3.4. Effect of Supplement on 5-km TT

Supplement had no impact on HR during the 5-km TT ($p = 0.89$, $\eta^2 = 0.01$, Figure 4A). Although there was a significant effect of running distance during the 5-km TT on GID (categorical scale) ($p = 0.00$, $\eta^2 = 0.58$), there was no significant effect of supplement or an interaction of supplement by distance on GID (categorical scale) during the 5-km TT (Figure 4B). RPE was not impacted by supplement ($p = 0.35$, $\eta^2 = 0.01$, Figure 4C). Running performance during the 5-km TT was unaffected by supplement (PLA, 21.6 ± 9.5; HGI, 23.0 ± 7.8; LGI, 24.1 ± 4.5 min, $p = 0.94$, $\eta^2 = 0.01$, Figure 4D).

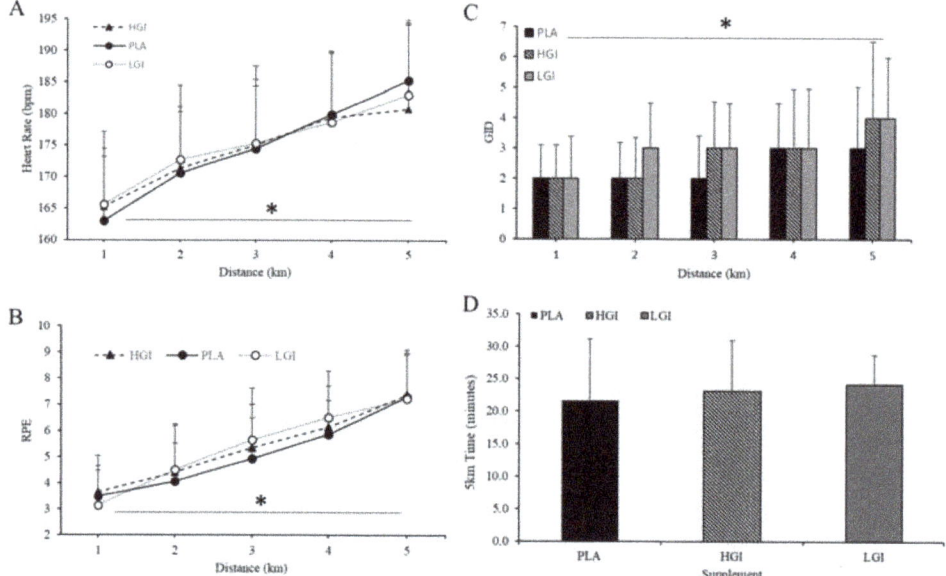

Figure 4. (**A**) Heart rate (HR), (**B**) gastrointestinal distress (GID, CS), (**C**) rating of perceived exertion (RPE) and (**D**) time (min) for 5-km time trial performance between placebo (PLA), high glycemic index (HGI), and low glycemic index (LGI) supplements ($n = 14$). Data expressed as means ± SD. * significant effect for distance $p < 0.05$.

3.5. Effect of Supplement on Perceptual Responses of GID and Satiety to Exercise

Supplement had no significant effect on satiety from pre- to post-experimental trial ($p = 0.39$, $\eta^2 = 0.08$; Figure 5A). There was no significant effect of supplement or time on pre- to post-experimental trial GID (VAS) (Figure 5B, $p = 0.56$, $\eta^2 = 0.03$).

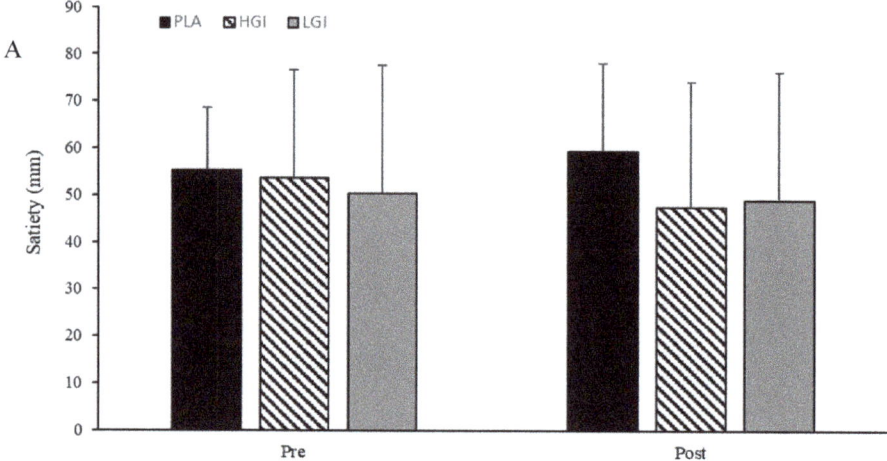

Figure 5. *Cont.*

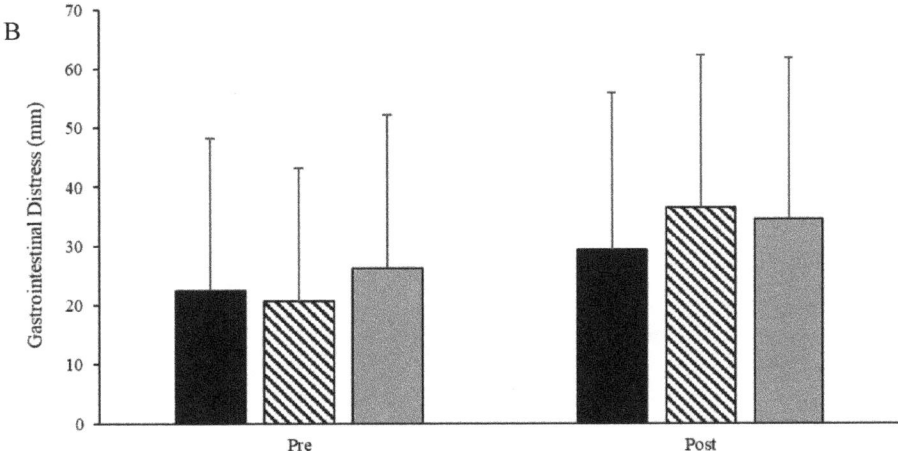

Figure 5. (**A**) Satiety (mm; VAS) and (**B**) gastrointestinal distress (GID; mm; VAS) at baseline (pre) and at conclusion (post) of running the 5-km time trial performance between placebo (PLA), high glycemic index (HGI), and low glycemic index (LGI) supplements ($n = 14$). Data expressed as means ± SD.

3.6. Blood Glucose (BG)

There were significant main effects for time ($p = 0.00$, $\eta^2 = 0.66$), where blood glucose at baseline (PLA, 97.7 ± 8.1; HGI, 99.4 ± 8.8; LGI, 98.4 ± 9.3 mg·dL^{-1}) was significantly increased immediately post-exercise (PLA, 127.2 ± 19.4; HGI, 131.0 ± 28.8; LGI, 124.4 ± 27.9 mg·dL^{-1}, $p = 0.00$) and ten minutes post-exercise (PLA, 127.6 ± 23.9; HGI, 133.3 ± 24.6; LGI, 126.7 ± 23.3 mg·dL^{-1}, $p = 0.00$; Figure 6), but no differences were observed between immediate and ten minutes post exercise. There were no significant differences in BG between supplements ($p = 0.54$, $\eta^2 = 0.04$) at any time point or an interaction ($p = 0.87$, $\eta^2 = 0.02$).

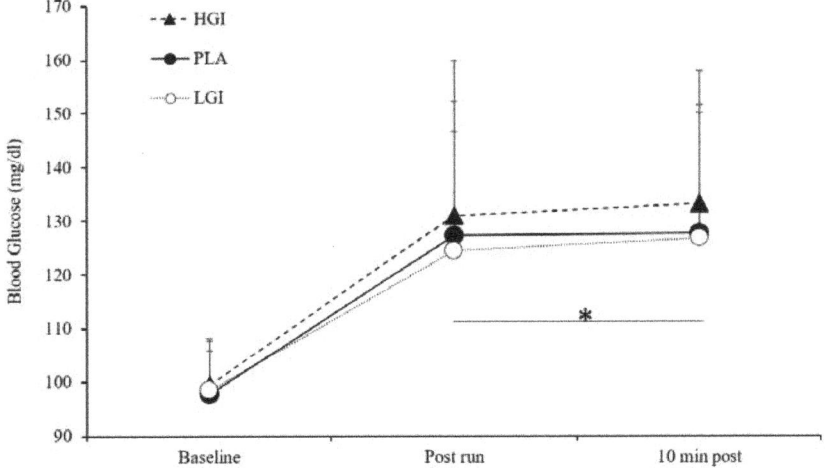

Figure 6. Blood glucose levels (mg·dL^{-1}) at baseline, 1 min post 5-km TT run, and 10 min post 5-km TT run trial between placebo (PLA), high glycemic index (HGI), and low glycemic index (LGI) supplements ($n = 14$). Data expressed as means ± SD. * significant effect of time, $p = 0.00$.

4. Discussion

The present study is the first to assess the effects of pre-sleep supplementation with a novel LGI CHO as compared to HGI CHO or placebo control on next-morning (~8 h later) exercise metabolism, GID, and endurance performance in male and female endurance athletes. It was hypothesized that the nighttime pre-sleep consumption of LGI CHOs would increase fat utilization during morning exercise, decrease GID, and improve 5-km TT performance. The primary findings were as follows: (1) supplementation had no significant effect on REE, CHO, or FAT utilization at rest, though females tended to utilize more CHO in the HGI and LGI supplement at rest; (2) supplementation had no significant effect on substrate utilization during graded submaximal exercise; (3) blood glucose was not different among supplements at any point during the trial; (4) perceptions of GID were not different among supplements; (5) supplementation had no discernable significant effect on 5-km TT performance. Although our data do not support our original hypothesis, the present study suggests that there are no detrimental effects of supplementing with either LGI or HGI CHO pre-sleep in endurance athletes and thus, they may be utilized as a feeding window and fueling strategy to ingest adequate daily energy intake.

The gastrointestinal tract can be very sensitive to the foods and beverages we consume. Unfortunately, nutrient ingestion prior to and during exercise may lead to GID. Baur and colleagues (2016) reported that GID increased after the consumption of the same hydrothermally modified starch (HMS) LGI supplement that our current study used [15]. Baur et al. (2016) compared the HMS to an HGI CHO supplement when ingested prior to, and during, prolonged cycling in ten trained male cyclists and triathletes [15]. It was reported that there were likely large correlations between mean sprint nausea ($r = -0.51$) and total GID ($r = -0.53$) and exercise trial, showing that GID contributed to reduced cycling performance [15]. Further, there was a HMS-associated increase in GID negatively effecting sprint cycling performance [15]. Given that HMS is slow releasing under normal digestion supplements, malabsorption may be the explanation for the primary pathophysiologic mechanism of LGI CHO-induced GID during exercise. Unlike the findings of Baur et al. (2016), the present study found no effect (positive or negative) on GID and performance. Perhaps the pre-sleep ingestion of LGI CHO avoids the LGI CHO-induced increase in GID in morning endurance performance. This is likely because the body can digest the LGI CHO during the overnight period. Participants in the Baur et al. (2016) study consumed LGI CHO during the exercise as well, which likely caused the incidences of GID with HMS ingestion [15].

An LGI CHO may still be an optimal source of CHO for athletes given its previously reported low osmolality, low insulin impact, slow release factor, and maintenance of blood glucose levels [5,24–26]. In general, elevated insulin levels attenuate lipolysis and fat metabolism, thus increasing utilization of CHO. Even though it is well documented that consuming LGI carbohydrates before exercising results in enhanced fat oxidation, or at least maintaining euglycemia during exercise [17,18,21,39–43], and possibly improved performance [44], though not all agree [16,20]. Data from the present study, albeit in a different methodological approach, do not support these findings, as we found no effect of LGI CHO, or HGI CHO for that matter. When comparing LGI to HGI, some studies have reported enhanced exercise performance [19,39,43,45,46] while other studies report no differences [41,42,47–50]. For example, Baur et al. (2016) reported an increase in total FAT oxidation and reduction in CHO oxidation with LGI supplementation 30 min before as well as during exercise [15], which disagrees with the findings of the present study utilizing pre-sleep supplementation of LGI. These inconsistencies may be explained by, principally, time but other methodological differences, such as timing or dose of CHO supplementation, type of exercise protocol (i.e., cycling versus running), or sample size should also be considered. Researchers have reported muscle glycogen sparing with LGI compared to HGI CHO [47], which may be explained by improved fat oxidation. Our findings are in accordance with previous literature that LGI and HGI CHO do not improve running TT performances [21,28].

Glycemic control is extremely important for those training and competing in endurance competitions and increasing fat oxidation could potentially benefit performance by preserving glycogen stores [51]. To maximize glucose fueling, the timing of pre-exercise consumption of CHO is essential, along with the type/amount of exercise being performed. The time of consumption may alter the metabolic effects. Studies have shown that CHO consumed one to four hours prior to exercise resulted in a decline in glucose and insulin basal levels prior to exercise [2,52]. Further research has reported that CHO consumed ≤ 60 min before exercise leads to elevated blood glucose and insulin levels immediately prior to exercise [47,53–55]. These findings emphasize the importance of nutrient timing and the exploring how the body performs from nutrient consumption solely the night before exercise takes place.

The trend towards higher CHO utilization during exercise after pre-sleep consumption of HGI or LGI CHO, perhaps more so in LGI, might suggest that pre-sleep LGI CHO supplementation increases morning CHO availability or more stable bioavailability, though more research is needed as this was not directly investigated in the present study. Due to the exercise paradigm used in the current study, the 5-km TT run lasting ~20–30 min could present itself as a higher intensity glycolytic exercise than longer endurance exercise performance trials. Research on the effects of CHO feeding for endurance exercise indicates that some measures of performance are more sensitive than others, and short duration exercises may not be long enough to cause CHO depletion and reveal potential effects of pre-sleep CHO supplementation [12]. This might explain the insignificant differences in 5-km TT performance in the current study, and perhaps longer bouts, and/or larger sample sizes, are required to reveal an effect. There was, however, a significant effect between supplement and sex for resting CHO and FAT oxidation in this study, where females utilized more CHO with LGI and HGI (PLA was consistent between sexes). This suggests females resting fuel selection may respond differently to pre-sleep LGI or HGI CHO supplementation, but further work is needed.

In the present study, which utilized a graded and shorter duration endurance event, we found no benefit with pre-sleep ingestion on enhancing exercise performance. A contributing factor for the lack of significant positive impact on exercise performance may be attributed to the relatively short duration of the exercise stimulus incorporated in the present study [12], the amount of CHO, and/or sample size. When exercise is prolonged in a moderately intense state, CHO oxidation gradually decreases while fat oxidation increases [51,56]. Muscle glycogen utilization decreases due to reduced muscle glycogen availability [57] hence why CHO supplementation is vital for exercise of longer duration since the body relies on CHO as fuel [13]. The exercise module that was used in the present study was based on previous literature that found an effect of nighttime feeding altering morning metabolism in a 10-km run [57], and was preceded by an incremental exercise trial of three five-minute stages at 55, 65, and 75% VO_{2peak} [57]. That protocol was altered to test a 5-km timed trial with an IET comprised of three three-minute stages at the same intensities. A main reason why those times were chosen include efficiency and time restraints. Additionally, not measuring substrate utilization during the 5-km TT limited the current study's understanding of substrate metabolism to only the initial nine-minute incremental test but this was intentional to allow the athletes to give their best efforts and be minimally distracted. Contrary to our hypothesis, we found that pre-sleep supplementation with LGI CHO tended to the lowest FAT oxidation as compared to HGI and placebo control. In the present study, we cannot ascertain the mechanisms responsible such as altered intramuscular CHO availability, or altered bloods level of glucoregulatory hormones (i.e., insulin and glucagon).

Experimental Considerations

Future studies should consider measuring exercise performance in live race scenarios, such as overland 5-km running events with performance feedback, for longer duration endurance bouts (e.g., 10 km, half-, or full-marathon), and explore optimal dosing strategies. Additionally, future work should determine if CHO availability is altered with pre-sleep CHO feeding by examining muscle glycogen, and with further consideration for sex differences, as females were shown to have higher CHO utilization than males at rest following both HGI and LGI pre-sleep supplementation. This observation contrasts with relatively established findings, but several factors could have contributed to females utilizing more CHO in the morning; we would like to acknowledge that the study was not designed to test sex differences and there were fewer female participants ($n = 6$) and larger studies may prove otherwise. Females also had, on average, lower VO_{2peak} value (49.9 ± 4.3 mL/kg/min vs. males at 59.5 ± 5.5 mL/kg/min), and lower body weight and thus higher relative CHO loading and thus fitness level and body weight may play a role. Another consideration of this study could be the dose of CHO that was administered; 66 g of CHO may not be enough to last the ~eight hours to the exercise trial. Future studies should investigate different dosages, dosing approaches (e.g., g/kg), and/or timings of nighttime CHO supplementation for next-morning endurance performance in a larger sample, with measurements of circulating glucoregulatory hormones or muscle glycogen which could provide greater mechanistic insight.

5. Conclusions

The present study is the first to assess the effects of pre-sleep LGI versus HGI CHO supplementation on next-morning exercise metabolism, GID, and endurance performance in male and female endurance athletes. The data indicate that pre-sleep supplementation with LGI, HGI, or PLA did not differ in GID response during exercise. There were no differences between supplements for resting REE or RER, BG, or TT performance. In a secondary analysis, there was an interaction of supplement and sex for FAT and CHO utilization at baseline with females utilizing more CHO with the pre-sleep LGI and HGI, which should be explored further. In this study, consuming a CHO supplement pre-sleep, and not within a couple of hours of exercise, might reduce GID, allowing for adequate digestion and absorption. Future studies should investigate the effect of pre-sleep CHO supplementation on the endurance performance of the following morning.

Author Contributions: Conceptualization, M.J.O., M.D.D., and S.J.I.; methodology, M.D.D., M.J.O., S.J.I.; formal analysis, M.D.D., E.D.B., K.R.F., R.A.B., M.M.C., N.R.M., M.J.O., S.J.I.; investigation, M.D.D., E.D.B., K.R.F., R.A.B., M.M.C., N.R.M., M.J.O., S.J.I.; resources, M.J.O., S.J.I.; data curation, M.D.D., E.D.B., K.R.F., R.A.B., M.M.C., N.R.M., M.J.O., S.J.I.; writing—original draft preparation, M.D.D., E.D.B., K.R.F., R.A.B., S.J.I.; writing—review and editing, M.D.D., E.D.B., K.R.F., R.A.B., M.M.C., N.R.M., M.J.O., S.J.I.; visualization, M.D.D., E.D.B., K.R.F., R.A.B., M.M.C., N.R.M.; supervision, S.J.I., M.J.O.; project administration, S.J.I., M.J.O. All authors have read and agreed to the published version of the manuscript.

Funding: This research received no external funding.

Acknowledgments: Foremost, the authors deeply appreciate and thank all study participants. We thank UCAN for the donation of the UCAN superstarch to MJO for this study and the Skidmore Student Opportunity Fund for providing modest financial assistance to help with the completion of this study.

Conflicts of Interest: The authors declare no conflict of interest.

References

1. Chryssanthopoulos, C.; Williams, C. Pre-exercise carbohydrate meal and endurance running capacity when carbohydrates are ingested during exercise. *Int. J. Sports Med.* **1997**, *18*, 543–548. [CrossRef] [PubMed]
2. Chryssanthopoulos, C.; Williams, C.; Nowitz, A.; Kotsiopoulou, C.; Vleck, V. The effect of a high carbohydrate meal on endurance running capacity. *Int. J. Sport Nutr. Exerc. Metab.* **2002**, *12*, 157. [CrossRef] [PubMed]
3. Heung-Sang Wong, S.; Sun, F.; Chen, Y.; Li, C.; Zhang, Y.; Ya-Jun Huang, W. Effect of pre-exercise carbohydrate diets with high vs low glycemic index on exercise performance: A meta-analysis. *Nutr. Rev.* **2017**, *75*, 327–338. [CrossRef] [PubMed]
4. Neufer, P.D.; Costill, D.L.; Flynn, M.G.; Kirwan, J.P.; Mitchell, J.B.; Houmard, J. Improvements in exercise performance: Effects of carbohydrate feedings and diet. *J. Appl. Physiol.* **1987**, *62*, 983–988. [CrossRef]
5. Thomas, D.; Brotherhood, J.; Brand, J. Carbohydrate feeding before exercise: Effect of glycemic index. *Int. J. Sports Med.* **1991**, *12*, 180–186. [CrossRef] [PubMed]
6. Wright, D.A.; Sherman, W.M.; Dernbach, A.R. Carbohydrate feedings before, during, or in combination improve cycling endurance performance. *J. Appl. Physiol.* **1991**, *71*, 1082–1088. [CrossRef] [PubMed]
7. Ho, G.W.K. Lower gastrointestinal distress in endurance athletes. *Curr. Sports Med. Rep.* **2009**, *8*, 85–91. [CrossRef] [PubMed]

8. Peters, H.P.; Bos, M.; Seebregts, L.; Akkermans, L.M.; Henegouwen, G.v.B.; Bol, E.; Mosterd, W.L.; Vries, W.R. Gastrointestinal symptoms in long-distance runners, cyclists, and triathletes: Prevalence, medication, and etiology. *Am. J. Gastroenterol.* **1999**, *94*, 1570–1581. [CrossRef]
9. Peters, H.P.; Zweers, M.; Backx, F.; Bol, E.; Hendriks Mosterd, W.L.; De Vries, W.R. Gastrointestinal symptoms during long-distance walking. *Med. Sci. Sports Exerc.* **1999**, *31*, 767–773. [CrossRef]
10. Pfeiffer, B.; Stellingwerff, T.; Hodgson, A.B.; Randell, R.; Pöttgen, K.; Res, P.; Jeukendrup, A.E. Nutritional intake and gastrointestinal problems during competitive endurance events. *Med. Sci. Sports Exerc.* **2012**, *44*, 344–351. [CrossRef]
11. Rehrer, N.J.; van Kemenade, M.; Meester, W.; Brouns, F.; Saris, W.H. Gastrointestinal complaints in relation to dietary intake in triathletes. *Int. J. Sport Nutr. Exerc. Metab.* **1992**, *2*, 48–59. [CrossRef] [PubMed]
12. Jeukendrup, A.E. Carbohydrate intake during exercise and performance. *Nutrition* **2004**, *20*, 669–677. [CrossRef] [PubMed]
13. Halson, S.L.; Lancaster, G.I.; Achten, J.; Gleeson, M.; Jeukendrup, A.E. Effects of carbohydrate supplementation on performance and carbohydrate oxidation after intensified cycling training. *J. Appl. Physiol.* **2004**, *97*, 1245–1253. [CrossRef]
14. Lehmann, U.; Robin, F. Slowly digestible starch—Its structure and health implications: A review. *Trends Food Sci. Technol.* **2007**, *18*, 346–355. [CrossRef]
15. Baur, D.A.; de Vargas Fernanda, C.S.; Bach, C.W.; Garvey, J.A.; Ormsbee, M.J. Slow-absorbing modified starch before and during prolonged cycling increases fat oxidation and gastrointestinal distress without changing performance. *Nutrients* **2016**, *8*, 392. [CrossRef]
16. Bennard, P.; Doucet, E. Acute effects of exercise timing and breakfast meal glycemic index on exercise-induced fat oxidation. *Appl. Physiol. Nutr. Metab.* **2006**, *31*, 502–511. [CrossRef]
17. Roberts, M.D.; Lockwood, C.; Dalbo, V.J.; Volek, J.; Kerksick, C.M. Ingestion of a high-molecular-weight hydrothermally modified waxy maize starch alters metabolic responses to prolonged exercise in trained cyclists. *Nutrition* **2011**, *27*, 659–665. [CrossRef]
18. Sun, F.; O'Reilly, J.; Li, L.; Wong, S.H. Effect of the glycemic index of pre-exercise snack bars on substrate utilization during subsequent exercise. *Int. J. Food Sci. Nutr.* **2013**, *64*, 1001–1006. [CrossRef]
19. Moore, L.J.S.; Midgley, A.W.; Thurlow, S.; Thomas, G.; Mc Naughton, L.R. Effect of the glycaemic index of a pre-exercise meal on metabolism and cycling time trial performance. *J. Sci. Med. Sport* **2009**, *13*, 182–188. [CrossRef]
20. Backhouse, S.H.; Williams, C.; Stevenson, E.; Nute, M. Effects of the glycemic index of breakfast on metabolic responses to brisk walking in females. *Eur. J. Clin. Nutr.* **2007**, *61*, 590–596. [CrossRef]
21. Baur, D.A.; Willingham, B.D.; Smith, K.A.; Kisiolek, J.N.; Morrissey, M.C.; Saracino, P.G.; Ragland, T.J.; Ormsbee, M.J. Adipose Lipolysis Unchanged by Preexercise Carbohydrate Regardless of Glycemic Index. *Med. Sci. Sports Exerc.* **2018**, *50*, 827–836. [CrossRef] [PubMed]
22. Stevenson, E.; Williams, C.; Nute, M.; Humphrey, L.; Witard, O. Influence of the glycaemic index of an evening meal on substrate oxidation following breakfast and during exercise the next day in healthy women. *Eur. J. Clin. Nutr.* **2008**, *62*, 608–616. [CrossRef] [PubMed]
23. Stevenson, E.; Williams, C.; Nute, M.; Swaile, P.; Tsui, M. The effect of the glycemic index of an evening meal on the metabolic responses to a standard high glycemic index breakfast and subsequent exercise in men. *Int. J. Sport Nutr. Exerc. Metab.* **2005**, *15*, 308–322. [CrossRef] [PubMed]
24. The UCAN Company. SuperStarch®. Available online: https://www.generationucan.com/superstarch/ (accessed on 22 April 2019).
25. Bhattacharya, K.; Orton, R.; Qi, X.; Mundy, H.; Morley, D.; Champion, M.; Eaton, S.; Tester, R.; Lee, P. A novel starch for the treatment of glycogen storage diseases. *J. Inherit. Metab. Dis.* **2007**, *30*, 350–357. [CrossRef]
26. Correia, C.E.; Bhattacharya, K.; Lee, P.J.; Shuster, J.J.; Theriaque, D.W.; Shankar, M.N.; Smit, G.P.A.; Weinstein, D.A. Use of modified cornstarch therapy to extend fasting in glycogen storage disease types Ia and Ib. *Am. J. Clin. Nutr.* **2008**, *88*, 1272–1276. [PubMed]
27. Johannsen, N.M.; Sharp, R.L. Effect of pre-exercise ingestion of modified cornstarch on substrate oxidation during endurance exercise. *Int. J. Sport Nutr. Exerc. Metab.* **2007**, *17*, 232. [CrossRef]
28. Ormsbee, M.J.; Contreras, R.J.; Spicer, M.T.; Miller, E.A.; Eckel, L.A.; Baur, D.A.; Gorman, K.A.; Panton, L.B. Nighttime feeding likely alters morning metabolism but not exercise performance in female athletes. *Appl. Physiol. Nutr. Metab.* **2016**, *41*, 719–727. [CrossRef]

29. Tseh, W.; Caputo, J.L.; Keefer, D.J. Validity and reliability of the BOD POD® S/T tracking system. *Int. J. Sports Med.* **2010**, *10*, 704–708. [CrossRef]
30. Crouter, S.E.; Antczak, A.; Hudak, J.R.; DellaValle, D.M.; Haas, J.D. Accuracy and reliability of the ParvoMedics TrueOne 2400 and MedGraphics VO2000 metabolic systems. *Eur. J. Appl. Physiol.* **2006**, *98*, 139–151. [CrossRef]
31. Averbuch, M.; Katzper, M. Assessment of visual analog versus categorical scale for measurement of osteoarthritis pain. *J. Clin. Pharm.* **2004**, *44*, 368–372. [CrossRef]
32. Bijur, P.E.; Silver, W.; Gallagher, E.J. Reliability of the visual analog scale for measurement of acute pain. *Acad. Emerg. Med.* **2001**, *8*, 1153–1157. [CrossRef] [PubMed]
33. Gallagher, E.J.; Bijur, P.E.; Latimer, C.; Silver, W. Reliability and validity of a visual analog scale for acute abdominal pain in the ED. *Am. J. Emerg. Med.* **2002**, *20*, 287–290. [CrossRef] [PubMed]
34. Frayn, K.N. Calculation of substrate oxidation rates in vivo from gaseous exchange. *J. Appl. Physiol.* **1983**, *55*, 628–634. [CrossRef]
35. Halldorsdottir, S.; Warchal-Windham, M.E.; Wallace, J.F.; Pardo, S.; Parkes, J.L.; Simmons, D.A. Accuracy evaluation of five blood glucose monitoring systems: The north american comparator trial. *J. Diabetes Sci. Technol.* **2013**, *7*, 1294–1304. [CrossRef]
36. Jäger, R.; Kerksick, C.M.; Campbell, B.I.; Cribb, P.J.; Wells, S.D.; Skwiat, T.M.; Purpura, M.; Ziegenfuss, T.N.; Ferrando, A.A.; Arent, S.M.; et al. International society of sports nutrition position stand: Protein and exercise. *J. Int. Soc. Sports Nutr.* **2017**, *14*, 20. [CrossRef]
37. Laursen, P.B.; Francis, G.T.; Abbiss, C.R.; Newton, M.J.; Nosaka, K. Reliability of time-to-exhaustion versus time-trial running tests in runners. *Med. Sci. Sports Exerc.* **2007**, *39*, 1374–1379. [CrossRef]
38. Jones, A.M.; Doust, J.H. A 1% treadmill grade most accurately reflects the energetic cost of outdoor running. *J. Sports Sci.* **2007**, *14*, 321–327. [CrossRef] [PubMed]
39. Kirwan, J.P.; Cyr-Campbell, D.; Campbell, W.W.; Scheiber, J.; Evans, W.J. Effects of moderate and high glycemic index meals on metabolism and exercise performance. *Metabolism* **2001**, *50*, 849–855. [CrossRef]
40. Sherman, W.M.; Peden, M.C.; Wright, D.A. Carbohydrate feedings 1 h before exercise improves cycling performance. *Am. J. Clin. Nutr.* **1991**, *54*, 866–870. [CrossRef]
41. Sparks, M.; Selig, S.; Febbraio, M. Pre-exercise carbohydrate ingestion: Effect of the glycemic index on endurance exercise performance. *Med. Sci. Sports Exerc.* **1998**, *30*, 844–849. [CrossRef]
42. Wee, S.L.; Williams, C.; Gray, S.; Horabin, J. Influence of high and low glycemic index meals on endurance running capacity. *Med. Sci. Sports Exerc.* **1999**, *31*, 393–399. [CrossRef] [PubMed]
43. Wu, C.; Williams, C. A low glycemic index meal before exercise improves endurance running capacity in men. *Int. J. Sport Nutr. Exerc. Metab.* **2006**, *16*, 510–527. [CrossRef] [PubMed]
44. Moore, L.J.S.; Midgley, A.W.; Thomas, G.; Thurlow, S.; McNaughton, L.R. The effects of low- and high-glycemic index meals on time trial performance. *Int. J. Sports Physiol. Perform.* **2009**, *4*, 331–344. [CrossRef]
45. DeMarco, H.M.; Sucher, K.P.; Cisar, C.J.; Butterfield, G.E. Pre-exercise carbohydrate meals: Application of glycemic index. *Med. Sci. Sports Exerc.* **1999**, *31*, 164–170. [CrossRef] [PubMed]
46. Wong, S.H.S.; Siu, P.M.; Lok, A.; Chen, Y.J.; Morris, J.; Lam, C.W. Effect of the glycaemic index of pre-exercise carbohydrate meals on running performance. *Eur. J. Sport Sci.* **2008**, *8*, 23–33. [CrossRef]
47. Febbraio, M.A.; Keenan, J.; Angus, D.J.; Campbell, S.E.; Garnham, A.P. Pre-exercise carbohydrate ingestion, glucose kinetics, and muscle glycogen use: Effect of the glycemic index. *J. Appl. Physiol.* **2000**, *89*, 1845–1851. [CrossRef]
48. Jentjens, R.; Jeukendrup, A. Effects of pre-exercise ingestion of trehalose, galactose and glucose on subsequent metabolism and cycling performance. *Eur. J. Appl. Physiol.* **2003**, *88*, 459–465. [CrossRef]
49. Kern, M.; Heslin, C.J.; Rezende, R.S. Metabolic and performance effects of raisins versus sports gel as pre-exercise feedings in cyclists. *J. Strength Cond. Res.* **2007**, *21*, 1204.
50. Stannard, S.R.; Constantini, N.W.; Miller, J.C. The Effect of Glycemic Index on Plasma Glucose and Lactate Levels during Incremental Exercise. *Int. J. Sport Nutr. Exerc. Metab.* **2000**, *10*, 51–61. [CrossRef]
51. Romijn, J.A.; Coyle, E.F.; Sidossis, L.S.; Gastaldelli, A.; Horowitz, J.F.; Endert, E.; Wolfe, R.R. Regulation of endogenous fat and carbohydrate metabolism in relation to exercise intensity and duration. *Am. J. Physiol. Endocrinol. Metab.* **1993**, *265*, E380–E391. [CrossRef]

52. Chen, Y.J.; Wong, S.H.S.; Chan, C.O.W.; Wong, C.K.; Lam, C.W.; Siu, P.M.F. Effects of glycemic index meal and CHO-electrolyte drink on cytokine response and run performance in endurance athletes. *J. Sci. Med. Sport* **2008**, *12*, 697–703. [CrossRef] [PubMed]
53. Chryssanthopoulos, C.; Hennessy, L.C.; Williams, C. The influence of pre-exercise glucose ingestion on endurance running capacity. *Br. J. Sports Med.* **1994**, *28*, 105–109. [CrossRef] [PubMed]
54. Koivisto, V.A.; Karonen, S.L.; Nikkila, E.A. Carbohydrate ingestion before exercise: Comparison of glucose, fructose, and sweet placebo. *J. Appl. Physiol.* **1981**, *51*, 783–787. [CrossRef] [PubMed]
55. Marmy-Conus, N.; Fabris, S.; Proietto, J.; Hargreaves, M. Pre-exercise glucose ingestion and glucose kinetics during exercise. *J. Appl. Physiol.* **1996**, *81*, 853–857. [CrossRef] [PubMed]
56. Ahlborg, G.; Felig, P.; Hagenfeldt, L.; Hendler, R.; Wahren, J. Substrate turnover during prolonged exercise in man. Splanchnic and leg metabolism of glucose, free fatty acids, and amino acids. *J. Clin. Investig.* **1974**, *53*, 1080–1090. [CrossRef] [PubMed]
57. Gollnick, P.D.; Piehl, K.; Saltin, B. Selective glycogen depletion pattern in human muscle fibres after exercise of varying intensity and at varying pedalling rates. *J. Physiol.* **1974**, *241*, 45–57. [CrossRef] [PubMed]

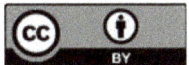

© 2020 by the authors. Licensee MDPI, Basel, Switzerland. This article is an open access article distributed under the terms and conditions of the Creative Commons Attribution (CC BY) license (http://creativecommons.org/licenses/by/4.0/).

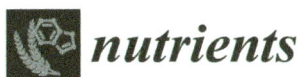

Review

Gut Microbiota, Probiotics and Physical Performance in Athletes and Physically Active Individuals

Maija Marttinen *, Reeta Ala-Jaakkola, Arja Laitila and Markus J. Lehtinen

DuPont Nutrition & Biosciences, Danisco Sweeteners Oy, Sokeritehtaantie 20, 02460 Kantvik, Finland; reeta.ala-jaakkola@dupont.com (R.A.-J.); arja.laitila@dupont.com (A.L.); markus.lehtinen@dupont.com (M.J.L.)
* Correspondence: maija.marttinen@dupont.com; Tel.: +358-40-820-6151

Received: 25 August 2020; Accepted: 24 September 2020; Published: 25 September 2020

Abstract: Among athletes, nutrition plays a key role, supporting training, performance, and post-exercise recovery. Research has primarily focused on the effects of diet in support of an athletic physique; however, the role played by intestinal microbiota has been much neglected. Emerging evidence has shown an association between the intestinal microbiota composition and physical activity, suggesting that modifications in the gut microbiota composition may contribute to physical performance of the host. Probiotics represent a potential means for beneficially influencing the gut microbiota composition/function but can also impact the overall health of the host. In this review, we provide an overview of the existing studies that have examined the reciprocal interactions between physical activity and gut microbiota. We further evaluate the clinical evidence that supports the effects of probiotics on physical performance, post-exercise recovery, and cognitive outcomes among athletes. In addition, we discuss the mechanisms of action through which probiotics affect exercise outcomes. In summary, beneficial microbes, including probiotics, may promote health in athletes and enhance physical performance and exercise capacity. Furthermore, high-quality clinical studies, with adequate power, remain necessary to uncover the roles that are played by gut microbiota populations and probiotics in physical performance and the modes of action behind their potential benefits.

Keywords: gut microbiota; probiotics; athletes; exercise; physical activity; physical performance; cognitive performance; recovery

1. Introduction

The human gastrointestinal (GI) tract harbors a vast number of microbial cells (10^{14}), which surpasses the number of cells that make up the human body [1]. Although many intestinal microbiota species are beneficial, others are potentially detrimental, or their functions remain unknown. These resident microbes are involved in many metabolic processes, such as the fermentation of undigested carbohydrates into short-chain fatty acids (SCFAs), lipid metabolism, and vitamin synthesis. Intestinal microbiota also stimulates the maturation of the immune system and protects against potentially pathogenic microbes [2]. Further, the microbiota may play a role in cognitive performance and stress tolerance [3,4].

A healthy adult gut is characterized by a high degree of microbial richness (diversity) [5], favoring health-promoting species, and features an intact epithelial barrier, which affects the inflammatory status and nutrient utilization of the host [6]. Genetic and environmental factors, in addition to diet and antibiotic use, have major influences on the gut microbiota composition, starting in early childhood and extending into adulthood [7]. Dysbiosis and the loss of diversity among gut microbiota species have been associated with various immune-regulated pathological conditions and diseases and may, in part, contribute to the risks of developing obesity-related disorders [7,8].

Gut microbiota populations with high degrees of microbial diversity have been associated with various health benefits in adults. Gut microbes have the potential to exert effects via metabolites, such as SCFAs and neurotransmitters, that can influence mucosal tissues locally or enter the circulation to affect extra-intestinal tissues. Recently, these findings have resulted in the conceptualization of a gut-brain axis (for review see [9]) and a gut-muscle axis (for review see [10]) indicating the existence of bidirectional communications between the gut microbiota and the peripheral tissues of the host.

Exercise has well-known effects on cardiorespiratory fitness, muscle strength, glucose metabolism, the immune system, and mental health [11]. Emerging evidence has indicated a plausible association between physical activity and the gut microbiota composition [12–14]. The particular features of gut microbiota compositions found in athletic individuals and the impacts of exercise on the gut microbiota compositions of sedentary populations have begun to be revealed. Intervention studies have supported the beneficial impacts of exercise and physical activity on the gut microbiota [15–17]. Furthermore, a growing interest has developed regarding whether the modification of the gut microbiota composition can affect the exercise and training outcomes of the host.

Probiotics are, by definition, "live micro-organisms that, when administered in adequate amounts, confer a health benefit on the host" [18]. Probiotic supplementation may modify the gut microbiota composition, promoting increased microbial diversity and supporting the growth of health-promoting species [19–21]. Probiotics may also help restore a disturbed gut microbiota [15] and support a microbiota under stress [22,23]. Although, many probiotics can support a general healthy GI and immune system function, the specific mechanisms underlying probiotic actions, such as the production of bioactive compounds, the inhibition of pathogen adhesion, the improvement of gut barrier function, and immune modulation, may be highly strain-specific, even within a single bacterial species [18].

Thus far, probiotic research has primarily focused on GI function and immune regulation; however, recent studies have targeted new research areas, such as metabolic and cognitive health. The well-established probiotic effects on gut health and immune system function may benefit endurance athletes, who train and perform at high intensities and often encounter physiological challenges associated with GI and immune health during and after a competition. Therefore, probiotic supplementation may indirectly improve the performance of an athlete by increasing the number of healthy training and competition days and maybe even benefit stamina. The benefits of probiotics for sports performance and training have been recognized, although the number of studies that have examined these issues remains limited. Recently, the International Society of Sports Nutrition (ISSN) provided a position stand on probiotics, concluding that probiotics have strain-specific effects in athletes [24]. In this review, we provide an overview of the current research on the relationships between exercise and gut microbiota and further evaluate the indirect and direct effects of probiotics on physical performance, in animal models and human subjects.

2. Gut Microbiota and Physical Performance

Exercise has well-known effects on metabolism and the immune system, but the effects of exercise on the gut microbiota have been less well studied. Compared with sedentary subjects, athletes and physically active subjects appear to have greater fecal microbial diversity and more health-associated microbial genera, such as *Akkermansia*, *Veillonella* and *Prevotella* [12–14]. However, the results of these observational studies can only confirm associations between training status and microbiota populations, without determining causality. In addition to physical activity patterns, sedentary subjects often differ from physically active subjects in dietary intake patterns [25], and diet has a strong impact on the gut microbiota composition [26].

The association between exercise and the gut microbiota composition appears to be bidirectional. Exercise intervention studies in humans have indicated that regular physical activity modulates the gut microbial composition [15–17]. Furthermore, growing evidence from animal studies has also suggested that the gut microbiota plays an important role in the physical performance of the host [27–29]. The composition and metabolic activity of gut microbiota may aid in the digestion of dietary compounds and improve energy harvest during exercise, which could provide metabolic benefits for an athlete during high-intensity exercise and recovery. Observational studies have demonstrated that the metabolic activity and pathways associated with amino acid and carbohydrate metabolism are increased among the athlete microbiome compared with those in sedentary subjects [13,14,30].

In the gut, bacteria ferment non-digestible carbohydrates, primarily into SCFAs acetate, propionate and butyrate. Training and regular exercise have been associated with increased fecal SCFA contents in humans [15,30], and specific SCFAs have been associated with improved physical performance in animal studies [14,29]. Most SCFAs are absorbed from the intestinal tract and contribute to the host's energy metabolism [31]. Butyrate is used primarily by epithelial cells in the colon, as an energy source. Acetate is metabolized in muscle tissue but can also cross the blood-brain barrier. Propionate can be used as a precursor for glucose synthesis in the liver [31]. Additionally, SCFAs improve intestinal barrier integrity, reducing local and systemic inflammation risk. Preclinical studies have strongly suggested that SCFAs may represent key modulators of physical performance.

Notably, the host may not be the only party to benefit from the symbiotic relationship with microbiota during exercise. A recent study suggested that lactate, produced by the host skeletal muscles during anaerobic exercise, enters the gut lumen through circulation, providing a selective advantage for lactate-utilizing species that reside in the colon [14]. The results from this seminal work imply that during high-intensity exercise, the host provides fuel, in the form of lactate, for specific bacteria, which, in turn, produce metabolites, such as propionate, that benefit the exercising host. Current research on the interactions between the gut microbiota and physical performance is reviewed below and summarized in Figure 1.

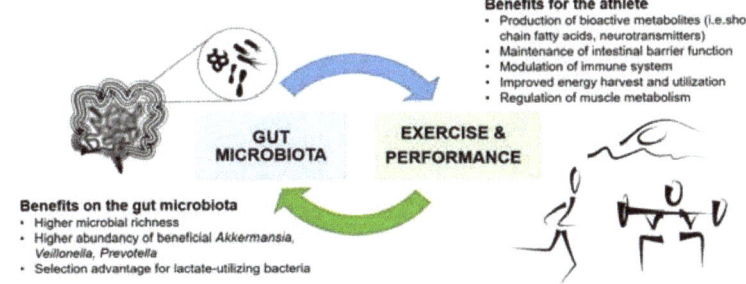

Figure 1. Interactions between gut microbiota and exercise.

2.1. Gut Microbiota in Athletes

Accumulating clinical evidence has suggested that exercise modifies the gut microbiota and that the gut microbiota composition in athletes differs from that in sedentary people, with athletes presenting with microbial populations that are enriched in health-promoting species and have greater diversity (Table 1). Diet and specific dietary components, such as dietary fiber, have been identified as major influencers of the gut microbiota composition [26]. In cross-sectional and longitudinal studies, the impacts of diet on gut microbiota cannot be excluded, especially because the dietary intake of an athlete can greatly differ from the intake of a sedentary individual, in terms of both caloric and nutrient contents. Most of the studies in Table 1 have reported dietary intake.

A study involving Irish, male professional rugby players showed a higher α-diversity (bacterial richness, such as how many bacterial species are identified in fecal samples) for the gut microbiota of athletes compared with those in sedentary controls [12]. Gut microbiota diversity correlated positively with protein consumption and plasma creatine kinase (CK) levels, a biomarker for exercise-induced muscle damage. A higher proportion of bacteria from the *Akkermansia* genus was detected in rugby players and controls with low body mass index (BMI) compared with the proportion in controls with high BMI. *Bacteroides* spp. were significantly less abundant in athletes than in controls with low BMI.

Table 1. Studies on exercise and gut microbiota conducted in athletes, physically active individuals and sedentary population.

Subjects	Training Regimen, Exercise Protocol	Dietary Intake	Main Results	Reference
Athletes:				
Rugby players vs. BMI-matched sedentary controls n = 86, males Age 29 ± 4 y	Habitual training and exercise	Self-reported intake by FFQ In athletes, higher total energy, macronutrient and fiber intake. Protein intake 22 E% in athletes, 16 E% in low-BMI and 15 E% in high-BMI controls	In athletes, higher α-diversity and *Akkermansia* spp. abundance vs. sedentary controls. Protein intake was positively correlated with microbial diversity.	[12]
Rugby players vs. BMI-matched sedentary controls n = 86, males Age 29 ± 4 y	Habitual training and exercise	Self-reported intake by FFQ In athletes, higher total energy, macronutrient and fiber intake. Protein intake 22 E% in athletes vs. 16 E% in low-BMI and 15 E% in high-BMI controls	In athletes, fecal SCFAs, microbial pathways for antibiotic biosynthesis, and amino acids and carbohydrate metabolism were increased.	[30]
Professional cyclists vs. amateur cyclists n = 33 (22/M, 11/F) Age 19–49 y	Habitual training	Dietary intake data collected by questionnaire, reported and analyzed as overall dietary patterns.	*Prevotella* spp. abundance was positively correlated with the amount of exercise and branched chain amino acid and carbohydrate metabolism pathways. Professional cyclists had increased *Methanobrevibacter smithii* transcripts and upregulated genes involved in the production of methane compared with amateur cyclists. No correlations between overall diet and gut microbiota clusters.	[13]
Cross-country runners n = 18, males Age: Control group 35.4 ± 9.0 y Protein group 34.9 ± 9.5 y	Habitual endurance training	Habitual diet by FFQ No differences in habitual dietary intake within or between groups, at baseline or after the intervention. Dietary intervention: habitual diet and whey isolate (10 g) + beef hydrolysate (10 g) or maltodextrin (control) for 10 weeks	After the intervention, higher Bacteroidetes and lower Firmicutes abundance in the protein group. *Bifidobacterium longum* was reduced after intervention in the protein group. No changes in microbiota composition in the control group, from pre- to post-intervention. No differences within or between groups in fecal SCFA, before or after the intervention.	[32]
Bodybuilders, long-distance runners vs. sedentary subjects n = 45, males Age: Bodybuilders 25 ± 3 y, distance runners 20 ± 1 y, sedentary 26 ± 2 y	Habitual training and exercise	Self-recorded 3-day food diary Bodybuilders had a high-protein and distance runners had a low-dietary-fiber dietary pattern. Dietary fiber intake was below recommendation in all groups.	Compositional differences in bodybuilders and runners associated with exercise type and diet. No difference in microbial diversity between groups. In distance runners, protein intake was negatively correlated with microbial diversity.	[33]
Highly trained ultra-endurance rowers n = 4, males Age 26.5 ± 1.3 y	ca. 5000 km rowing race over 34 days	Self-reported intake (FFQ), detailed daily record pre-race and during the race No fresh produce consumed during race. Pre-race fiber intake: 21.45 g/day, intra-race 23.1 g/day. Only small changes in intra-race macronutrient intake compared with pre-race	After the race, increased diversity and butyrate-producing species including *Roseburia hominis* and changes in microbial composition were observed.	[34]

Table 1. Cont.

Subjects	Training Regimen, Exercise Protocol	Dietary Intake	Main Results	Reference
Elite race walkers n = 21, males Age 20–35 y	3-week structured program of intensified training	Dietary intervention for 3 weeks with planned and individualized menus. Subjects allocated into High-carbohydrate diet (HCHO) Periodized-carbohydrate diet (PCHO), or Low-carbohydrate, high-fat diet (LCHF) (ketogenic) group	At baseline, microbiota profiles could be separated into *Prevotella*- or *Bacteroides*-dominating enterotypes. HCHO and PCHO resulted in minor changes, whereas LCHF resulted in stronger changes in microbial composition. LCHF was associated with reduced *Faecalibacterium*, *Bifidobacterium*, and *Veillonella* spp. Increased *Bacteroides* and *Dorea* spp. in the LCHF group was associated with decreased performance.	[35]
Marathon runners: n = 15 (4/M, 11/F) Mean age 27.1 y; Non-runners: n = 11 (5/M, 6/F) Mean age 29.2 y; Ultramarathon and rower athletes: n = 11 (5/M, 6/F) Age not reported	Habitual training and a marathon Type of exercise not reported for the cohort of ultra-marathon and rower athletes	Dietary intake data collected by questionnaire	In marathon runners, the relative abundance of *Veillonella* spp. increased post-marathon. In ultramarathon and rower athletes, the relative abundance of the methylmalonyl-CoA pathway (degrading lactate into propionate) in the gut microbiome increased post-exercise. No correlations between dairy, protein, grains, fruits, or vegetables and *Veillonella* spp. abundance was observed among marathon runners.	[14]
Non-athletes and sedentary subjects:				
Healthy subjects n = 39 (22/M, 17/F) Age 18–35 y	VO_2Peak test to assess CRF and to allocate subjects into groups (low, average, and high CRF)	24-h dietary recall interview No significant differences in dietary intake between groups.	CRF correlated with microbial diversity and butyrate production.	[36]
Active vs. sedentary women n = 40 Active: 30.7 ± 5.9 y, BMI 24.4 ± 4.5 kg/m²; Sedentary: 32.2 ± 8.7 y, BMI 22.9 ± 3.0 kg/m²	Habitual physical activity measured by accelerometer.	Self-reported food intake (FFQ) Fiber, fruit, and vegetable intake significantly higher in the active group.	Higher abundance of *Faecalibacterium prausnitzii*, *Roseburia hominis* and *Akkermansia muciniphila* in active women. Physical activity was not associated with differences in microbiota richness.	[37]
Lean and obese sedentary subjects n = 32 Lean: n = 18 (9/M, 9/F), mean age 25.10 y; Obese: n = 14 (3/M, 11/F), mean age 31.14 y	Exercise intervention study: 6 weeks of moderate-to-vigorous intensity aerobic exercise and 6 weeks without exercise	Maintenance of habitual diet during the intervention. A designed 3-day food menu, based on previous reported habitual diet, before fecal sample collection.	At baseline, the composition of gut microbiota differed between lean and obese subjects, but after exercise training, no difference was observed between lean and obese subjects. Exercise increased fecal SCFA and SCFA producing bacteria in lean subjects.	[15]

Table 1. Cont.

Subjects	Training Regimen, Exercise Protocol	Dietary Intake	Main Results	Reference
Children and teenagers n = 267 (178/M, 89/F) Age 7–18 y	Self-reported physical activity	Type of diet reported as omnivore or vegetarian.	Gut microbiota composition was affected by BMI, exercise frequency, and diet type. Firmicutes were significantly enriched in subjects with more frequent exercise.	[38]
Overweight sedentary women n = 17 Age 36.8 ± 3.9 y BMI 31.8 ± 4.4 kg/m^2	Habitual physical activity. Exercise intervention study: 6-week control period without exercise, 6-week programmed endurance exercise, on a bicycle ergometer	Habitual diet Self-reported 3-day food record No changes in intake of total energy, macronutrients or fiber from baseline, after control or exercise period. A modest increase in energy from starch	Exercise did not affect α-diversity. Exercise increased *Akkermansia* spp. and reduced Proteobacteria abundance. No significant changes in BMI or total fat mass after exercise. Significant reduction in android fat mass.	[16]
Healthy subjects n = 37 (20/M, 17/F) Age 25.7 ± 2.2 y	VO$_{2max}$ test to assess CRF	Habitual diet recorded for 7 days	CRF correlated with Firmicutes/Bacteroidetes ratio. No correlation between dietary factors or BMI and Firmicutes/Bacteroidetes ratio.	[39]
Elderly community-dwelling men n = 373 Age 78–98 y	Habitual physical activity, measured by activity sensor, for 5 days. Step count as primary physical activity variable	Self-reported food intake (FFQ) Step count was not associated with food or alcohol intake.	Physical activity was not associated with α-diversity but was positively associated with β-diversity. Increased physical activity was associated with greater *Faecalibacterium* and *Lachnospira* spp. prevalence.	[40]
Elderly sedentary women n = 29 Age 65–77 y	Exercise intervention study: resistance training (trunk muscles) or aerobic exercise (brisk walking) for 12 weeks	Self-reported food intake (FFQ) No changes in energy or nutrient intake after interventions.	Brisk walking increased the relative abundance of *Bacteroides* spp. *Bacteroides* spp. abundance was positively associated with improved CRF after aerobic training but not with improved CRF after resistance training.	[17]

BMI, body mass index; y, years; FFQ, food frequency questionnaire; E%, percentage of total energy intake; SCFA, short-chain fatty acid; M, males; F, females; VO$_{2Peak}$/VO$_{2Max}$, maximum rate of oxygen consumption; CRF, cardiorespiratory fitness.

Akkermansia sp. has been shown to inversely correlate with obesity [41] and *Bacteroides* spp. has been associated with a "Western" type of diet, with high protein and fat contents [42].

Differences between rugby players and sedentary controls were also detected in the microbial metabolism level, with increased amino acid and carbohydrate metabolism pathway activity detected in athletes [30]. Furthermore, higher fecal SCFA (acetate, propionate, and butyrate) levels were detected in rugby players compared with those in sedentary controls. SCFAs produced by gut bacteria have well-known health-promoting effects on the maintenance of intestinal barrier function, immune modulation, and the host's energy metabolism [43,44].

Similar to Clarke et al. [12], Petersen et al. [13] reported lower levels of *Bacteroides* spp. in competitive cyclists. Cyclists who trained >11 h/week had a higher relative abundance of *Prevotella* spp. than those who trained less often. In addition, a meta-transcriptomics analysis showed that *Prevotella* transcripts were positively correlated with branched-chain amino acid (BCAA) metabolism pathways in the microbiome. BCAAs, especially leucine, are essential amino acids that promote muscle protein synthesis and may enhance recovery after exercise. Further, more fecal *Methanobrevibacter smithii* transcripts were identified in professional cyclists compared with amateur cyclists. *M. smithii* was associated with upregulated methane metabolism, which correlated positively with upregulation of SCFA metabolism pathways in the gut microbiome [13]. However, the authors recognized the lack of dietary control and the absence of a non-athlete control group in the study. In line with the results observed in cyclists, fecal microbiotas were classified into *Prevotella*- or *Bacteroides*-dominant enterotypes in a small group of elite race walkers [35].

Scheiman et al. [14] demonstrated that the relative abundance of *Veillonella* spp. bacteria among marathon runners was significantly higher after the marathon, compared with the pre-exercise abundance. In addition, the same research group conducted metagenomic analyses using fecal samples from ultramarathoners and Olympic level rowers, which revealed the enrichment of genes associated with lactate and propionate metabolism in post-exercise compared with pre-exercise samples. A follow-up study, conducted in mice, demonstrated that treatment with a *Veillonella* sp. strain, which was isolated from a marathon runner, increased the treadmill running time of mice by 13% [14].

The chronological impact of prolonged, very-high-intensity exercise on the gut microbial composition was investigated in four well-trained men who participated in a trans-oceanic rowing competition [34]. All, except one rower, who required antibiotic treatment before mid-race, showed increased microbial α-diversity at mid-race, which continued until the end of the race. Baseline diversity was partially or completely restored three months after the competition. Although this study represents a very small sample size, the microbial metabolic pathways related to specific amino acids and medium and long-chain fatty acids tended to increase [34]. However, the diet differed considerably during the rowing race compared with the pre-race diet; therefore, dietary change may have also contributed to the microbial diversity findings.

In addition to the high-intense training that is practiced by professional or competitive athletes, exercise that is performed at the recommended minimum level, based on the World Health Organization (WHO) guidelines of 150 min of moderate-intensity exercise each week [45], appears to sufficiently modify the gut microbiota composition [37]. Premenopausal women who practiced continuous exercise at a low dose demonstrated increased abundance of *Akkermansia muciniphila*, *Faecalibacterium prausnitzii*, and *Roseburia hominis*, compared with those in sedentary women [37]. These all are bacterial species that are associated with health-promoting and anti-inflammatory effects [43]. Moreover, *Faecalibacterium* spp. and *Roseburia* spp. are among the most abundant butyrate-producers in the human gut [43,44]. Different dietary patterns between physically active and sedentary groups may have influenced the gut microbiota composition, as the intake of dietary fiber was significantly higher in active women compared with sedentary women (mean intake 30.9 g vs. 21.4 g), and the intake of processed meat was significantly higher in the sedentary group [37].

Associations between physical activity levels and gut microbiota compositions have also been demonstrated in children [38] and seniors [40]. In a study cohort of children, aged 7–18 years, from the American Gut Project, BMI, exercise frequency, and type of diet were individually associated with the gut microbiota composition, after controlling for covariates (age, gender, and the use of antibiotics and probiotics) [38]. Exercise frequency was associated with gut microbiota enriched with Firmicutes phylum. Furthermore, children who exercised daily showed an increase in genera within Clostridiales, Lachnospiraceae, and Erysipelotrichaceae. In older men, physical activity, measured based on step count and self-reported activity, was not associated with microbial α-diversity, but modest associations between physical activity level and *Faecalibacterium* spp. and *Lachnospira* spp. were found [40].

These studies indicated the existence of differences in the gut microbiota composition between athletes or physically active populations and sedentary populations. However, some of the characteristics of the microbiota composition in athletes and physically active people may be explained by diet, rather than the effects of exercise. Athletes often follow strict diets that support training and performance, and exercise extremes are often associated with dietary extremes [12]. Protein supplements are often consumed to meet the higher protein requirements of training individuals, although the popularity of protein supplements is likely also influenced by claims regarding increased muscle mass and improved performance and recovery [46]. Thus, protein intake can be substantially higher among athletes compared with the normal population. Following high protein intake, unabsorbed protein enters the colon and promotes the growth and selection of specific bacteria. Protein supplementation (whey isolate and beef hydrolysate) for 10 weeks increased the abundance of Bacteroidetes and decreased health-related taxa, including *Roseburia* spp., *Blautia* spp., and *Bifidobacterium longum*, in runners [32]. However, the long-term effects of such alterations in the gut microbiota composition on host health remain unclear.

Differences in dietary intake between study populations may explain some of the inconsistencies observed among the results of different studies. In a clinical study in Korea, total protein intake was inversely correlated with microbial diversity [33], whereas high protein intake was associated with increased microbial diversity among Irish professional rugby players [12]. Korean athletes did not meet the dietary recommendations for dietary fiber intake (recommendation ≥ 25 g/day; median intake in bodybuilders 19 g/day, endurance athletes 17 g/day), whereas Irish rugby players had fiber intake values at the recommended level (median intake 39 g/day). Undigested dietary fiber is an important energy and carbon source for the gut microbiota, acting as a substrate for SCFA synthesis, and representing a key contributor to microbial diversity. A high-protein diet, in combination with low-dietary-fiber diet, may be harmful for the gut microbiota composition, rather than high protein intake alone [47].

Limited data, derived primarily from animal studies, have suggested that popular sports nutrition supplements, such as caffeine, BCAAs, sodium bicarbonate, and carnitine, can modify the gut microbiota composition [48]. The effects of sports nutrition supplements on the gut microbiota remain understudied among athletes.

To summarize, exercise and training have been associated with compositional changes in the gut microbiota, including increased microbial diversity and increased abundance of health-promoting microbial species. Results from large study cohorts with recreationally active subjects suggest that exercise is associated with increases in genera within Clostridiales and Lachnospiraceae [38,40]. Although several studies have investigated small populations that likely lack sufficient statistical power, it is intriguing that they commonly identify genera such as *Akkermansia* [12,37] and *Prevotella* [12,13] at higher abundance in athletes and physically active subjects. However, because the number of clinical studies remains limited, with highly different participant demographics and dietary intake—dietary fiber intake in specific—conclusions should be drawn carefully. Observational studies that have compared trained athletes and physically active subjects with sedentary subjects have suggested long-term effects of exercise training on gut microbiota composition, wherein the diet plays an important role. Sedentary and physically active subjects differ not only in their exercise patterns but also in their dietary intake and body composition, which are both factors that are associated with the gut microbiota composition.

2.2. Impacts of Exercise Interventions on Gut Microbiota

Because athletes often adhere to special diets that may influence the gut microbiota, exercise intervention studies can provide a more diet-independent approach for examining whether exercise has an impact on the host gut microbiota (Table 1). A research group demonstrated that exercise training intervention modified the gut microbiota composition of sedentary, non-trained, Finnish women, without changes in dietary habits, weight, or body composition [16]. The authors demonstrated that endurance exercise altered the gut microbiome of overweight, sedentary women, who participated in an exercise intervention that consisted of performing a bicycle ergometer routine, three times a week, for six weeks. The study showed no differences in total energy intake or the intake of macronutrients or dietary fiber after the training intervention. Differences were not found in the gut microbiota α-diversity or phylum-level abundance between pre- and post-intervention samples; however, endurance exercise increased relative abundance of members of the genera *Verrucomicrobia* and *Akkermansia* and decreased the number of inflammation-associated Proteobacteria in the gut. Changes in *Akkermansia* spp. and genera and species within phyla Proteobacteria and Verrucomicrobia were responsive to exercise and were independent of age, weight, percent body fat, and food intake. Another study, performed by Morita et al. [17] found that a 12-week aerobic exercise training program significantly increased the relative abundance of *Bacteroides* spp. in elderly, sedentary women, without changes in nutrient intake.

A study by Allen et al. [15] supported these findings, showing that aerobic exercise induced changes in the gut microbiota composition, independent of dietary intake, among sedentary subjects; however, BMI may influence the response of gut microbiota to exercise. In their study, obese and lean individuals had different gut microbiota compositions at baseline, but after a 6-week aerobic exercise training program, no difference was found in microbiota community composition between obese and lean. In addition, aerobic exercise increased fecal SCFA concentrations and SCFA production capacity in lean subjects. The effects of exercise on gut microbiota were reversed after training was discontinued.

Overall, aerobic exercise training improves cardiorespiratory fitness (CRF), an effect that has been demonstrated in studies by Munukka et al. [16], Allen et al. [15] and Morita et al. [17]. CRF, which was measured as the maximum rate of oxygen consumption (VO$_{2max}$), has been observed to correlate with gut microbial diversity, fecal butyrate levels [36], and the Firmicutes-Bacteroidetes ratio [39]. The ratio between Firmicutes and Bacteroidetes phyla has been reported to be associated with body composition, with a higher fraction of Bacteroidetes associated with higher proportions of lean body mass, whereas lower levels have been associated with obesity [49].

In addition to human clinical studies, preclinical research in animal models has demonstrated that exercise changes the gut microbiota composition [50–55] and fecal SCFA concentrations, by increasing the production of butyrate [50,54], in particular. However, forced exercise, under stressful conditions, such as the exhaustive swimming test, may impact gut microbiota differently than voluntary activity, such as wheel running. In an overtraining mouse model, the gut microbial diversity was reduced in mice forced to swim to exhaustion compared with that in non-swimming mice [56].

2.3. Effects of Targeted Gut Microbiota Modulation on Physical Performance

Due to nutritional, genetic, and environmental factors, dissecting the exact role played by gut microbiota on exercise performance in human clinical studies can be difficult. Germ-free animal models overcome many of those challenges and have been used to demonstrate the roles played by gut microbiota on physical performance outcomes. Hsu et al. [27] studied the swimming capacities of specific pathogen-free (SPF), germ-free (GF), and *Bacteroides fragilis* gnotobiotic mice. The swim-to-exhaustion time was the shortest for GF mice and the longest for SPF mice, indicating decreased performance in the absence of gut microbiota. Similar findings regarding the reduced performance of GF mice compared with that in gnotobiotic and SPF mice were observed by Huang et al. [57].

In contrast to the above, Lahiri et al. [58] showed that GF mice and SPF mice did not differ in physical performance when exercising until exhaustion. However, GF mice demonstrated reduced muscle mass, fewer muscle fibers, and reduced muscle strength compared with SPF mice. Muscle atrophy in GF mice was associated with dysregulated mitochondrial biogenesis and reduced oxidative capacity. The transplantation of gut microbiota from SPF mice restored the muscle mass in GF mice, and treatment with a blend of SCFAs increased skeletal muscle mass and muscle strength in GF mice compared with those in untreated GF mice [58].

Antibiotic treatment drastically alters the composition of gut microbiota. Nay et al. [28] demonstrated that gut microbiota depletion, following a broad-spectrum antibiotic treatment, reduced the endurance running time of mice, and the endurance capacity was normalized after microbiota restoration through reseeding. Changes in endurance capacity were not related to changes in muscle mass, muscle fiber typology, or mitochondrial function but were associated with changes in muscle glycogen levels, which were restored after reseeding. Okamoto et al. [29] reported similar findings, in which the treadmill running time was shorter in mice treated with multiple antibiotics compared with that in non-treated controls. Okamoto et al. [29] also investigated the effects of SCFA production and its role on exercise performance, by feeding mice with fibers with differential substrate availability for microbial SCFA production in the gut. Mice fed with reduced fermentable fibers showed significantly shorter running times compared with mice fed with highly fermentable fibers, suggesting that microbiota and its substrates are both associated with physical performance. To further explore the putative role of SCFAs in performance capacity, antibiotic-treated mice were administered with a subcutaneous infusion of acetate or butyrate [29]. Acetate, but not butyrate, infusion improved the antibiotic-induced deterioration in running time.

Germ-free animals are of course an extreme model and may not explain the more subtle difference observed in the microbiota of humans. Nevertheless, studies in germ-free animal models have established a cause-effect relationship between gut microbiota and physical performance. Overall, the normalization of gut microbiota dysbiosis appeared to effectively restore exercise capacity and skeletal muscle parameters in rodents [58]. In addition, differences in gut microbiota compositions or the lack of gut microbiota have been shown to modulate exercise capacity, associated with muscle structure, muscle strength, and/or energy utilization [25,28]. Thus, the host appears to benefit from microbes through improved performance. The effects of gut microbiota are at least partially mediated by the production of SCFAs, which impact the gut and can also affect peripheral target tissues, via circulation.

3. Probiotics as a Potential Ergogenic Aid to Enhance Physical Performance

Nutritional ergogenic aids are dietary supplements that are consumed to help an individual exercise, enhance exercise performance capacity, enhance training adaptations, and improve recovery from exercise [59]. The use of nutritional ergogenic supplements is popular among athletes and recreationally active individuals of all age groups; however, evidence that supports the efficacy of many supplements is very limited or lacking. Performance-enhancing supplements with good or strong evidence have been identified by the International Olympic Committee and include the following: caffeine, creatine, nitrate, sodium bicarbonate, and beta-alanine [60]. Even when associated with only marginal improvements in performance, safe, proven, ergogenic dietary supplements may provide competitive benefits for an athlete.

Probiotic supplementation has been demonstrated to beneficially modify and support the gut microbiota composition [19–21]. Probiotics comprise many bacterial species, with the most studied probiotics belonging to the genera *Lactobacillus* (and associated genera) or *Bifidobacterium*. Associations between probiotics and physical performance and plausible mechanisms underlying these actions have been addressed in animal studies, which have suggested that probiotic supplementation protects against undesirable physiological changes that may be induced by strenuous exercise. Preclinical studies have demonstrated that probiotics can improve gut barrier properties [61] and the antioxidative status [62] and attenuate inflammatory response [63–65] in rodents after exhaustive exercise. However, how these protective effects are associated with physical performance outcomes has not been determined.

To date, the effects of probiotic supplementation have been studied in a variety of athletic and physically active populations, examining a variety of probiotic strains. Because the number of clinical studies on the association between probiotics and physical performance remains very low, with each study generally including a small number of participants and utilizing different exercise protocols, conclusions should be drawn carefully. The training status and training history of the participants can also influence the outcomes of exercise interventions [66]. Trained athletes and untrained individuals differ in their physiological responses to exercise [66], which can result in controversial results among different study populations. The use of resistance training programs alone during exercise intervention studies can contribute to changes in body composition and skeletal muscle organization that may supersede the impacts associated with probiotic supplementation, especially among previously sedentary populations.

The studies that have examined the effects of probiotics on physical performance have generally focused on mid- to long-term benefits, with supplementation periods varying from 2 weeks to 3 months (Table 2). The examined probiotic strains, formulas, and doses vary from study to study, which creates controversy among the obtained results. The most studied species are members of genera *Lactobacillus* (and associated genera) and *Bifidobacterium*; however, the benefits of probiotics, even within a single species, are often strain-specific. Furthermore, studies have been performed using both live and inactivated bacteria, which may have different modes of action. To comply with the definition, probiotics need to be alive microbes [18]. The proposed mode-of-action for probiotics and the benefits they provide to athletes are summarized in Figure 2.

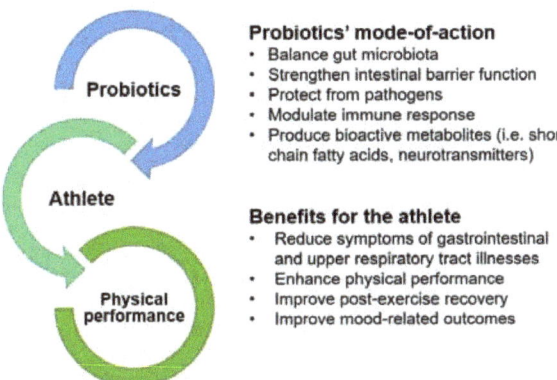

Figure 2. Proposed mechanisms and benefits of probiotic use in athletes.

3.1. Reduction of Gastrointestinal and Upper Respiratory Tract Symptoms

The beneficial effects of probiotics on GI health and upper respiratory tract (URT) illness symptoms among the general population have been well-acknowledged and reviewed extensively, elsewhere [67,68]. Because the exercise performance capacity of an athlete can be greatly influenced by overall health and resistance to infections, we have briefly highlighted the main findings, here.

Several studies have shown the potential of probiotic use to shorten the duration of GI disturbance episodes and relieve GI symptoms in athletes [69–74]. GI symptoms are common in athletes and can be influenced by the type of exercise performed [75]. GI challenges are most prominent in endurance athletes, among whom the prevalence of symptoms varies from 30% to up to 90%, depending on the individual athlete and the type and the extremes of the exercise [75]. Typically, endurance athletes suffer from mild to severe symptoms, including nausea, vomiting, abdominal angina, and bloody diarrhea, which are caused, in part, by reduced blood circulation in the splanchnic region during intensive exercise [75]. Reduced circulation can result in oxygen deprivation in the gut epithelial cells, which damages the cells and causes changes in the gut permeability, a phenomenon known as "leaky gut syndrome." Metabolites, such as SCFAs, and other effector molecules, which are produced by beneficial bacteria, may improve the intestinal barrier function by increasing the expression of tight junction proteins in the epithelia, which reduces mucosal permeability [43]. Clinical results regarding the effects of probiotic administration on gut permeability in athletes are scarce and controversial, showing positive effects [72,73] or no effects [76,77].

Prolonged high-intensity exercise has been associated with transient immune dysfunction and increased illness risk [78]. Due to the transient suppression of mucosal and systemic immune responses, athletes are especially susceptible to viral respiratory infections, which affect the quality of training and physical performance [79,80]. In contrast, moderate exercise appears to protect against infections, whereas a sedentary lifestyle increases the risk [78,79]. Several studies have investigated whether probiotic supplementation can reduce the risks of respiratory tract illness episodes, alleviate symptoms, and reduce the duration of episodes among athletes and recreationally active subjects. The study results have not shown consistent effects for all of the aforementioned benefits; however, beneficial effects on incidence, duration, and the number of symptoms have been reported [69,81–85]. Consequently, the positive impacts of probiotic supplementation on URT symptoms and illness may facilitate an earlier return to normal activity levels, references [83,85] increasing the hours spent on training, which can positively influence overall athletic performance. The administration of a two-strain probiotic supplement (*Lactobacillus acidophilus* NCFM and *Bifidobacterium animalis* subsp. *lactis* Bi-07) delayed the occurrence of URT illness and significantly increased the training load during a 5-month intervention period compared with placebo [83].

Reducing the incidence or severity of illness has positive impacts on performance during training and competition. Thus, probiotics may indirectly enhance physical performance.

3.2. Enhancement of Physical Performance

Depending on the sport and exercise type, physical performance can be measured as outcomes related to endurance, strength, speed, flexibility, or psychological performance (concentration, motivation) [86]. Exercise capacity often refers to exercise time to fatigue or exhaustion, at a given intensity or workload [87]. The potential for probiotics to improve physical performance has been recognized during exercise interventions and training studies involving athletes, recreational athletes, and sedentary individuals. Table 2 summarizes the studies examining the associations between physical performance and probiotic use, including preclinical and clinical studies, in which the used supplementation protocol fulfills the definition of a probiotic as a live organism.

Probiotic supplementation has been shown to increase the time to fatigue in both preclinical studies [88–90] and clinical studies, among both athletes and non-athletes [77,91,92]. *Lactiplantibacillus plantarum* TWK10 is among the most studied probiotic strains in terms of physical performance outcomes. A preclinical animal study demonstrated a dose-dependent increase in forelimb grip strength and endurance swimming time in mice supplemented with TWK10 [88]. Mice supplemented with TWK10 also showed an increased number of type I (slow-twitch) muscle fibers in the gastrocnemius muscle compared with control mice. These performance benefits were further confirmed in clinical studies. Endurance performance in an exhaustive treadmill exercise was improved in healthy, untrained adult males, who were supplemented daily with TWK10 for 6 weeks, compared with those who received a placebo [91]. In addition to significantly longer time to exhaustion (58% longer running time in the probiotic vs. placebo groups), the post-exercise blood glucose level was higher in TWK10 group compared with the placebo group suggesting improved energy harvest from gluconeogenic precursors during exhaustive exercise. No significant improvements in perceived exertion during exhaustive exercise were reported by the probiotic supplementation group compared with the placebo group.

A more recent clinical study from the same research group demonstrated a dose-dependent improvement in endurance performance (time to exhaustion) following TWK10 supplementation

(3×10^{10} or 9×10^{10} colony forming units, CFU, per day) in untrained subjects [92]. A higher dose of TWK10 significantly increased muscle mass compared with placebo treatment during the 6-week supplementation period. Further, blood lactate levels were significantly lower at the end of the exercise bout after both doses of probiotic supplementation compared with placebo treatment.

A double-blind, cross-over, exercise study examining trained male runners demonstrated that supplementation with a multi-strain probiotic (*L. acidophilus*, *Lacticaseibacillus rhamnosus*, *Lacticaseibacillus casei*, *L. plantarum*, *Limosilactobacillus fermentum*, *Bifidobacterium lactis*, *B. breve*, *B. bifidum*, and *Streptococcus thermophilus*) for 4 weeks significantly increased the time to fatigue on a treadmill running exercise performed in the heat compared with placebo, resulting in an average 16% longer running time [77]. No differences were observed in the severity of GI symptoms or GI permeability between the probiotic and placebo groups during exercise [77].

However, not all studies have shown enhancements in endurance performance following probiotic use in highly trained subjects or athletes [81,84,85,93]. Performance measurements related to exhaustive endurance exercise were not affected in endurance-trained males, after 4 weeks of *L. fermentum* VRI-003 supplementation [81], or in trained subjects, after *Lactobacillus helveticus* Lafti L10 [84]. A multi-species probiotic formulation (*B. bifidum* W23, *B. lactis* W51, *Enterococcus faecium* W54, *L. acidophilus* W22, *Levilactobacillus brevis* W63, and *Lactococcus lactis* W58) for 3 months did not have benefit in endurance performance in highly trained athletes [85]. In female swimmers, a multi-strain probiotic (*L. acidophilus* SPP, *L. bulgaricus*, *B. bifidum*, and *S. thermophilus*) yogurt improved the VO_{2max} (calculated using a Harvard step test) but had no impact on the 400-m swimming time after a 2-month intervention [82]. The 6-week supplementation with *B. longum* 35,624 in competitive, high-level, female swimmers did not enhance aerobic or anaerobic swimming performance or improve power or force production measurements [93]. Marshall et al. [94] found no effects for a 12-week multistrain probiotic or probiotic + glutamine supplementation protocol on the time to complete an ultra-marathon race compared with controls.

A few clinical studies have addressed the impacts of probiotic supplementation on sprint and power performance showing no clear benefits. *Bacillus subtilis* DE111 did not improve either strength or performance in male [95] or female athletes [96] when combined with a training protocol involving resistance exercises. Multi-strain probiotic supplementation for 12 weeks, combined with circuit-training, which involved resistance exercises, improved muscular performance to a similar degree as circuit-training alone in healthy, sedentary males [97], confirming the positive effects of resistance training on muscular outcomes, which is a result that has been demonstrated by other probiotic and exercise interventions among athletes [95,96]. The effects of probiotic supplementation on muscle strength and power production may be superseded by the effects of the resistance training protocols used by these studies. Regular resistance exercise strongly induces physiological changes in skeletal muscles and improves muscular strength in the long term

A recent trend in the field of gut microbiota and exercise research has been to isolate gut bacteria from the feces of elite athletes, to study the performance benefits of athlete-derived gut bacteria in animals. Recently, the oral administration of either *B. longum* subsp. *longum* OLP-01 [98] or *Ligilactobacillus salivarius* subsp. *salicinius* SA-03 [99], isolated from a female weightlifting Olympic medalist, was demonstrated to significantly increase forelimb grip strength and endurance capacity in a swim-to-exhaustion test in mice. Both OLP-01 and SA-03 significantly decreased blood lactate, ammonia, and CK levels after an acute exercise bout, and increased hepatic and muscle glycogen stores at autopsy and decreased which indicated improved energy utilization and the attenuation of fatigue-related biomarkers in mice.

The inoculation of *Veillonella atypica,* isolated from a marathon runner, increased the treadmill running time in mice compared with that of control mice [14]. In a subsequent experiment, the intracolonic infusion of propionate also improved running times until exhaustion in mice. *Veillonella* species are known to metabolize lactate into propionate and acetate. Notably, a series of experiments by this research group also showed that $^{13}C_3$-lactate injected into the mouse tail vein could be found in the contents of colon and cecum, post-injection, indicating that circulating lactate can pass through the intestinal epithelium into the gut lumen. This seminal work in mice implies that lactate that is produced by skeletal muscles during prolonged anaerobic exercise may enter the colon from the circulation, which can serve as fuel for certain bacteria in the gut, providing a selection advantage [14]. These findings suggested that both the host and gut microbes may benefit from a symbiotic relationship; however, clinical evidence remains necessary to provide additional proof of these beneficial effects. Although athlete-originating microbes, such as *Veillonella,* sp. may show benefits in preclinical settings, the development of clinically proven commercial probiotics that can provide health benefits in humans requires further research.

Thus far, the number of human clinical studies investigating the impacts of probiotics on physical performance remains low, and those that have been performed have examined limited exercise types and performance measures. Clinical data have suggested that probiotics may improve the time to exhaustion during endurance exercise; however, these data are scarce and contradictory results exist. Studies have been conducted using a variety of probiotic strains that may differ in their efficacy. Further research remains necessary to determine the direct effects of probiotic supplementation on performance outcomes.

Table 2. Probiotic studies on physical performance, post-exercise recovery and cognitive outcomes.

Subjects	Design	Exercise Protocol and/or Intervention	Probiotic Supplementation	Main Results	Reference
Animal studies:					
6-week-old male ICR mice 3 groups n = 8/group	Animal study	Forelimb grip strength Forced swim-to-exhaustion test, with loads 15-min swim test to determine recovery and fatigue-related biomarkers	*L. plantarum* TWK10 (LP10) Dosing per group: 0, 2.05×10^8, or 1.03×10^9 CFU/kg/day for 6 weeks	PRO improved forelimb grip strength and exhaustive swimming time. Blood lactate, ammonia, and CK levels were lower in PRO mice after a 15-min swim compared with those in control mice. Type I muscle fiber type increased, and relative muscle weight increased in PRO mice vs. control mice.	[88]
6-week-old male ICR mice 4 groups n = 8/group	Animal study	Forelimb grip strength Forced swim-to-exhaustion test with loads 10-min and 90-min swim tests, to determine recovery and fatigue-related biomarkers	A kefir drink with *L. fermentum* DSM 32,784 (LF26), *L. helveticus* DSM 32,787 (LH43), *L. paracasei* DSM 32,785 (LPC12), *L. rhamnosus* DSM 32,786 (LRH10), and *S. thermophilus* DSM 32,788 (ST30) Kefir dosing per group: 0, 2.15, 4.31, or 10.76 g/kg/day for 4 weeks	Kefir supplementation increased time-to-exhaustion, and improved forelimb grip strength. Blood lactate, ammonia, blood urea nitrogen, and CK levels were lower after exercise in kefir-fed mice compared with control mice, in a dose-dependent manner. Glycogen contents in the liver and muscle were higher in kefir-supplemented mice compared with control mice.	[89]
11-week-old male Wistar rats 2 groups n = 13/group	Animal study	Incremental speed exercise on a treadmill, until exhaustion Treadmill chamber, coupled with gas-analyzer, to assess VO_{2max}	*Saccharomyces boulardii* (strain not reported) 3×10^8 CFU/kg/day for 10 days	PRO supplementation moderately improved aerobic performance. PRO mice ran approx. 8 min longer than control mice (until exhaustion) and had higher maximal speed.	[90]
7-week-old male ICR mice 4 groups n = 10/group	Animal study	Forelimb grip strength Forced swim-to-exhaustion test, with loads 10-min and 90-min swim tests, to determine recovery and fatigue-related biomarkers	*B. longum* subsp. *longum* OLP-01 isolated from a female weightlifter Dosing per group: 0, 2.05×10^9, 4.10×10^9, or 1.03×10^{10} CFU/kg/day for 4 weeks	PRO improved forelimb grip strength and swim-to-exhaustion time, in a dose-dependent manner. Blood lactate and ammonia levels were lower after the acute swim test in PRO vs. control mice. After a 90-min swim test, blood urea nitrogen and CK levels were lower in PRO mice compared with those in control mice. PRO increased hepatic and muscular glycogen contents, observed at autopsy.	[98]
6-week-old male ICR mice 4 groups n = 10/group	Animal study	Forelimb grip strength Forced swim-to-exhaustion test, with loads 10-min and 90-min swim tests, to determine recovery and fatigue-related biomarkers	*L. salivarius* subsp. *salicinius* SA-03, isolated from a female weightlifter's gut microbiota Dosing per group: 0, 2.05×10^9, 4.10×10^9, or 1.03×10^{10} CFU/kg/day for 4 weeks	PRO improved forelimb grip strength and swim-to-exhaustion time, in a dose-dependent manner. Blood lactate and ammonia levels were lower and blood glucose levels were higher after acute tests in the PRO groups vs. control group. After a 90-min swim, blood CK levels were lower in PRO groups compared to the control group. PRO increased hepatic and muscular glycogen contents, observed at autopsy.	[99]

Table 2. Cont.

Subjects	Design	Exercise Protocol and/or Intervention	Probiotic Supplementation	Main Results	Reference
Clinical studies:					
Swimmers					
Highly trained competitive swimmers n = 17, females Age not reported	Randomized, double-blind, placebo-controlled	6 weeks of intensified off-season training, including swimming and resistance exercise. **Performance assessment:** Vertical jump force plate test, aerobic and anaerobic swim performance test **Cognitive assessment:** stress and recovery during the intensified exercise training load (the Recovery-Stress Questionnaire for Athletes)	B. longum 35,624; 1×10^9 CFU bacteria/day for 6 weeks	No significant differences in exercise performance or systemic inflammation markers (at rest) between PRO and PLA. Differences in cognitive outcomes were detected showing more favorable sport recovery related scores in the PRO group.	[93]
Swimmers n = 46, females Age 13.8 ± 1.8 y	Randomized, placebo-controlled	Normal exercise regimen **Performance assessment:** 400-m free-swimming record, Harvard step test to, measure VO_{2max}	L. acidophilus SPP, L. delbrueckii subsp. bulgaricus, B. bifidum, and S. salivarus subsp. thermophilus, strains not reported 400 mL of probiotic yogurt/day with 4×10^{10} CFU/mL for 8 weeks	Significant improvement in VO_{2max} in the PRO group. No differences in 400-m swimming times between PRO and PLA groups.	[82]
Endurance runners					
Elite distance runners n = 20, males Age 27.3 ± 6.4 y	Randomized, double-blind, placebo-controlled, crossover	Habitual winter-season training **Performance assessment:** A treadmill running test until exhaustion, at the start of the study period and the end of each study month	L. fermentum VRI-003; 1.2×10^{10} CFU bacteria/day for 4 weeks Cross-over study, with 1-month wash-out	No difference in performance outcomes with PRO compared to PLA. The number of illness days during PRO supplementation was significantly lower than with PLA (30 vs. 72 days). IFN-γ response was moderately higher with the PRO than with PLA.	[81]
Endurance-trained runners n = 8, males Age 26 ± 6 y	Randomized, blinded, placebo-controlled, cross-over	Habitual training **Bout of exercise:** 2-h running exercise at 60% VO_{2max} in hot ambient conditions	L. casei (strain not reported) 1×10^{11} CFU/day for 7 days Cross-over study, with 1-month wash-out	No differences in hydration status between PRO and PLA. Inflammatory cytokine levels were not different between PRO and PLA, either pre-exercise or post-exercise (1, 2, 4, and 24 h after running).	[100]
Endurance-trained runners n = 8, males Age 26 ± 6 y	Randomized, blinded, placebo-controlled, cross-over	Habitual training **Bout of exercise:** 2-h running exercise at 60% VO_{2max}, in hot, ambient conditions	L. casei (strain not reported) 1×10^{11} CFU/day for 7 days Cross-over study, with 1-month wash-out	PRO and PLA did not differ in salivary anti-microbial protein or serum cortisol responses during the post-exercise period (1, 2, 4, and 24 h after running).	[101]
Runners n = 10, males Age 27 ± 2 y	Randomized, double-blind, placebo-controlled, cross-over	Normal training **Performance assessment:** Running to fatigue, at 80% of ventilatory threshold, at 35 °C and 40% humidity	Multispecies probiotic, strains not specified; L. acidophilus, L. rhamnosus, L. casei, L. plantarum, L. fermentum, B. lactis, B. breve, B. bifidum, and S. thermophilus 45×10^9 CFU/day for 4 weeks, cross-over study with a 3-week wash-out	PRO increased run time to fatigue (PRO 37:44 vs. PLA 33:00 min:sec). A moderate, non-significant reduction in pre-exercise and post-exercise serum lipopolysaccharide (LPS) levels for PRO compared to PLA. No differences between PRO and PLA in plasma IL-6, IL-10, and IL-1Ra or GI permeability after exercise in the heat.	[77]

Table 2. Cont.

Subjects	Design	Exercise Protocol and/or Intervention	Probiotic Supplementation	Main Results	Reference
Marathon runners n = 42, males Age 39.5 ± 9.4 y	Randomized, double-blind, placebo-controlled	Usual training Bout of exercise: marathon run	*L. casei* Shirota 40 × 10^9 CFU/day for 30 days	PRO maintained salivary immune protection and increased anti-inflammatory response on the upper airways, immediately after the marathon. Serum TNF-α level was significantly lower immediately post-marathon in the PRO group compared to that in the PLA group	[102]
Marathon runners n = 119 (105/M, 14/F) Average age 40 y	Randomized, double-blind, placebo-controlled	3-month training period, 6-day preparation period Bout of exercise: marathon run	*L. rhamnosus* GG 4.0 × 10^{10} bacteria in drink/day (or 1 × 10^{10} in tablet/day) for 3 months	PRO did not differ from PLA in ox-LDL or antioxidant activity, pre- or post-marathon.	[103]
Marathon runners n = 24 (20/M, 4/F) Age 22–50 y	Randomized, double-blind, placebo-controlled, matched-pairs	Habitual training routine Performance assessment/Bout of exercise: Marathon race (no baseline assessment)	*L. acidophilus* CUL60, *L. acidophilus* CUL21, *B. bifidum* CUL20, and *B. animalis* subsp. *lactis* CUL34 2.5 × 10^{10} CFU/day for 28 days	No difference in marathon times between PRO and PLA. During the final third of the race, the reduction in average relative speed was greater in PLA compared to PRO. GI symptoms were lower in PRO compared to PLA during the final third. No difference in post-race serum IL-6, IL-8, IL-10, and cortisol levels between groups.	[104]
Ultramarathon runners n = 32 (26/M, 6/F) Age 23–53 y	Randomized, controlled (single-blind for glutamine supplementation)	Training for a marathon, ultra-marathon race of 294 km Performance assessment: A graded exercise test, to maximal exhaustion, on a motorized treadmill, VO$_{2max}$ test, pre-marathon, time-to-completion in ultra-marathon race	PRO: Multi-strain probiotic, daily dose 30 × 10^9 CFU comprising of 10 × 10^9 CFU *L. acidophilus* CUL-60 (NCIMB 30,157), 10 × 10^9 CFU *L. acidophilus* CUL-21 (NCIMB 30,156), 9.5 × 10^9 CFU *B. bifidum* CUL-20 (NCIMB 30,172), and 0.5 × 10^9 CFU *B. animalis* subsp. *lactis* CUL-34 (NCIMB 30,153 + 55.8 g fructooligosaccharides PRO + glutamine: Daily dose 2 × 10^9 CFU *L. acidophilus* CUL-60 (NCIMB 30,157), 2 × 10^9 CFU *L. acidophilus* CUL-21 (NCIMB 30,156), 5 × 10^7 CFU *B. bifidum* CUL-20 (NCIMB 30,172), 9.5 × 10^8 CFU *B. animalis* subsp. *lactis* CUL-34 (NCIMB 30,153), and 5x 10^9 CFU *L. salivarius* CUL61 (NCIMB 30,211) + 0.9 g glutamine 12 weeks before the marathon	No difference in pre-race VO$_{2max}$ or in time-to-completion for ultra-marathon between PRO, PRO + glutamine, and control groups. PRO and PRO + glutamine had no effects on immune activation via extracellular heat-shock protein eHsp72 signaling at post-race.	[94]

Table 2. Cont.

Subjects	Design	Exercise Protocol and/or Intervention	Probiotic Supplementation	Main Results	Reference
Cyclists, triathletes					
Competitive cyclists n = 99 (64/M, 35/F) Age 35 ± 9 y/M and 36 ± 9 y/F	Randomized, double-blind, placebo-controlled	Habitual training (physical activity recorded) Performance assessment: an incremental cycle ergometer performance test (peak power output, VO_{2max})	*L. fermentum* VRI-003 PC 1×10^9 CFU/day for 11 weeks	PRO did not affect training patterns or performance in VO_{2max} testing. Acute exercise-induced changes in anti- and pro-inflammatory cytokines were attenuated with PRO.	[71]
Triathletes Study I: n = 18, Study II: n = 16 Sex not reported Age 19–26 y	Randomized, double-blind, placebo-controlled	8 weeks of programmed training before a sprint triathlon (Study I) or full triathlon competition (Study II) Performance assessment: Wingate and 85% VO_{2max} test (after full triathlon)	*L. plantarum* PS128 3×10^{10} CFU/day Study I: last 4 weeks of training Study II: last 3 weeks of training	In Study II, performance during recovery from a full triathlon was decreased in the PLA group and maintained at the pre-triathlon level in the PRO group. PRO group had lower blood TNF-α, IFN-γ, IL-6, and IL-8 levels compared to PLA, immediately after exercise (Study I/II), with levels significantly lower in PRO group 3 h after full triathlon (Study II). Anti-inflammatory IL-10 was higher in the PRO group, immediately after exercise (Study II) compared with that in the PLA group. No differences in muscle damage or fatigue markers detected between groups (Study I/II) except, lower CK in PRO vs. PLA, 3 h after full triathlon (Study II). Oxidative stress marker (MPO) was lower in PRO after exercise, with no differences 3 h post-exercise.	[105]
Elite athletes (badminton, triathlon, cycling, alpinism, karate, savate, kayak, judo, tennis, and swimming) n = 50 (36/M, 14/F) Age 18–28 y	Randomized, double-blind, placebo-controlled	Habitual training >11 h/week, self-reported training loads Performance assessment: VO_{2max} by a graded cardiopulmonary test, on a treadmill Cognitive assessment: Profile of mood and state (POMS) questionnaire	*L. helveticus* Lafti L10 2×10^{10} CFU/day for 14 weeks	No difference in VO_{2max} and treadmill performance between PRO and PLA. Increase in the subjective feeling of vigor in the PRO group, but no difference in other cognitive scores between groups.	[84]
Recreational triathletes n = 30 (25/M, 5/F) Age 35 ± 1 y	Randomized, double-blind, placebo-controlled	Standardized training program for the previous 6 months Performance assessment/Bout of exercise: a long-distance triathlon (no baseline assessment)	Multistrain probiotic, daily dose 30×10^9 CFU (10×10^9 CFU *L. acidophilus* CUL-60 (NCIMB 30,157), 10×10^9 CFU *L. acidophilus* CUL-21 (NCIMB 30,156), 9.5×10^9 CFU *B. bifidum* CUL-20 (NCIMB 30,172), 0.5×10^9 CFU *B. animalis* subsp. *lactis* CUL-34 (NCIMB 30,153)) + 55.8 g fructo-oligosaccharides, alone or in combination with 600 mg N-acetyl carnitine + 400 mg α-lipoic acid for 12 weeks before and 6 days after triathlon	Non-significantly faster times were reported for PRO during swim and cycle stages, and a trend towards an overall faster time was reported compared to PLA (−86 min faster). No baseline measurements on performance were assessed. PRO reduced post-race plasma endotoxin levels, whereas PLA had no effect.	[73]

Table 2. Cont.

Subjects	Design	Exercise Protocol and/or Intervention	Probiotic Supplementation	Main Results	Reference
Team sports					
Division I volleyball and soccer athletes n = 23, females Age 19.6 ± 1.0 y	Randomized, double-blind, placebo-controlled	Offseason resistance training protocol Performance assessment: 1RM testing (bench press, squat, deadlift), isometric midthigh pull, vertical jump height, pro-agility test	*Bacillus subtilis* DE111 5×10^9 CFU/day for 10 weeks	PRO had no effect on strength or athletic performance but significantly reduced percentage of body fat percentage.	[96]
Division I baseball athletes n = 25, males Age 20.1 ± 1.5 y	Randomized, double-blind, placebo-controlled	Resistance training program Performance assessment: 1RM testing (squat, deadlift), pro-agility test, 10-yard sprint, standing long jump	*Bacillus subtilis* DE111 1×10^9 CFU/day for 12 weeks	No differences between PRO and PLA in strength, performance, or body composition. PRO reduced TNF-α levels, but no differences in IL-10, cortisol, zonulin, or testosterone levels observed between PRO and PLA.	[95]
Highly trained athletes n = 29 (13/M, 16/F) Age 20–35 years	Randomized, double-blind, placebo-controlled	Normal training Performance assessment: Cycle ergometer exercise test until exhaustion	*B. bifidum* W23, *B. lactis* W51, *Enterococcus faecium* W54, *L. acidophilus* W22, *L. brevis* W63, and *L. lactis* W58 1×10^{10} CFU/day for 12 weeks	No difference in performance between groups. Weekly training loads were significantly higher in PRO compared to PLA (8.0 ± 2.3 vs. 6.6. ± 4.3 h/week). Exercise-induced reduction in tryptophan levels in PLA but not in the PRO group. PRO reduced the incidence of URI infections.	[85]
Active non-athletes					
Resistance trained subjects n = 15, males Age 25 ± 4 y	Randomized, double-blind, placebo-controlled, crossover	Muscle-damaging eccentric exercise bout Performance assessment: isometric peak torque, after muscle damaging-exercise	*S. thermophilus* FP4, and *B. breve* BR03 5×10^9 CFU of each/day for 21 days	PRO attenuated performance decrements caused by muscle-damaging exercise during the recovery period. No effects of PRO on muscle soreness, range of motion, or plasma creatine kinase. PRO lowered resting IL-6 concentrations that were sustained until 48 h post-exercise.	[106]
Recreational exercisers n = 29, males Age 21.5 ± 2.8 y	Single-blind, crossover (casein first, after washout, PRO+casein)	Single-leg exercise bout Performance assessment: Anaerobic power by modified Wingate test, single-leg vertical jump, strength, by 1RM testing in the one-legged leg press, after muscle damaging-exercise	*Bacillus coagulans* BC30 1×10^9 CFU/day + 20 g casein for 14 days	PRO + casein increased perceived recovery status and reduced muscle soreness after exercise compared with casein alone. PRO + casein maintained post-exercise Wingate peak power at the pre-exercise level, whereas casein alone demonstrated reduced post-exercise performance. For 1RM leg-press and vertical jump power, no differences between groups in post-exercise performance.	[107]
Physically active subjects n = 27, females Age 18–25 y	Controlled, randomized	Habitual moderate exercise Performance assessment: treadmill running until exhaustion, VO_{2max} test (Bruce test)	Probiotic not specified 450 g of probiotic yogurt/day for 2 weeks	No difference in VO_{2max} between PRO and PLA. PRO yogurt increased antioxidant enzyme activities and reduced MMP2 and MMP9 levels before and after exhaustive exercise. No significant differences between PRO and PLA in high-sensitivity CRP, IL-6, and TNF-α after intense exercise.	[108]

Table 2. Cont.

Subjects	Design	Exercise Protocol and/or Intervention	Probiotic Supplementation	Main Results	Reference
Physically active students n = 11, sex not reported Age 22 ± 1 y	Non-controlled	Habitual training including endurance exercise **Bout of exercise**: 2-h cycling at 60% of VO_{2max}	*L. acidophilus, L. delbrueckii* subsp. *bulgaricus, Lactococcus lactis* subsp. *lactis, L. casei, L. helveticus, L. plantarum, L. rhamnosus, L. salivarius* subsp. *salivarius, B. breve, B. bifidum, B. infantis, B. longum, Bacillus subtilis, S. thermophilus* minimum 2×10^9 CFU/capsule, 3 capsules/day for 30 days	Rating of perceived exertion during exercise was not different between PRO and PLA. PRO did not affect salivary antimicrobial proteins at rest or in response to an acute bout of prolonged exercise.	[109]
Students n = 67, males and females (n not specified by sex) Age 18–24 y	Controlled	The exercise groups completed structured, long-distance, endurance run training, whereas the active group maintained their usual exercise routine. **Performance assessment**: 1.5-mile (2.41 km) walk or run	Probiotic kefir, probiotic strain and dose not specified 15 weeks	No effect of PRO on 1.5-mile completion time. PRO attenuated exercise-induced inflammation, measured as serum CRP levels.	[110]
Students of physical education n = 30, males Average age: PRO 21.56 y, PLA 21.28 y	Randomized, matched pairs	Habitual training and training program by the study **Performance assessment**: Cooper test, maximum aerobic power, using Bulk test on a laboratory treadmill	Probiotic strains unspecified, included *S. thermophilus* and/or *L. delbrueckii* subsp. *bulgaricus* 1×10^5 CFU/g in 200 mL yogurt/day for 10 weeks	PRO improved VO_{2max} and aerobic performance. PRO decreased serum high-sensitivity CRP and increased HDL levels.	[111]
Healthy participants n = 16, males Age 20–40 y	Randomized, double-blind, placebo-controlled	Habitual exercise **Performance assessment**: Treadmill running at 85% VO_{2max} workload, until exhaustion.	*L. plantarum* TWK10 1×10^{11} CFU/day for 6 weeks	PRO improved time-to-exhaustion (PLA vs. PRO: 817 ± 79 vs. 1292 ± 204 s). Blood glucose was higher in PRO vs. PLA after exhaustive exercise. No differences in post-exercise blood lactate, free fatty acid, CK levels between PRO and PLA.	[91]
Healthy participants n = 54, (27/M, 27/F) Age 20–30 y	Double-blind, placebo-controlled	Habitual exercise **Performance assessment**: treadmill running, at 60% VO_{2max} and 85% VO_{2max} workload, until exhaustion	*L. plantarum* TWK10 3×10^{10} CFU/day or 9×10^{10} CFU/day for 6 weeks	Exhaustion time was increased in both PRO groups and were longer compared to PLA. Improvement in exercise capacity was dose-dependent. PRO reduced serum lactate during and after exercise compared to PLA. Muscle mass increased in the high-dose PRO group.	[92]
Healthy sedentary individuals n = 41, males Age 19–26 y	Randomized, parallel, placebo-controlled	Circuit training protocol, including resistance exercises, 3 times a week **Performance assessment**: muscular strength (peak torque) and power via an isokinetic dynamometer	*L. acidophilus* BCMC 12,130, *L. casei* BCMC 12,313, *L. lactis* BCMC 12,451, *B. bifidum* BCMC 02,290, *B. infantis* BCMC 02,129 and *B. longum* BCMC 02,120 6×10^{10} CFU/day for 12 weeks	PRO did not show superior effects to PLA on muscular strength (peak torque) and power. PRO alone and exercise alone increased post-intervention serum IL-10 concentrations from pre-intervention levels. PRO and PLA with or without exercise, had no effects on serum IL-6 concentration.	[97]

Table 2. Cont.

Subjects	Design	Exercise Protocol and/or Intervention	Probiotic Supplementation	Main Results	Reference
Healthy elderly individuals with stretching experience n = 29 (14/M, 25/F) Age > 65 y	Randomized, double-blind, placebo-controlled	Moderate resistance exercise training, in instructed classes and at home **Cognitive assessment:** General cognitive performance (incl. tests for accuracy, reaction time), mental state (scoring for depression, anxiety, and overall mental state)	*B. longum* BB536, *B. infantis* M-63, *B. breve* M-16V and *B. breve* B-3 5×10^{10} CFU/day (1.25×10^{10} CFU each probiotic/day) for 12 weeks	An increase in the general cognitive function scores was observed in PRO and PLA groups, at 12 weeks. PRO group showed a decrease in anxiety-depression scores, body weight, BMI and body fat.	[112]

ICR mice, Institute of Cancer Research mice; L., *Lactobacillus* (or related genera); B., *Bifidobacterium*; S., *Streptococcus*; CFU, colony-forming units; PRO, probiotic supplementation; PLA, placebo supplementation; CK, creatine kinase; VO$_{2max}$, maximum rate of oxygen consumption; M, males, F, females; IFN-γ, interferon γ; IL, interleukin; GI, gastrointestinal; TNF-α = tumor necrosis factor α; ox-LDL, oxidized low-density lipoprotein; MPO, myeloperoxidase; 1RM, 1 repetition maximum; MMP2/9, matrix metalloproteinase 2/9; CRP, C-reactive protein; HDL, high-density lipoprotein; BMI, body mass index.

3.3. Improvement in Post-Exercise Recovery

Recovery from exercise represents an important determinant of performance enhancement that enables adaptation to training. Strategies for optimizing recovery may prevent under-recovery, overtraining syndrome, injuries, or illnesses [86]. Exercise-induced muscle damage, inflammation, metabolic responses, and fatigue are part of the recovery process and are, therefore, important contributors to training adaptation. In addition to physical performance outcomes, biochemical markers and the athlete's subjective perception of fatigue and readiness to perform can be assessed, to evaluate the subject's recovery state after exercise.

The impacts of probiotic supplementation on health outcomes, performance measurements, and/or biochemical markers in athletes have been addressed in numerous studies, comparing post-intervention and pre-intervention resting levels after a training period. Endpoints and markers that are measured directly after acute exercise sessions and during recovery periods provide a more defined approach to the evaluation of post-exercise recovery status. The effects of probiotics on biochemical and immune markers during the post-exercise recovery state after an exercise session have been reported in several studies (Table 2). The effects of probiotic supplementation on performance capacity during the recovery period after exercise were studied in triathletes by Huang et al. [105], who assessed anaerobic (Wingate test) and aerobic (85% VO_{2max} test) exercise capacities, 48 and 72 h after a triathlon race. Probiotic supplementation (*L. plantarum* PS128) for 3 weeks significantly improved maximal power, the fatigue index, and endurance indices during the recovery period after the triathlon race compared with those in the placebo group. The probiotic group also maintained aerobic performance, when measured during the recovery period at the resting level, whereas the placebo group reached exhaustion significantly sooner during the recovery period

High-intensity training acutely increases muscle damage, fatigue, and soreness, which contributed to decreased athletic performance. Excess mechanical load creates micro-damage to skeletal muscle tissues, causing local inflammation and decreasing muscle function. Inflammation that occurs in the muscle tissue is a mechanism of muscular adaptation to exercise, through which the muscle can regenerate and repair itself [113]. Mechanical overload has been associated with increased systemic levels of muscle-derived proteins, such as creatine kinase (CK) and myoglobin [107]. Interleukin (IL)-6 is a cytokine that is produced by contracting muscles during exercise and increases in the plasma after strenuous exercise. Changes in muscle-damage-related biomarkers are associated with delayed-onset muscle soreness (DOMS) and muscle recovery [114].

In athletes who participated in a full triathlon championship competition, the *L. plantarum* PS128 probiotic group and the placebo group did not differ in blood CK values immediately after competition [105]. However, in the probiotic group, the CK level was significantly lower 3 h post-exercise compared with that in the placebo group. No differences in post-exercise lactate dehydrogenase, myoglobin, or free fatty acids were observed between the probiotic and placebo groups. After less-demanding sprint triathlon, supplementation with *L. plantarum* PS128 had no effects compared with placebo on post-exercise CK or blood lactate measurements [105]. In sedentary subjects who participated in exhaustive exercise, *L. plantarum* TWK10 improved blood lactate clearance during a 1-h post-exercise recovery period [92]. Blood lactate and lactate clearance are often measured to assess recovery. However, the suitability of these variables to evaluate fatigue and recovery is controversial and not agreed on [86].

In the triathlete study performed by Huang et al. [105], the levels of exercise-induced serum pro-inflammatory cytokines, tumor necrosis factor (TNF)-α, interferon (IFN)-γ, IL-6, and IL-8, were significantly lower in the probiotic group compared with those in the placebo group, both immediately and 3 h after the triathlon competition. The investigators also found increased anti-inflammatory IL-10 levels after the exercise, but not at the 3-h time point. Prolonged, high-intensity exercise is well-known to be associated with transient inflammation, immune dysfunction, and oxidative stress [78]. Lamprecht et al. [72] and Mazani et al. [108] both demonstrated a trend towards reduced circulating TNF-α levels in the probiotic group compared with the placebo, immediately after exhaustive exercise, supporting the findings reported by Huang et al. [105]. Probiotic interventions were found to increase antioxidant capacity [108], reduce oxidated molecules [72], and decrease myeloperoxidase and increase thioredoxin activity [105], suggesting overall benefits associated with reduced exercise-induced oxidative stress levels. However, some probiotic intervention studies have not found any effects on inflammation [93,100,101,104]; thus, further investigations are warranted to understand the effects of probiotics on post-exercise immune function and inflammation.

Increased levels of inflammatory cytokines may result from damaged muscle tissue but may also be caused by the disruption of intestinal barrier function after prolonged, intense, endurance exercise. Reduced intestinal blood flow causes the acute disruption of epithelial barrier function and increased leakage, resulting in endotoxemia, during which microbial lipopolysaccharides enter the blood circulation. The resulting systemic inflammation compromises the athlete's ability to recover and perform. Lamprecht et al. [72] showed that a 14-week, multi-strain, probiotic supplementation protocol reduced fecal zonulin and TNF-α levels significantly compared with those supplemented with placebo, indicating improved intestinal barrier integrity and reduced systemic inflammation, respectively. Probiotic supplementation of shorter duration for 4 weeks resulted in reduced gastrointestinal permeability and improved exercise capacity under heat conditions, with no impacts on circulating cytokine levels [77]. Moreover, probiotic supplementation did not attenuate exertional heat stress-induced blood endotoxemia or inflammation [100], the salivary antimicrobial protein response [101], or extracellular heat shock protein 72 (eHsp72) concentrations [94], when monitored during the recovery stage, post-exercise. Under normal ambient conditions, a 30-day supplementation protocol using a multi-strain probiotic did not demonstrate differences in the salivary antimicrobial peptides during post-exercise recovery after 2 h of cycling at 60% of VO_{2max} [109].

The benefits of probiotic use during recovery from muscle-damaging exercise have been demonstrated in two clinical studies [106,107]. A study performed in resistance-trained men, demonstrated that a 3-week supplementation with *S. thermophilus* FP4 and *B. breve* BR03 moderately attenuated post-exercise decreases in muscle performance, as assessed by isometric average peak torque, 24 to 72 h after a muscle-damaging exercise [106]. In addition, circulating IL-6 concentrations were reduced after the 3-week probiotic supplementation protocol but were not affected by the treatment during the post-exercise recovery period. Beneficial effects were observed in the resting arm angle after probiotic supplementation, whereas no differences in flexed arm angle, CK levels, or muscle soreness were observed during the recovery period, between the probiotic and placebo groups.

A 2-week supplementation of casein combined with *Bacillus coagulans* BC30, increased perceived recovery status scores at 24 and 72 h after muscle-damaging exercise compared with casein supplementation alone in recreationally trained men [107]. Probiotic combined with casein also reduced perceived muscle soreness compared with casein alone, 72 h post-exercise. Trends toward reduced circulating CK levels and improved performance, as measured by the Wingate test, were observed after the muscle-damaging exercise following probiotics combined with casein supplementation compared with casein supplementation alone. The amounts of muscle swelling and blood urea nitrogen levels did not differ between the groups. The effects of *B. coagulans* BC30 have also been studied among soldiers, who are known to train intensively, on a daily basis, with limited time to recover. β-Hydroxy-β-methylbutyrate calcium (CaHMB) combined with BC30 maintained muscle integrity during an intensive 40-day military training period better than CaHMB alone [115]. Treatment with both CaHMB combined with BC30 and CaHMB alone significantly attenuated resting serum IL-1β, IL-2, and TNF-α concentrations after the 40-day supplementation period, whereas CaHMB that was combined with BC30 significantly reduced serum IL-6 and IL-10 during the post-intervention period compared with control. However, the acute effects on biochemical marker levels during the recovery state were not evaluated. Probiotics have been proposed to enhance recovery and to shorten the time necessary for muscle repair by improving the absorption and utilization of dietary nutrients [107,115,116].

To date, studies that have assessed performance and exercise capacity during the post-exercise recovery period remain low in number. Studies that have investigated the probiotic effects on biochemical and immune markers during the post-exercise recovery period have shown somewhat controversial results, due to large variations in study designs, training protocols, analytical methods, athletic populations, and investigated probiotic strains. These results also warrant longer follow-up measurements during the recovery period. Thus, conclusions cannot be drawn regarding probiotics' potential to improve recovery and attenuate exercise-induced physiological responses, which are, in part, necessary for training adaptations and performance enhancement. Furthermore, the relationships between physiological recovery processes and improvements in performance should be established more clearly before further conclusions can be made regarding the ergogenic potential of probiotics.

3.4. Improvements in Mood-Related Outcomes

Good physical condition, accompanied by good mental condition, are part of a continuum that enables the optimal training and performance of competitive athletes. Fatigue and mood disturbances during performance are common among athletes during the training season and in competition [4]. Intensive exercise causes both physical and psychological stress responses, which can often be difficult to differentiate between.

Results from preclinical and clinical studies suggest that probiotic administration may have positive effects in mental responses [117,118]. Few studies have investigated the effects of probiotic supplementation on the cognitive outcomes of athletes or physically active subjects [84,93,112] (Table 2). In a group of highly trained, elite athletes, the self-rated sense of vigor (Profile of Mood States, POMS questionnaire) was significantly increased among the probiotic group, who ingested *L. helveticus* Lafti for 14 weeks, compared with the placebo group, with no difference in the total mood disturbance scores between groups detected [84]. Decreased vigor is related to an individual's feelings of possessing the necessary physical strength to perform.

In a study involving highly trained, female, competitive swimmers, probiotic supplementation (*B. longum* 35,624) during a 6-week intensive training period improved the cognitive functions of the athletes [93]. At the end of the intensive training period, significant differences in the scores related to sport recovery categories (the Recovery-Stress Questionnaire for Athletes) were detected between groups, showing that the scores of the probiotic group were more favorable compared with those in the placebo group. A training intervention performed in healthy, elderly, Japanese individuals demonstrated that a 12-week resistance training program induced beneficial effects on the general cognitive functions of both the placebo and probiotic groups [112]. The 12-week supplementation with multi-strain bifidobacteria significantly decreased overall mental state scores compared with baseline scores, with lower scores indicating lower depression and anxiety symptoms [112].

Probiotics are, by definition, live microorganisms. In addition to viable bacteria, studies have been performed using inactivated bacteria. Two studies have investigated the effects of supplementation with inactivated *Lactobacillus* on mood related measurements [119,120]. A 4-week supplementation period, using heat-inactivated *L. gasseri* OLL2809, reduced tension-anxiety scores after a 1-h cycle ergometer exercise, compared with baseline scores [119]. The 12-week administration of heat-inactivated *L. gasseri* CP2305 significantly decreased scores that measured physical fatigue, anxiety, and depression in male university student-athletes [120]. Salivary cortisol and chromogranin A serve as biochemical markers for stress. In the above-mentioned studies, salivary chromogranin A was significantly reduced in the inactivated *Lactobacillus* group compared with that in the placebo group [120], whereas no changes in salivary cortisol levels were detected after the intervention period [119,120].

Probiotics appear to have benefits on cognitive outcomes in athletes, as measured by self-reported scores. Several potential mechanisms exist for the gut bacteria to interact with the brain, through the gut-brain axis. Messages to the brain can be delivered by gut-derived cytokines, hormones, and bacterial metabolites, including neurotransmitters, or via the vagus nerve [4]. Probiotic studies that focus on the mental health of athletes represent an emerging area in the field of sports nutrition and exercise performance. The number of probiotic studies remains very low, with studies often including a low number of subjects, and a wide variety of questionnaires have been used to assess cognitive outcomes. Despite limited evidence, cognitive health remains an intriguing area of sports nutrition research.

4. Conclusions

Overall, growing evidence from animal and human studies has indicated that the gut microbiota composition plays an important role in host physiology and can affect physical performance. The microbial community of the gut and its potential health benefits are highly impacted by individual life choices, including dietary patterns and activity levels. Probiotics are known for their potential to reduce GI and URT symptoms and infection episodes and thus may benefit the athlete by increasing the numbers of healthy training days and completed races. Further, probiotics may support athletic performance by enhancing training adaptations, attenuating physiological responses during post-exercise recovery periods, and improving mood and mental responses after intense exercise. Therefore, probiotics can be considered to act as indirect ergogenic aids; however, the causal impacts of indirect effects on performance remain to be established in good-quality, long-term studies of adequate size that consider the diet, and the training and competition seasons of the athletes. The functions of probiotics in enhancing performance, as direct ergogenic aids, require additional research that targets the mode of action that underlies their potential benefits.

Author Contributions: Conceptualization, M.M., R.A.-J., A.L., and M.J.L.; writing—original draft preparation, M.M. and R.A.-J.; writing—review and editing, M.M., R.A.-J., A.L., and M.J.L.; visualization, M.M. and R.A.-J. All authors have read and agreed to the published version of the manuscript.

Funding: This research received no external funding.

Acknowledgments: Arthur Ouwehand and Johanna Maukonen are acknowledged for their comments during the manuscript preparation.

Conflicts of Interest: The authors are employees of Danisco Sweeteners Oy, legal entity of DuPont Nutrition & Biosciences that manufactures probiotics.

References

1. Sender, R.; Fuchs, S.; Milo, R. Revised Estimates for the Number of Human and Bacteria Cells in the Body. *PLoS Biol.* **2016**, *14*, e1002533. [CrossRef] [PubMed]
2. Cheng, H.Y.; Ning, M.X.; Chen, D.K.; Ma, W.T. Interactions Between the Gut Microbiota and the Host Innate Immune Response Against Pathogens. *Front. Immunol.* **2019**, *10*, 607. [CrossRef] [PubMed]
3. Dinan, T.G.; Cryan, J.F. Regulation of the stress response by the gut microbiota: Implications for psychoneuroendocrinology. *Psychoneuroendocrinology* **2012**, *37*, 1369–1378. [CrossRef] [PubMed]
4. Clark, A.; Mach, N. Exercise-induced stress behavior, gut-microbiota-brain axis and diet: A systematic review for athletes. *J. Int. Soc. Sports Nutr.* **2016**, *13*, 43. [CrossRef]
5. Larsen, O.F.; Claassen, E. The mechanistic link between health and gut microbiota diversity. *Sci. Rep.* **2018**, *8*, 1–5. [CrossRef]
6. Neish, A.S.J.G. Microbes in gastrointestinal health and disease. *Gastroenterology* **2009**, *136*, 65–80. [CrossRef]
7. Lozupone, C.A.; Stombaugh, J.I.; Gordon, J.I.; Jansson, J.K.; Knight, R.J.N. Diversity, stability and resilience of the human gut microbiota. *Nature* **2012**, *489*, 220–230. [CrossRef]
8. Valdes, A.M.; Walter, J.; Segal, E.; Spector, T.D. Role of the gut microbiota in nutrition and health. *BMJ* **2018**, *361*, k2179. [CrossRef]

9. Dinan, T.G.; Cryan, J.F. The microbiome-gut-brain axis in health and disease. *Gastroenterol. Clin. N. Am.* **2017**, *46*, 77–89. [CrossRef]
10. Grosicki, G.J.; Fielding, R.A.; Lustgarten, M.S. Gut microbiota contribute to age-related changes in skeletal muscle size, composition, and function: Biological basis for a gut-muscle axis. *Calcif. Tissue Int.* **2018**, *102*, 433–442. [CrossRef]
11. McKinney, J.; Lithwick, D.J.; Morrison, B.N.; Nazzari, H.; Isserow, S.H.; Heilbron, B.; Krahn, A.D. The health benefits of physical activity and cardiorespiratory fitness. *Br. Columbia Med. J.* **2016**, *58*, 131–137.
12. Clarke, S.F.; Murphy, E.F.; O'Sullivan, O.; Lucey, A.J.; Humphreys, M.; Hogan, A.; Hayes, P.; O'Reilly, M.; Jeffery, I.B.; Wood-Martin, R.; et al. Exercise and associated dietary extremes impact on gut microbial diversity. *Gut* **2014**, *63*, 1913–1920. [CrossRef] [PubMed]
13. Petersen, L.M.; Bautista, E.J.; Nguyen, H.; Hanson, B.M.; Chen, L.; Lek, S.H.; Sodergren, E.; Weinstock, G.M. Community characteristics of the gut microbiomes of competitive cyclists. *Microbiome* **2017**, *5*, 98. [CrossRef] [PubMed]
14. Scheiman, J.; Luber, J.M.; Chavkin, T.A.; MacDonald, T.; Tung, A.; Pham, L.-D.; Wibowo, M.C.; Wurth, R.C.; Punthambaker, S.; Tierney, B.T.; et al. Meta-omics analysis of elite athletes identifies a performance-enhancing microbe that functions via lactate metabolism. *Nat. Med.* **2019**, *25*, 1104–1109. [CrossRef]
15. Allen, J.M.; Mailing, L.J.; Niemiro, G.M.; Moore, R.; Cook, M.D.; White, B.A.; Holscher, H.D.; Woods, J.A. Exercise Alters Gut Microbiota Composition and Function in Lean and Obese Humans. *Med. Sci. Sports Exerc.* **2018**, *50*, 747–757. [CrossRef]
16. Munukka, E.; Ahtiainen, J.P.; Puigbo, P.; Jalkanen, S.; Pahkala, K.; Keskitalo, A.; Kujala, U.M.; Pietila, S.; Hollmen, M.; Elo, L.; et al. Six-Week Endurance Exercise Alters Gut Metagenome That Is not Reflected in Systemic Metabolism in Over-weight Women. *Front. Microbiol.* **2018**, *9*, 2323. [CrossRef]
17. Morita, E.; Yokoyama, H.; Imai, D.; Takeda, R.; Ota, A.; Kawai, E.; Hisada, T.; Emoto, M.; Suzuki, Y.; Okazaki, K. Aerobic exercise training with Brisk walking increases intestinal Bacteroides in healthy elderly women. *Nutrients* **2019**, *11*, 868. [CrossRef]
18. Hill, C.; Guarner, F.; Reid, G.; Gibson, G.R.; Merenstein, D.J.; Pot, B.; Morelli, L.; Canani, R.B.; Flint, H.J.; Salminen, S. The International Scientific Association for Probiotics and Prebiotics consensus statement on the scope and appropriate use of the term probiotic. *Nat. Rev. Gastroenterol. Hepatol.* **2014**, *11*, 506–514. [CrossRef]
19. Sánchez, B.; Delgado, S.; Blanco-Míguez, A.; Lourenço, A.; Gueimonde, M.; Margolles, A. Probiotics, gut microbiota, and their influence on host health and disease. *Mol. Nutr. Food Res.* **2017**, *61*, 1600240. [CrossRef]
20. Korpela, K.; Salonen, A.; Vepsäläinen, O.; Suomalainen, M.; Kolmeder, C.; Varjosalo, M.; Miettinen, S.; Kukkonen, K.; Savilahti, E.; Kuitunen, M. Probiotic supplementation restores normal microbiota composition and function in antibiotic-treated and in caesarean-born infants. *Microbiome* **2018**, *6*, 1–11. [CrossRef]
21. Hibberd, A.; Yde, C.; Ziegler, M.; Honoré, A.H.; Saarinen, M.T.; Lahtinen, S.; Stahl, B.; Jensen, H.; Stenman, L. Probiotic or synbiotic alters the gut microbiota and metabolism in a randomised controlled trial of weight management in overweight adults. *Benef. Microbes* **2019**, *10*, 121–135. [CrossRef] [PubMed]
22. Eutamene, H.; Bueno, L. Role of probiotics in correcting abnormalities of colonic flora induced by stress. *Gut* **2007**, *56*, 1495–1497. [CrossRef] [PubMed]
23. Kim, N.; Yun, M.; Oh, Y.J.; Choi, H.-J. Mind-altering with the gut: Modulation of the gut-brain axis with probiotics. *J. Microbiol.* **2018**, *56*, 172–182. [CrossRef] [PubMed]
24. Jäger, R.; Mohr, A.E.; Carpenter, K.C.; Kerksick, C.M.; Purpura, M.; Moussa, A.; Townsend, J.R.; Lamprecht, M.; West, N.P.; Black, K.; et al. International Society of Sports Nutrition Position Stand: Probiotics. *J. Int. Soc. Sports Nutr.* **2019**, *16*, 62. [CrossRef] [PubMed]
25. Charreire, H.; Kesse-Guyot, E.; Bertrais, S.; Simon, C.; Chaix, B.; Weber, C.; Touvier, M.; Galan, P.; Hercberg, S.; Oppert, J.-M.J.B.J.o.N. Associations between dietary patterns, physical activity (leisure-time and occupational) and television viewing in middle-aged French adults. *Brit. J. Nutr.* **2011**, *105*, 902–910. [CrossRef] [PubMed]
26. Sheflin, A.M.; Melby, C.L.; Carbonero, F.; Weir, T.L. Linking dietary patterns with gut microbial composition and function. *Gut Microbes* **2017**, *8*, 113–129. [CrossRef]
27. Hsu, Y.J.; Chiu, C.C.; Li, Y.P.; Huang, W.C.; Te Huang, Y.; Huang, C.C.; Chuang, H.L. Effect of intestinal microbiota on exercise performance in mice. *J. Strength. Cond. Res.* **2015**, *29*, 552–558. [CrossRef]

28. Nay, K.; Jollet, M.; Goustard, B.; Baati, N.; Vernus, B.; Pontones, M.; Lefeuvre-Orfila, L.; Bendavid, C.; Rué, O.; Mariadassou, M. Gut bacteria are critical for optimal muscle function: A potential link with glucose homeostasis. *Am. J. Physiol. Endocrinol. Metab.* **2019**, *317*, E158–E171. [CrossRef]
29. Okamoto, T.; Morino, K.; Ugi, S.; Nakagawa, F.; Lemecha, M.; Ida, S.; Ohashi, N.; Sato, D.; Fujita, Y.; Maegawa, H. Microbiome potentiates endurance exercise through intestinal acetate production. *Am. J. Physiol. Endocrinol. Metab.* **2019**, *316*, E956–E966. [CrossRef]
30. Barton, W.; Penney, N.C.; Cronin, O.; Garcia-Perez, I.; Molloy, M.G.; Holmes, E.; Shanahan, F.; Cotter, P.D.; O'Sullivan, O. The microbiome of professional athletes differs from that of more sedentary subjects in composition and particularly at the functional metabolic level. *Gut* **2018**, *67*, 625–633. [CrossRef]
31. LeBlanc, J.G.; Chain, F.; Martín, R.; Bermúdez-Humarán, L.G.; Courau, S.; Langella, P. Beneficial effects on host energy metabolism of short-chain fatty acids and vitamins produced by commensal and probiotic bacteria. *Microb. Cell. Fact.* **2017**, *16*, 79. [CrossRef] [PubMed]
32. Moreno-Pérez, D.; Bressa, C.; Bailén, M.; Hamed-Bousdar, S.; Naclerio, F.; Carmona, M.; Pérez, M.; González-Soltero, R.; Montalvo-Lominchar, M.G.; Carabaña, C. Effect of a protein supplement on the gut microbiota of endurance athletes: A randomized, controlled, double-blind pilot study. *Nutrients* **2018**, *10*, 337. [CrossRef] [PubMed]
33. Jang, L.G.; Choi, G.; Kim, S.W.; Kim, B.Y.; Lee, S.; Park, H. The combination of sport and sport-specific diet is associated with characteristics of gut microbiota: An observational study. *J. Int. Soc. Sports Nutr.* **2019**, *16*, 21. [CrossRef] [PubMed]
34. Keohane, D.M.; Woods, T.; O'Connor, P.; Underwood, S.; Cronin, O.; Whiston, R.; O'Sullivan, O.; Cotter, P.; Shanahan, F.; Molloy, M.G. Four men in a boat: Ultra-endurance exercise alters the gut microbiome. *J. Sci. Med. Sport* **2019**, *22*, 1059–1064. [CrossRef]
35. Murtaza, N.; Burke, L.M.; Vlahovich, N.; Charlesson, B.; O'Neill, H.; Ross, M.L.; Campbell, K.L.; Krause, L.; Morrison, M. The effects of dietary pattern during intensified training on stool microbiota of elite race walkers. *Nutrients* **2019**, *11*, 261. [CrossRef]
36. Estaki, M.; Pither, J.; Baumeister, P.; Little, J.P.; Gill, S.K.; Ghosh, S.; Ahmadi-Vand, Z.; Marsden, K.R.; Gibson, D.L. Cardiorespiratory fitness as a predictor of intestinal microbial diversity and distinct metagenomic functions. *Microbiome* **2016**, *4*, 42. [CrossRef] [PubMed]
37. Bressa, C.; Bailén-Andrino, M.; Pérez-Santiago, J.; González-Soltero, R.; Pérez, M.; Montalvo-Lominchar, M.G.; Maté-Muñoz, J.L.; Domínguez, R.; Moreno, D.; Larrosa, M. Differences in gut microbiota profile between women with active lifestyle and sedentary women. *PLoS ONE* **2017**, *12*, e0171352. [CrossRef]
38. Bai, J.; Hu, Y.; Bruner, D. Composition of gut microbiota and its association with body mass index and lifestyle factors in a cohort of 7–18 years old children from the American Gut Project. *Pediatr. Obes.* **2019**, *14*, e12480. [CrossRef]
39. Durk, R.P.; Castillo, E.; Márquez-Magaña, L.; Grosicki, G.J.; Bolter, N.D.; Lee, C.M.; Bagley, J.R. Gut microbiota composition is related to cardiorespiratory fitness in healthy young adults. *Int. J. Sport. Nutr. Exerc. Metab.* **2019**, *29*, 249–253. [CrossRef]
40. Langsetmo, L.; Johnson, A.; Demmer, R.; Fino, N.; Orwoll, E.; Ensrud, K.; Hoffman, A.R.; Cauley, J.A.; Shmagel, A.; Meyer, K. The Association between Objectively Measured Physical Activity and the Gut Microbiome among Older Community Dwelling Men. *J. Nutr. Health Aging* **2019**, *23*, 538–546. [CrossRef]
41. Cani, P.D.; de Vos, W.M. Next-Generation Beneficial Microbes: The Case of Akkermansia muciniphila. *Front. Microbiol.* **2017**, *8*, 1765. [CrossRef] [PubMed]
42. Xu, Z.; Knight, R. Dietary effects on human gut microbiome diversity. *Br. J. Nutr.* **2015**, *113*, S1–S5. [CrossRef]
43. Hiippala, K.; Jouhten, H.; Ronkainen, A.; Hartikainen, A.; Kainulainen, V.; Jalanka, J.; Satokari, R. The potential of gut commensals in reinforcing intestinal barrier function and alleviating inflammation. *Nutrients* **2018**, *10*, 988. [CrossRef] [PubMed]
44. Koh, A.; De Vadder, F.; Kovatcheva-Datchary, P.; Bäckhed, F. From dietary fiber to host physiology: Short-chain fatty acids as key bacterial metabolites. *Cell* **2016**, *165*, 1332–1345. [CrossRef] [PubMed]
45. WHO. Global recommendations on physical activity for health. *Geneva World Health Organ.* **2010**, *60*.
46. Cintineo, H.P.; Arent, M.A.; Antonio, J.; Arent, S.M. Effects of Protein Supplementation on Performance and Recovery in Resistance and Endurance Training. *Front. Nutr.* **2018**, *5*, 83. [CrossRef]

47. Russell, W.R.; Gratz, S.W.; Duncan, S.H.; Holtrop, G.; Ince, J.; Scobbie, L.; Duncan, G.; Johnstone, A.M.; Lobley, G.E.; Wallace, R.J.; et al. High-protein, reduced-carbohydrate weight-loss diets promote metabolite profiles likely to be detrimental to colonic health. *Am. J. Clin. Nutr.* **2011**, *93*, 1062–1072. [CrossRef]
48. Donati Zeppa, S.; Agostini, D.; Gervasi, M.; Annibalini, G.; Amatori, S.; Ferrini, F.; Sisti, D.; Piccoli, G.; Barbieri, E.; Sestili, P. Mutual Interactions among Exercise, Sport Supplements and Microbiota. *Nutrients* **2020**, *12*, 17. [CrossRef]
49. Ley, R.E.; Turnbaugh, P.J.; Klein, S.; Gordon, J.I. Human gut microbes associated with obesity. *Nature* **2006**, *444*, 1022–1023. [CrossRef]
50. Matsumoto, M.; Inoue, R.; Tsukahara, T.; Ushida, K.; Chiji, H.; Matsubara, N.; Hara, H. Voluntary running exercise alters microbiota composition and increases n-butyrate concentration in the rat cecum. *Biosci. Biotechnol. Biochem.* **2008**, *72*, 572–576. [CrossRef]
51. Choi, J.J.; Eum, S.Y.; Rampersaud, E.; Daunert, S.; Abreu, M.T.; Toborek, M. Exercise attenuates PCB-induced changes in the mouse gut microbiome. *Environ. Health Perspect.* **2013**, *121*, 725–730. [CrossRef]
52. Queipo-Ortuño, M.I.; Seoane, L.M.; Murri, M.; Pardo, M.; Gomez-Zumaquero, J.M.; Cardona, F.; Casanueva, F.; Tinahones, F.J. Gut microbiota composition in male rat models under different nutritional status and physical activity and its association with serum leptin and ghrelin levels. *PLoS ONE* **2013**, *8*, e65465. [CrossRef]
53. Liu, F.; Zhang, N.; Li, Z.; Wang, X.; Shi, H.; Xue, C.; Li, R.W.; Tang, Q. Chondroitin sulfate disaccharides modified the structure and function of the murine gut microbiome under healthy and stressed conditions. *Sci. Rep.* **2017**, *7*, 1–14. [CrossRef] [PubMed]
54. Evans, C.C.; LePard, K.J.; Kwak, J.W.; Stancukas, M.C.; Laskowski, S.; Dougherty, J.; Moulton, L.; Glawe, A.; Wang, Y.; Leone, V. Exercise prevents weight gain and alters the gut microbiota in a mouse model of high fat diet-induced obesity. *PLoS ONE* **2014**, *9*, e92193. [CrossRef] [PubMed]
55. Carbajo-Pescador, S.; Porras, D.; García-Mediavilla, M.V.; Martínez-Flórez, S.; Juarez-Fernández, M.; Cuevas, M.J.; Mauriz, J.L.; González-Gallego, J.; Nistal, E.; Sánchez-Campos, S. Beneficial effects of exercise on gut microbiota functionality and barrier integrity, and gut-liver crosstalk in an in vivo model of early obesity and non-alcoholic fatty liver disease. *Dis. Model Mech.* **2019**, *12*, dmm039206. [CrossRef] [PubMed]
56. Yuan, X.; Xu, S.; Huang, H.; Liang, J.; Wu, Y.; Li, C.; Yuan, H.; Zhao, X.; Lai, X.; Hou, S. Influence of excessive exercise on immunity, metabolism, and gut microbial diversity in an overtraining mice model. *Scand. J. Med. Sci. Sports* **2018**, *28*, 1541–1551. [CrossRef] [PubMed]
57. Huang, W.-C.; Chen, Y.-H.; Chuang, H.-L.; Chiu, C.-C.; Huang, C.-C. Investigation of the Effects of Microbiota on Exercise Physiological Adaption, Performance, and Energy Utilization Using a Gnotobiotic Animal Model. *Front. Microbiol.* **2019**, *10*, 1906. [CrossRef]
58. Lahiri, S.; Kim, H.; Garcia-Perez, I.; Reza, M.M.; Martin, K.A.; Kundu, P.; Cox, L.M.; Selkrig, J.; Posma, J.M.; Zhang, H. The gut microbiota influences skeletal muscle mass and function in mice. *Sci. Transl. Med.* **2019**, *11*, eaan5662. [CrossRef]
59. Kerksick, C.M.; Wilborn, C.D.; Roberts, M.D.; Smith-Ryan, A.; Kleiner, S.M.; Jäger, R.; Collins, R.; Cooke, M.; Davis, J.N.; Galvan, E. ISSN exercise & sports nutrition review update: Research & recommendations. *J. Int. Soc. Sports Nutr.* **2018**, *15*, 38. [CrossRef]
60. Maughan, R.J.; Burke, L.M.; Dvorak, J.; Larson-Meyer, D.E.; Peeling, P.; Phillips, S.M.; Rawson, E.S.; Walsh, N.P.; Garthe, I.; Geyer, H. IOC consensus statement: Dietary supplements and the high-performance athlete. *Int. J. Sport Nutr. Exerc. Metab.* **2018**, *28*, 104–125. [CrossRef]
61. Ducray, H.; Globa, L.; Pustovyy, O.; Roberts, M.; Rudisill, M.; Vodyanoy, V.; Sorokulova, I. Prevention of excessive exercise-induced adverse effects in rats with Bacillus subtilis BSB3. *J. Appl. Microbiol.* **2020**, *128*, 1163. [CrossRef] [PubMed]
62. Ünsal, C.; Ünsal, H.; Ekici, M.; Koc Yildirim, E.; Üner, A.; Yildiz, M.; Güleş, Ö.; Ekren Aşici, G.; Boyacioğlu, M.; Balkaya, M. The effects of exhaustive swimming and probiotic administration in trained rats: Oxidative balance of selected organs, colon morphology, and contractility. *Physiol. Int.* **2018**, *105*, 309–324. [CrossRef]
63. Lollo, P.; Cruz, A.; Morato, P.; Moura, C.; Carvalho-Silva, L.; Oliveira, C.A.F.d.; Faria, J.; Amaya-Farfan, J. Probiotic cheese attenuates exercise-induced immune suppression in Wistar rats. *J. Dairy Sci.* **2012**, *95*, 3549–3558. [CrossRef]
64. Lollo, P.C.B.; de Moura, C.S.; Morato, P.N.; Cruz, A.G.; de Freitas Castro, W.; Betim, C.B.; Nisishima, L.; José de Assis, F.F.; Junior, M.M.; Fernandes, C.O. Probiotic yogurt offers higher immune-protection than probiotic whey beverage. *Food Res. Int.* **2013**, *54*, 118–124. [CrossRef]

65. Appukutty, M.; Ramasamy, K.; Rajan, S.; Vellasamy, S.; Ramasamy, R.; Radhakrishnan, A. Effect of orally administered soy milk fermented with Lactobacillus plantarum LAB12 and physical exercise on murine immune responses. *Benef. Microbes* **2015**, *6*, 491–496. [CrossRef]
66. Coffey, V.G.; Hawley, J.A. Concurrent exercise training: Do opposites distract? *J. Physiol.* **2017**, *595*, 2883–2896. [CrossRef] [PubMed]
67. Rondanelli, M.; Faliva, M.A.; Perna, S.; Giacosa, A.; Peroni, G.; Castellazzi, A.M. Using probiotics in clinical practice: Where are we now? A review of existing meta-analyses. *Gut Microbes* **2017**, *8*, 521–543. [CrossRef]
68. Hao, Q.; Dong, B.R.; Wu, T. Probiotics for preventing acute upper respiratory tract infections. *Cochrane Database Syst. Rev.* **2015**, CD006895. [CrossRef]
69. Gleeson, M.; Bishop, N.C.; Oliveira, M.; Tauler, P. Daily probiotic's (Lactobacillus casei Shirota) reduction of infection incidence in athletes. *Int. J. Sport Nutr. Exerc. Metab.* **2011**, *21*, 55–64. [CrossRef]
70. Kekkonen, R.A.; Vasankari, T.J.; Vuorimaa, T.; Haahtela, T.; Julkunen, I.; Korpela, R. The effect of probiotics on respiratory infections and gastrointestinal symptoms during training in marathon runners. *Int. J. Sport Nutr. Exerc. Metab.* **2007**, *17*, 352–363. [CrossRef]
71. West, N.P.; Pyne, D.B.; Cripps, A.W.; Hopkins, W.G.; Eskesen, D.C.; Jairath, A.; Christophersen, C.T.; Conlon, M.A.; Fricker, P.A. Lactobacillus fermentum (PCC(R)) supplementation and gastrointestinal and respiratory-tract illness symptoms: A randomised control trial in athletes. *Nutr. J.* **2011**, *10*, 30. [CrossRef] [PubMed]
72. Lamprecht, M.; Bogner, S.; Schippinger, G.; Steinbauer, K.; Fankhauser, F.; Hallstroem, S.; Schuetz, B.; Greilberger, J.F. Probiotic supplementation affects markers of intestinal barrier, oxidation, and inflammation in trained men; a randomized, double-blinded, placebo-controlled trial. *J. Int. Soc. Sports Nutr.* **2012**, *9*, 45. [CrossRef] [PubMed]
73. Roberts, J.D.; Suckling, C.A.; Peedle, G.Y.; Murphy, J.A.; Dawkins, T.G.; Roberts, M.G. An Exploratory Investigation of Endotoxin Levels in Novice Long Distance Triathletes, and the Effects of a Multi-Strain Probiotic/Prebiotic, Antioxidant Intervention. *Nutrients* **2016**, *8*, 733. [CrossRef] [PubMed]
74. Haywood, B.A.; Black, K.E.; Baker, D.; McGarvey, J.; Healey, P.; Brown, R.C. Probiotic supplementation reduces the duration and incidence of infections but not severity in elite rugby union players. *J. Sci. Med. Sport* **2014**, *17*, 356–360. [CrossRef]
75. De Oliveira, E.P.; Burini, R.C.; Jeukendrup, A. Gastrointestinal complaints during exercise: Prevalence, etiology, and nutritional recommendations. *Sports Med.* **2014**, *44* (Suppl. 1), S79–S85. [CrossRef]
76. West, N.P.; Pyne, D.B.; Cripps, A.; Christophersen, C.T.; Conlon, M.A.; Fricker, P.A. Gut Balance, a synbiotic supplement, increases fecal Lactobacillus paracasei but has little effect on immunity in healthy physically active individuals. *Gut Microbes* **2012**, *3*, 221–227. [CrossRef]
77. Shing, C.M.; Peake, J.M.; Lim, C.L.; Briskey, D.; Walsh, N.P.; Fortes, M.B.; Ahuja, K.D.; Vitetta, L. Effects of probiotics supplementation on gastrointestinal permeability, inflammation and exercise performance in the heat. *Eur. J. Appl. Physiol.* **2014**, *114*, 93–103. [CrossRef]
78. Nieman, D.C.; Wentz, L.M. The compelling link between physical activity and the body's defense system. *J. Sport Health Sci.* **2019**, *8*, 201–217. [CrossRef]
79. Nieman, D.C. Exercise, upper respiratory tract infection, and the immune system. *Med. Sci. Sports Exerc.* **1994**, *26*, 128–139. [CrossRef]
80. Colbey, C.; Cox, A.J.; Pyne, D.B.; Zhang, P.; Cripps, A.W.; West, N.P. Upper Respiratory Symptoms, Gut Health and Mucosal Immunity in Athletes. *Sports Med.* **2018**, *48*, 65–77. [CrossRef]
81. Cox, A.J.; Pyne, D.B.; Saunders, P.U.; Fricker, P.A. Oral administration of the probiotic Lactobacillus fermentum VRI-003 and mucosal immunity in endurance athletes. *Br. J. Sports Med.* **2010**, *44*, 222–226. [CrossRef] [PubMed]
82. Salarkia, N.; Ghadamli, L.; Zaeri, F.; Sabaghian Rad, L. Effects of probiotic yogurt on performance, respiratory and digestive systems of young adult female endurance swimmers: A randomized controlled trial. *Med. J. Islam. Repub. Iran* **2013**, *27*, 141–146.
83. West, N.P.; Horn, P.L.; Pyne, D.B.; Gebski, V.J.; Lahtinen, S.J.; Fricker, P.A.; Cripps, A.W. Probiotic supplementation for respiratory and gastrointestinal illness symptoms in healthy physically active individuals. *Clin. Nutr.* **2014**, *33*, 581–587. [CrossRef] [PubMed]

84. Michalickova, D.; Minic, R.; Dikic, N.; Andjelkovic, M.; Kostic-Vucicevic, M.; Stojmenovic, T.; Nikolic, I.; Djordjevic, B. Lactobacillus helveticus Lafti L10 supplementation reduces respiratory infection duration in a cohort of elite athletes: A randomized, double-blind, placebo-controlled trial. *Appl. Physiol. Nutr. Metab.* **2016**, *41*, 782–789. [CrossRef] [PubMed]
85. Strasser, B.; Geiger, D.; Schauer, M.; Gostner, J.M.; Gatterer, H.; Burtscher, M.; Fuchs, D. Probiotic Supplements Beneficially Affect Tryptophan-Kynurenine Metabolism and Reduce the Incidence of Upper Respiratory Tract Infections in Trained Athletes: A Randomized, Double-Blinded, Placebo-Controlled Trial. *Nutrients* **2016**, *8*, 752. [CrossRef]
86. Kellmann, M.; Bertollo, M.; Bosquet, L.; Brink, M.; Coutts, A.J.; Duffield, R.; Erlacher, D.; Halson, S.L.; Hecksteden, A.; Heidari, J.; et al. Recovery and Performance in Sport: Consensus Statement. *Int. J. Sports Physiol. Perform.* **2018**, *13*, 240–245. [CrossRef]
87. EFSA Panel on Nutrition; Novel Foods and Food Allergens (EFSA NDA Panel); Turck, D.; Castenmiller, J.; De Henauw, S.; Hirsch-Ernst, K.; Kearney, J.; Knutsen, H.; Maciuk, A.; Mangelsdorf, I.; et al. Guidance on the scientific requirements for health claims related to muscle function and physical performance. *EFSA J.* **2018**, *16*. [CrossRef]
88. Chen, Y.M.; Wei, L.; Chiu, Y.S.; Hsu, Y.J.; Tsai, T.Y.; Wang, M.F.; Huang, C.C. Lactobacillus plantarum TWK10 Supplementation Improves Exercise Performance and Increases Muscle Mass in Mice. *Nutrients* **2016**, *8*, 205. [CrossRef] [PubMed]
89. Hsu, Y.J.; Huang, W.C.; Lin, J.S.; Chen, Y.M.; Ho, S.T.; Huang, C.C.; Tung, Y.T. Kefir Supplementation Modifies Gut Microbiota Composition, Reduces Physical Fatigue, and Improves Exercise Performance in Mice. *Nutrients* **2018**, *10*, 862. [CrossRef]
90. Soares, A.D.N.; Wanner, S.P.; Morais, E.S.S.; Hudson, A.S.R.; Martins, F.S.; Cardoso, V.N. Supplementation with Saccharomyces boulardii Increases the Maximal Oxygen Consumption and Maximal Aerobic Speed Attained by Rats Subjected to an Incremental-Speed Exercise. *Nutrients* **2019**, *11*, 2352. [CrossRef]
91. Huang, W.C.; Hsu, Y.J.; Li, H.; Kan, N.W.; Chen, Y.M.; Lin, J.S.; Hsu, T.K.; Tsai, T.Y.; Chiu, Y.S.; Huang, C.C. Effect of Lactobacillus Plantarum TWK10 on Improving Endurance Performance in Humans. *Chin. J. Physiol.* **2018**, *61*, 163–170. [CrossRef] [PubMed]
92. Huang, W.C.; Lee, M.C.; Lee, C.C.; Ng, K.S.; Hsu, Y.J.; Tsai, T.Y.; Young, S.L.; Lin, J.S.; Huang, C.C. Effect of Lactobacillus plantarum TWK10 on Exercise Physiological Adaptation, Performance, and Body Composition in Healthy Humans. *Nutrients* **2019**, *11*, 2836. [CrossRef] [PubMed]
93. Carbuhn, A.F.; Reynolds, S.M.; Campbell, C.W.; Bradford, L.A.; Deckert, J.A.; Kreutzer, A.; Fry, A.C. Effects of Probiotic (Bifidobacterium longum 35624) Supplementation on Exercise Performance, Immune Modulation, and Cognitive Outlook in Division I Female Swimmers. *Sports* **2018**, *6*, 116. [CrossRef] [PubMed]
94. Marshall, H.; Chrismas, B.C.R.; Suckling, C.A.; Roberts, J.D.; Foster, J.; Taylor, L. Chronic probiotic supplementation with or without glutamine does not influence the eHsp72 response to a multi-day ultra-endurance exercise event. *Appl. Physiol. Nutr. Metab.* **2017**, *42*, 876–883. [CrossRef]
95. Townsend, J.R.; Bender, D.; Vantrease, W.C.; Sapp, P.A.; Toy, A.M.; Woods, C.A.; Johnson, K.D. Effects of Probiotic (Bacillus subtilis DE111) Supplementation on Immune Function, Hormonal Status, and Physical Performance in Division I Baseball Players. *Sports* **2018**, *6*, 70. [CrossRef] [PubMed]
96. Toohey, J.C.; Townsend, J.R.; Johnson, S.B.; Toy, A.M.; Vantrease, W.C.; Bender, D.; Crimi, C.C.; Stowers, K.L.; Ruiz, M.D.; VanDusseldorp, T.A.; et al. Effects of Probiotic (Bacillus subtilis) Supplementation During Offseason Resistance Training in Female Division I Athletes. *J. Strength. Cond. Res.* **2018**, *10*. [CrossRef]
97. Ibrahim, N.S.; Muhamad, A.S.; Ooi, F.K.; Meor-Osman, J.; Chen, C.K. The effects of combined probiotic ingestion and circuit training on muscular strength and power and cytokine responses in young males. *Appl. Physiol. Nutr. Metab.* **2018**, *43*, 180–186. [CrossRef] [PubMed]
98. Lee, M.C.; Hsu, Y.J.; Chuang, H.L.; Hsieh, P.S.; Ho, H.H.; Chen, W.L.; Chiu, Y.S.; Huang, C.C. In Vivo Ergogenic Properties of the Bifidobacterium longum OLP-01 Isolated from a Weightlifting Gold Medalist. *Nutrients* **2019**, *11*, 2003. [CrossRef]
99. Lee, M.C.; Hsu, Y.J.; Ho, H.H.; Hsieh, S.H.; Kuo, Y.W.; Sung, H.C.; Huang, C.C. Lactobacillus salivarius Subspecies salicinius SA-03 is a New Probiotic Capable of Enhancing Exercise Performance and Decreasing Fatigue. *Microorganisms* **2020**, *8*, 545. [CrossRef]

100. Gill, S.K.; Allerton, D.M.; Ansley-Robson, P.; Hemmings, K.; Cox, M.; Costa, R.J. Does Short-Term High Dose Probiotic Supplementation Containing Lactobacillus casei Attenuate Exertional-Heat Stress Induced Endotoxaemia and Cytokinaemia? *Int. J. Sport Nutr. Exerc. Metab.* **2016**, *26*, 268–275. [CrossRef]
101. Gill, S.K.; Teixeira, A.M.; Rosado, F.; Cox, M.; Costa, R.J. High-Dose Probiotic Supplementation Containing Lactobacillus casei for 7 Days Does Not Enhance Salivary Antimicrobial Protein Responses to Exertional Heat Stress Compared With Placebo. *Int. J. Sport Nutr. Exerc. Metab.* **2016**, *26*, 150–160. [CrossRef]
102. Vaisberg, M.; Paixao, V.; Almeida, E.B.; Santos, J.M.B.; Foster, R.; Rossi, M.; Pithon-Curi, T.C.; Gorjao, R.; Momesso, C.M.; Andrade, M.S.; et al. Daily Intake of Fermented Milk Containing Lactobacillus casei Shirota (Lcs) Modulates Systemic and Upper Airways Immune/Inflammatory Responses in Marathon Runners. *Nutrients* **2019**, *11*, 1678. [CrossRef] [PubMed]
103. Valimaki, I.A.; Vuorimaa, T.; Ahotupa, M.; Kekkonen, R.; Korpela, R.; Vasankari, T. Decreased training volume and increased carbohydrate intake increases oxidized LDL levels. *Int. J. Sports Med.* **2012**, *33*, 291–296. [CrossRef] [PubMed]
104. Pugh, J.N.; Sparks, A.S.; Doran, D.A.; Fleming, S.C.; Langan-Evans, C.; Kirk, B.; Fearn, R.; Morton, J.P.; Close, G.L. Four weeks of probiotic supplementation reduces GI symptoms during a marathon race. *Eur. J. Appl. Physiol.* **2019**, *119*, 1491–1501. [CrossRef] [PubMed]
105. Huang, W.C.; Wei, C.C.; Huang, C.C.; Chen, W.L.; Huang, H.Y. The Beneficial Effects of Lactobacillus plantarum PS128 on High-Intensity, Exercise-Induced Oxidative Stress, Inflammation, and Performance in Triathletes. *Nutrients* **2019**, *11*, 353. [CrossRef] [PubMed]
106. Jager, R.; Purpura, M.; Stone, J.D.; Turner, S.M.; Anzalone, A.J.; Eimerbrink, M.J.; Pane, M.; Amoruso, A.; Rowlands, D.S.; Oliver, J.M. Probiotic Streptococcus thermophilus FP4 and Bifidobacterium breve BR03 Supplementation Attenuates Performance and Range-of-Motion Decrements Following Muscle Damaging Exercise. *Nutrients* **2016**, *8*, 642. [CrossRef] [PubMed]
107. Jager, R.; Shields, K.A.; Lowery, R.P.; De Souza, E.O.; Partl, J.M.; Hollmer, C.; Purpura, M.; Wilson, J.M. Probiotic Bacillus coagulans GBI-30, 6086 reduces exercise-induced muscle damage and increases recovery. *PeerJ* **2016**, *4*, e2276. [CrossRef]
108. Mazani, M.; Nemati, A.; Baghi, A.N.; Amani, M.; Haedari, K.; Alipanah-Mogadam, R. The effect of probiotic yoghurt consumption on oxidative stress and inflammatory factors in young females after exhaustive exercise. *J. Pak. Med. Assoc.* **2018**, *68*, 1748–1754.
109. Muhamad, A.; Gleeson, M. Effects of a 14-strain probiotics supplement on salivary antimicrobial proteins at rest and in response to an acute bout of prolonged exercise. *Int. J. Sports Sci.* **2014**, *4*, 7. [CrossRef]
110. O'Brien, K.V.; Stewart, L.K.; Forney, L.A.; Aryana, K.J.; Prinyawiwatkul, W.; Boeneke, C.A. The effects of postexercise consumption of a kefir beverage on performance and recovery during intensive endurance training. *J. Dairy Sci.* **2015**, *98*, 7446–7449. [CrossRef]
111. Salehzadeh, K. The effects of probiotic yogurt drink on lipid profile, CRP and record changes in aerobic athletes. *Int. J. Life Sci.* **2015**, *9*, 32–37. [CrossRef]
112. Inoue, T.; Kobayashi, Y.; Mori, N.; Sakagawa, M.; Xiao, J.Z.; Moritani, T.; Sakane, N.; Nagai, N. Effect of combined bifidobacteria supplementation and resistance training on cognitive function, body composition and bowel habits of healthy elderly subjects. *Benef. Microbes* **2018**, *9*, 843–853. [CrossRef] [PubMed]
113. Peake, J.M.; Neubauer, O.; Della Gatta, P.A.; Nosaka, K. Muscle damage and inflammation during recovery from exercise. *J. Appl. Physiol.* **2017**, *122*, 559–570. [CrossRef] [PubMed]
114. Dupuy, O.; Douzi, W.; Theurot, D.; Bosquet, L.; Dugue, B. An Evidence-Based Approach for Choosing Post-exercise Recovery Techniques to Reduce Markers of Muscle Damage, Soreness, Fatigue, and Inflammation: A Systematic Review with Meta-Analysis. *Front. Physiol.* **2018**, *9*, 403. [CrossRef]
115. Gepner, Y.; Hoffman, J.R.; Shemesh, E.; Stout, J.R.; Church, D.D.; Varanoske, A.N.; Zelicha, H.; Shelef, I.; Chen, Y.; Frankel, H.; et al. Combined effect of Bacillus coagulans GBI-30, 6086 and HMB supplementation on muscle integrity and cytokine response during intense military training. *J. Appl. Physiol.* **2017**, *123*, 11–18. [CrossRef] [PubMed]
116. Jager, R.; Zaragoza, J.; Purpura, M.; Iametti, S.; Marengo, M.; Tinsley, G.M.; Anzalone, A.J.; Oliver, J.M.; Fiore, W.; Biffi, A.; et al. Probiotic Administration Increases Amino Acid Absorption from Plant Protein: A Placebo-Controlled, Randomized, Double-Blind, Multicenter, Crossover Study. *Probiotics Antimicrob. Proteins* **2020**. [CrossRef]

117. Foster, J.A.; Rinaman, L.; Cryan, J.F. Stress & the gut-brain axis: Regulation by the microbiome. *Neurobiol. Stress* **2017**, *7*, 124–136. [CrossRef]
118. Vitellio, P.; Chira, A.; De Angelis, M.; Dumitrascu, D.L.; Portincasa, P. Probiotics in Psychosocial Stress and Anxiety. A Systematic Review. *J. Gastrointestin. Liver Dis.* **2020**, *29*, 77–83. [CrossRef]
119. Sashihara, T.; Nagata, M.; Mori, T.; Ikegami, S.; Gotoh, M.; Okubo, K.; Uchida, M.; Itoh, H. Effects of Lactobacillus gasseri OLL2809 and α-lactalbumin on university-student athletes: A randomized, double-blind, placebo-controlled clinical trial. *Appl. Physiol. Nutr. Metab.* **2013**, *38*, 1228–1235. [CrossRef]
120. Sawada, D.; Kuwano, Y.; Tanaka, H.; Hara, S.; Uchiyama, Y.; Sugawara, T.; Fujiwara, S.; Rokutan, K.; Nishida, K. Daily intake of Lactobacillus gasseri CP2305 relieves fatigue and stress-related symptoms in male university Ekiden runners: A double-blind, randomized, and placebo-controlled clinical trial. *J. Funct. Foods* **2019**, *57*, 465–476. [CrossRef]

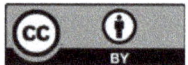

© 2020 by the authors. Licensee MDPI, Basel, Switzerland. This article is an open access article distributed under the terms and conditions of the Creative Commons Attribution (CC BY) license (http://creativecommons.org/licenses/by/4.0/).

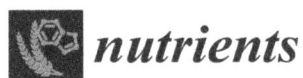

Article

High Salt Diet Impacts the Risk of Sarcopenia Associated with Reduction of Skeletal Muscle Performance in the Japanese Population

Yasuko Yoshida [1,2,*], Keisei Kosaki [3,4,5], Takehito Sugasawa [2], Masahiro Matsui [5,6], Masaki Yoshioka [6], Kai Aoki [6], Tomoaki Kuji [6], Risuke Mizuno [7], Makoto Kuro-o [8], Kunihiro Yamagata [9], Seiji Maeda [4] and Kazuhiro Takekoshi [2]

1. Department of Clinical Laboratory Science, Faculty of Health Sciences, Tsukuba International University, Ibarak 300-0051, Japan
2. Laboratory of Sports Medicine, Division of Clinical Medicine, Faculty of Medicine, University of Tsukuba, Ibaraki 305-8577, Japan; take0716@krf.biglobe.ne.jp (T.S.); K-takemd@md.tsukuba.ac.jp (K.T.)
3. Faculty of Sport Sciences, Waseda University, Saitama 359-1192, Japan; kosaki.keisei.gm@u.tsukuba.ac.jp
4. Faculty of Health and Sport Sciences, University of Tsukuba, Ibaraki 305-8577, Japan; maeda.seiji.gn@u.tsukuba.ac.jp
5. Japan Society for the Promotion of Science, Tokyo 102-0083, Japan; masahiromatsui0708@gmail.com
6. Graduate School of Comprehensive Human Sciences, University of Tsukuba, Ibaraki 305-8577, Japan; masakiyoshioka1129@gmail.com (M.Y.); fineday0126@gmail.com (K.A.); s1930394@s.tsukuba.ac.jp (T.K.)
7. Faculty of Veterinary Medicine, Okayama University of Science, Ehime 794-8555, Japan; r-mizuno@vet.ous.ac.jp
8. Division of Anti-aging Medicine, Center for Molecular Medicine, Jichi Medical University, Tochigi 329-0431, Japan; mkuroo@jichi.ac.jp
9. Department of Nephrology, Faculty of Medicine, University of Tsukuba, Ibaraki 305-8577, Japan; k-yamaga@md.tsukuba.ac.jp
* Correspondence: y-yoshida@tius.ac.jp; Tel.: +81-29-826-6000

Received: 16 October 2020; Accepted: 5 November 2020; Published: 12 November 2020

Abstract: The World Health Organization has recommended 5 g/day as dietary reference intakes for salt. In Japan, the averages for men and women were 11.0 g/day and 9.3 g/day, respectively. Recently, it was reported that amounts of sodium accumulation in skeletal muscles of older people were significantly higher than those in younger people. The purpose of this study was to investigate whether the risk of sarcopenia with decreased muscle mass and strength was related to the amount of salt intake. In addition, we investigated its involvement with renalase. Four groups based on age and salt intake ("younger low-salt," "younger high-salt," "older low-salt," and "older high-salt") were compared. Stratifying by age category, body fat percentage significantly increased in high-salt groups in both younger and older people. Handgrip strength/body weight and chair rise tests of the older high-salt group showed significant reduction compared to the older low-salt group. However, there was no significant difference in renalase concentrations in plasma. The results suggest that high-salt intake may lead to fat accumulation and muscle weakness associated with sarcopenia. Therefore, efforts to reduce salt intake may prevent sarcopenia.

Keywords: salt; sarcopenia; renalase; body fat percentage; knee extensor muscle strength; single-leg stance time; maximum gait speed; long seat type body anteflexion; chair rise test

1. Introduction

Japan has a large aging population; the 2019 White Paper on Aging Society reported that 28.1% of the population is over the age of 65 years [1]. In addition, soaring medical costs have become a social problem. One of the causes is that there is a discrepancy between the average life expectancy and the period of healthy life expectancy during which a person can live an independent life [1]. Frailty, the decline in motor and cognitive function in individuals with advanced age, is one of the reasons healthy life expectancy remains lower than average life expectancy. The main cause for frailty is sarcopenia, a progressive age-related weakness of the muscles. The definition of sarcopenia was based on the criteria of the European Working Group on Sarcopenia in Older People (EWGSOP) in 2010 [2]. In Japan, the criteria of the Asian Working Group for Sarcopenia (AWGS) are generally recommended for diagnosis, and in 2017 the Japanese Association on Sarcopenia and Frailty created the sarcopenia clinical practice guidelines [3–5].

The main cause of sarcopenia is aging [2–4,6]. Secondary factors include physical inactivity, illness, and nutrition, and it is likely that multiple factors overlap to cause sarcopenia. Specifically, with regard to nutrition, reports indicate that deficiency of protein and vitamin D intake increases the risk of sarcopenia [7–21]. The leading problem regarding nutrients in Japanese people is high-salt intake. The World Health Organization (WHO) has recommended an intake of no more than 5 g of salt/day [22]. In Japan, there is an average salt intake of 11.0 g/day for men and 9.3 g/day for women. Recently in Japan, salt intake has been declining slightly each year [23].

Many studies report that excessive salt intake is one of the causes of various diseases, such as hypertension [24,25], where sodium in the skeletal muscle accumulates more in older people than in younger people, and patients with refractory hypertension have increased tissue sodium(Na (+)) content when compared with normotensive controls [26]. In addition, the sodium-potassium-chloride symporter 1 (NKCC1) is highly expressed in mammalian skeletal muscle. The physiologic function of NKCC1 in myogenesis is unclear. However, NKCC1 protein levels increased skeletal myoblast differentiation, and NKCC1 inhibitors markedly suppressed skeletal myoblast differentiation [27]. It has also been reported that excess sodium leads to a downregulation of expression of NKCC [28]. Therefore, we hypothesized that the risk of sarcopenia, which is associated with decreased muscle mass and strength, is related to the amount of salt intake, because Na (+) is stored in tissues and NKCC1 is involved in muscle hypertrophy and suppression.

Incidentally, renalase, a recently discovered enzyme released by the kidneys, may break down blood-derived catecholamine and regulate blood pressure. A report of loss of renalase function can result in increased blood pressure (hypertension), increased heart rate (tachycardia), increased vascular resistance (vasoconstriction), and increased catecholamine response [29]. Human and animal studies have suggested that high levels of dietary salt may lower blood and renal renalase levels. Due to blood pressure increasing with salt intake, the renalase levels that breaks down catecholamines, may also be reduced [30–32]. For the relationship between renalase and skeletal muscle, exercise load increased blood levels of renalase, independent of renal secretion, and increased gene expression of renalase in skeletal muscles [33–35]. In a study based on disuse atrophy, there was a study that showed muscle proteolysis decreased and muscle mass increased in renalase knockout mice [36]. On the other hand, skeletal muscle has β2 adrenergic receptors involved in catecholamines, and β2-adrenergic receptor stimulation increases muscle mass by promoting muscle protein synthesis and/or attenuating protein degradation. However, excessive stimulation of -adrenergic receptors negates their beneficial effects [37]. By these reports, we considered that renalase, which is related to catecholamines that increase with salt intake, may also be involved in skeletal muscle atrophy. Therefore, we speculated that the decreased level of renalase might be a marker for sarcopenia.

We aimed to clarify the relationship between salt intake, blood renalase concentrations, and sarcopenia risk for Japanese adults.

2. Materials and Methods

2.1. Study Design

Healthy adult volunteers (n = 122, age (standard deviation [SD]): 56.3 (12.3) years) were recruited from the community using local advertisements, and participants were selected from Tsukuba and nearby urban areas (Ibaraki, Japan). Participants with an estimated glomerular filtration rate of 90 mL/min/1.73 m^2 or less were excluded because renal function is involved in sodium uptake and renalase levels [24,30–32,38–40]. In addition, eight participants who showed more than four times the standard deviation of the mean blood test of all 122 participants were excluded, because there was a possibility of other diseases. The items are renalase, Interleukin-6 (IL-6), triglyceride (TG), insulin, glucose (Glu), glycosylated hemoglobin (HbA1c), aspartate transaminase (AST), and alanine aminotransferase (ALT). Therefore, 114 participants were analyzed.

We calculated estimated salt intake using spot urine testing and divided the participants into two groups with an average estimated salt intake of 9.37 g/day [1]. The participants with lower salt intake than average was designated as "low-salt," and the participants with a higher intake were designated as "high-salt." Furthermore, since the age range of the selection criteria for this study is 20 years and over, volunteers from a very wide range of age groups participated, we also analyzed after stratifying by age. Participants were divided according to the overall average age (56.3 (12.3)) designated "younger" and "older." That is, "younger" is younger than the average age of participants and "older" is older than the average age. Overall, the participants were divided into four groups ("younger low-salt," "younger high-salt," "older low-salt," "older high-salt") and blood test results, anthropometric measurements, and assessment of physical performance were compared.

This study was approved by the Ethical Review Board of University of Tsukuba, and all participants provided written, informed consent as per the requirements of the Declaration of Helsinki (IRB approval No. H30-161).

2.2. Data Collection

2.2.1. Blood Test and Urinalysis

Participants were asked to avoid strenuous exercise, live a normal life the day before and were banned from eating and drinking except water after 20:00 p.m., before testing to control for exercise and nutrition. They were asked to arrive at the laboratory between 8:00 a.m. and 11:00 a.m.

First, participants provided urine samples. We conducted urinalysis to measure the concentration of sodium and creatinine at Tsukuba i-Laboratory Limited Liability Partnership (Ibaraki, Japan), using the ion-selective electrode method to measure urinary sodium and the enzyme method to measure urinary creatinine. We calculated the 24-h salt intake using the following formula [41,42]:

$$\text{Estimated 24 h Creatinine (mg/day)} = -2.04 \times \text{age} + 14.89 \times \text{weight (kg)} + 16.14 \times \text{height (cm)} - 2244.45, \quad (1)$$

$$\text{Estimated 24 h urinary sodium (mEq/day)} = 21.98 \times \text{urinary sodium}/10/(1)^{0.392}, \quad (2)$$

$$\text{Estimated 24-h salt intake (g/day)} = (2)/17. \quad (3)$$

Next, blood samples were collected from the antecubital vein. In this study, we measured some parameters in the blood that could pose a risk for sarcopenia. IL-6 (pg/mL) for inflammation, urea nitrogen (UN) (mg/dL) and cystatin C (CysC) (mg/L) for renal function, TG (mg/dL) for fat accumulation that causes obesity, albumin (Alb) (g/dL) for nutritional status, Glu (mg/dL), insulin (μU/mL) and HbA1c (%), for glucose metabolism, and AST (U/L) and ALT (U/L) for liver function. In addition, since renalase (mg/L) has been reported to be involved in blood pressure control function and skeletal muscle atrophy by metabolizing catecholamines, it was measured as a marker candidate for sarcopenia. Whole blood was used to measure HbA1c, which was measured using the enzyme method. The remaining blood was brought to room temperature of 20 to 25 °C and then centrifuged at

3000 rpm for 10 min to obtain a serum. It was then stored at −80 °C until measurement. Serum was used for measurement of concentrations of the following parameters: IL-6, UN, CysC, TG, Alb, insulin, Glu, AST, ALT, and renalase. The measurement was carried out at Tsukuba i-Laboratory Limited Liability Partnership (Ibaraki, Japan) by chemiluminescent enzyme immunoassay (insulin), ultraviolet (UN, Glu), latex coagulating nephelometry (CysC), the enzyme method (TG), the bromocresol purple method (Alb), and the Japan Society of Clinical Chemistry (JSCC) Standardization Corresponding Method (AST, ALT). IL-6 was measured by Chemiluminescent Enzyme Immunoassay at Jichi Medical University Hospital. Renalase was measured by enzyme-linked immunosorbent assay (ELISA) using the FAD-Dependent Amine Oxidase ELISA Kit (Cloud-Clone Corp, Houston, TX, USA). In addition, the estimated glomerular filtration value (eGFR) was calculated using the renal function presumption formula and serum CysC concentrations to evaluate kidney function. Moreover, eGFR using the serum CysC concentration was calculated using the equation for Japanese people as shown in the chronic kidney disease (CKD) clinical practice guidelines [40] as follows: eGFR (mL/min/1.73 m^2) = (104 × [Concentration of serum CysC (mg/dL)]$^{-1.019}$ × $0.996^{(Age)}$ − 8″.

2.2.2. Anthropometric Measurements

Heights were measured using a stadiometer. Weight and body compositions were then measured using bioelectrical impedance analysis (Inbody 770; Inbody, Tokyo, Japan). The body composition measurement included skeletal muscle mass index (SMI; kg/m^2), body fat percentage (BFP; %), and mass of muscle of upper limbs (ULMM; kg) and lower limbs (LLMM; kg) [43,44]. Then we calculated the body mass index (BMI; kg/m^2)

2.2.3. Assessment of Physical Performance

Handgrip strength (HGS) (kg), knee extensor muscle strength (KES) (kg), single-leg stance time (SLT) (s), maximum gait speed (MGS) (m/s), long seat type body anteflexion (FleX) (cm), and the chair rise test (30CS) (number of repetitions) were used as indices of physical performance [3–5,45–51]. HGS was determined using a handheld dynamometer (T.K.K.5401; Takei Kiki Kogyo, Niigata, Japan). The participants being tested alternated between their left and right hand and were measured twice. The mean of the maximal values for each hand was used for analysis [49,50]. Then, the HGS was divided by body weight (BW). KES was determined using a handheld dynamometer (μTas F-1; ANIMA, Tokyo, Japan). Both lower limbs were measured twice, and the average of their highest score was registered as the result. Then, the KES was divided by body weight [48,50]. SLT was measured as an indicator of balance performance. Participants balanced as long as possible on one leg with their eyes open. The participant could choose which foot on which to balance. The maximum value was 60 s. If the maximum value was achieved, it was completed once; if not, the test was carried out twice and the longest time was used [47,50]. MGS was calculated using the time to cover a distance of 10 m on a straight walking course. To ensure that the participants reached their maximal walking speed, the 10 m was measured within a 16-m track [46,50]. FleX was determined using the long seat type body anteflexion measurement device (T.K.K.5412; Takei Kiki Kogyo, Niigata, Japan) [45]. The measurement was performed twice, and the largest value was used as the data. Muscular function of lower extremities was measured by 30CS as described by Jones et al. [51]. Participants were instructed to stand up as often as possible within 30 s. The score was the total number of stands executed correctly (stretched knee and hip) within 30 s. The measurement was performed only once.

2.3. Statistical Analysis

Data were analyzed using SPSS Statistics 26.0 (IBM, Armonk, IL, USA). Significance was set at $p < 0.05$. All values are expressed as mean (standard deviation) or median [interquartile range] unless stated otherwise. A chi-square test was performed to confirm that there was no difference in the ratio of males and females in each group. Normal distribution was confirmed by a Kolmogorov–Smirnov test. In the comparison between two groups, an independent t-test was performed in the case of normal distribution, and the Mann–Whitney U test was performed in other cases. For unequal variance, Welch's correction was applied. The correlation was analyzed by Pearson's correlation coefficient and Spearman's correlation coefficient. In the comparison between the four groups, one-way analysis of variance (ANOVA) for normality was performed, and Kruskal–Wallis for non - normality testing was performed otherwise. If there was a significant difference, either the Tukey test or the Bonferroni test was applied as a post hoc test. For multiple analysis, multiple linear regression analysis was performed with salt intake as the dependent variable.

3. Results

3.1. Comparison with Estimated Daily Salt Intake

The normality of each parameter is shown in Table 1. All parameters except BFP, HGS/BW, KES/BW, Flex, UN, Alb, HbA1c, and AST showed a non-normal distribution. The comparison between the "low-salt" and "high-salt" groups is shown in Table 1. There were no significant differences in sex ratio, age, and height. However, there were significant differences in SBP, DBP, weight, BMI, BFP, HGS/BW, Flex, 30CS, IL-6, TG, insulin, and ALT.

Table 1. Comparison of sarcopenia-related parameters by estimated salt intake.

	Low—Salt	High—Salt	Normality p Value	T Test p Value
Sample size (n)	57	57	-	-
Salt intake (g/day)	7.62(1.31)	11.11(1.16)	0.63	<0.01 *
Male/Female (n/n)	11/46	8/49	-	0.45 †
Age (year) §	56.00[49.00–63.00]	56.00[50.5–65.00]	<0.01 *	0.60
SBP (mmHg) §	113.00[104.33–122.00]	117.33[110.33–128.00]	<0.01 *	0.05 *
DBP (mmHg) §	65.67[60.00–73.00]	70.33[66.17–76.00]	0.04 *	0.01 *
Height (m) §	1.59 [1.53–1.66]	1.57[1.52–1.61]	<0.01 *	0.28
Weight (kg) §	51.20[45.30–58.30]	57.60[48.75–66.25]	<0.01 *	0.01 *
BMI (kg/m^2) §	20.61[18.88–21.89]	22.69[20.28–25.58]	<0.01 *	<0.01 *
SMI (kg/m^2) §	6.10[5.50–6.90]	6.20[5.80–6.85]	<0.01 *	0.34
ULMM (kg) §	3.56[2.95–4.32]	3.67[3.24–4.35]	<0.01 *	0.24
LLMM (kg) §	11.69[10.04–14.19]	11.78[10.44–12.82]	<0.01 *	0.88
BFP (%)	23.21(7.15)	29.91(8.65)	0.10	<0.01 *
HGS/BW (kg/BW)	0.54(0.10)	0.46(0.12)	0.23	<0.01 *
KES/BW (kg/BW)	0.62(0.17)	0.57(0.16)	0.16	0.13
SLT (sec) §	60.00[48.05–60.00]	60.00[38.24–60.00]	<0.01 *	0.72
MGS (m/sec) §	2.28[2.04–2.61]	2.18[1.99–2.44]	<0.01 *	0.14
Flex (m)	0.39(9.08)	0.36(7.54)	0.75	0.04 *
30CS (time) §	24.00[19.00–29.00]	18.00[16.00–23.00]	<0.01 *	<0.01 *
Renalase (mg/L) §	4.26[2.93–5.46]	4.24[3.30–5.38]	<0.01 *	0.90
IL-6 (pg/mL) §	1.00[0.65–1.20]	1.20[0.90–1.90]	<0.01 *	<0.01 *
UN (mg/dL)	14.04(2.81)	13.07(2.61)	0.10	0.06
CysC (mg/L) §	0.65[0.61–0.69]	0.67[0.62–0.70]	<0.01 *	0.27
TG (mg/dL) §	61.00[46.00–78.00]	83.00[59.50–100.50]	<0.01 *	<0.01 *
Alb (g/dL)	4.53(0.30)	4.51(0.26)	0.10	0.77
Glu (mg/dL) §	96.00[91.00–106.00]	99.00[92.50–104.00]	<0.01 *	0.28
Insulin (μU/mL) §	3.90[2.90–6.10]	4.90[3.75–7.15]	<0.01 *	0.02 *
HbA1c (%)	5.61(0.33)	5.69(0.38)	0.11	0.27
AST (U/L)	22.93(4.93)	24.11(5.03)	0.70	0.21
ALT (U/L) §	17.00[14.00–19.00]	18.00[15.00–27.00]	<0.01 *	0.05 *

These data are shown as mean (standard deviation) or median [interquartile range]. For the normality test, the Kolmogorov—Smirnov test was performed. Two-group comparison is the result of the independent T test or Mann—Whitney-U test [§]. The statistics of male and female is the chi-square test [†]. *: $p < 0.05$. sec: seconds, BW: body weight, SBP: systolic blood pressure, DBP: diastolic blood pressure, BMI: body mass index, SMI: skeletal muscle mass index, ULMM: mass of muscle of upper limbs, LLMM: mass of muscle of lower limbs, BFP: body fat percentage, HGS/BW: handgrip strength/weight, KES: knee extensor muscle strength, SLT: single-leg stance time, MGS: maximum gait speed, Flex: long seat type body anteflexion, 30CS: chair rise test, IL-6: Interleukin-6, UN: urea nitrogen, CysC: cystatin C, TG: triglyceride, Alb: albumin, Glu: glucose, HbA1c: Glycosylated hemoglobin, AST: Aspartate transaminase, ALT: Alanine aminotransferase.

3.2. Correlation with Estimated Salt Intake

The correlations between estimated salt intake and sarcopenia-related parameters are shown in Table 2. As for the correlation coefficient, the correlation coefficient of Pearson was analyzed in the case of normality, and the correlation coefficient of spearman was analyzed in the case of non-normality. There were significant differences in SBP, Weight, BMI, SMI, ULMM, BFP, HGS/BW, Flex, 30Cs, IL-6, TG, Insulin, and ALT. SBP, Weight, SMI, ULMM, HGS/BW, Flex, 30CS, IL-6, TG, Insulin, and ALT was weakly correlated and BMI and BFP was moderately correlated.

Table 2. Correlation of sarcopenia-related parameters based on estimated salt intake.

	Correlation Coefficient	
	p Value	r Value
Age (year) [§]	0.54	-
SBP (mmHg) [§]	0.03 *	0.21
DBP (mmHg) [§]	0.07	-
Height (m) [§]	0.74	-
Weight (kg) [§]	<0.01 *	0.39
BMI (kg/m^2) [§]	<0.01 *	0.49
SMI (kg/m^2) [§]	0.03 *	0.21
ULMM (kg) [§]	0.01 *	0.24
LLMM (kg) [§]	0.42	-
BFP (%)	<0.01 *	0.49
HGS/BW (kg/BW)	<0.01 *	−0.38
KES/BW (kg/BW)	0.14	-
SLT (sec)[§]	0.46	-
MGS (m/sec) [§]	0.24	-
Flex (m)	0.03 *	−0.20
30CS (time) [§]	<0.01 *	−0.32
Renalase (mg/L) [§]	0.67	-
IL-6 (pg/mL) [§]	<0.01 *	0.31
UN (mg/dL)	0.25	-
CysC (mg/L) [§]	0.15	-
TG (mg/dL) [§]	<0.01	0.34
Alb (g/dL)	0.67	-
Glu (mg/dL) [§]	0.11	-
Insulin (μU/mL) [§]	<0.01 *	0.27
HbA1c (%)	0.12	-
AST (U/L)	0.51	-
ALT (U/L) [§]	0.02 *	0.21

This table shows the correlation between estimated salt intake and sarcopenia-related parameters. As for the correlation coefficient, the Pearson correlation coefficient was shown in the case of normality, and the Spearman correlation coefficient was shown in the case of non-normality [§]. *: $p < 0.05$. sec: seconds, BW: body weight, SBP: systolic blood pressure, DBP: diastolic blood pressure, BMI: body mass index, SMI: skeletal muscle mass index, ULMM: mass of muscle of upper limbs, LLMM: mass of muscle of lower limbs, BFP: body fat percentage, HGS/BW: handgrip strength/weight, KES: knee extensor muscle strength, SLT: single-leg stance time, MGS: maximum gait speed, Flex: long seat type body anteflexion, 30CS: chair rise test, IL-6: Interleukin-6, UN: urea nitrogen, CysC: cystatin C, TG: triglyceride, Alb: albumin, Glu: glucose, HbA1c: Glycosylated hemoglobin, AST: Aspartate transaminase, ALT: Alanine aminotransferase.

3.3. Comparison of Estimated Salt Intake and Age

The comparison between the "younger low-salt," "younger high-salt," "older low-salt," and "older high-salt" groups is shown in Table 3. There were significant differences in SBP, DBP, weight, BMI, SMI, ULMM, LLMM, BFP, HGS/BW, 30CS, IL-6, UN, TG, Glu, HbA1c, and AST.

Table 3. Comparison of sarcopenia-related parameters by estimated salt intake and age.

	Younger Low—Salt	Younger High—Salt	Older Low—Salt	Older High—Salt	p Value
Sample size (n)	26	25	31	32	—
Salt intake (g/day)	7.56(1.19)	11.01(1.08)	7.67(1.42)	11.19(1.23)	—
Male/Female (n)	5/21	6/19	6/25	2/30	—
Age (year) §	48.50[37.75–53.00]	50.00[44.50–54.00]	62.00[58.00–71.00]	65.00[60.25–67.00]	—
SBP (mmHg) §	115.33[103.33–122.67]	112.67[103.83–119.83]	112.33[105.75–121.00]	122.50[113.67–130.75]	<0.01 *
DBP (mmHg) §	68.17[60.50–73.75]	68.33[64.17–72.50]	65.33[59.67–71.67]	72.67[67.83–81.50]	<0.01 *
Weight (kg) §	52.50[46.23–62.33]	61.50[52.80–69.00]	47.00[44.80–56.80]	51.15[47.83–62.13]	<0.01 *
BMI (kg/m²) §	20.61[19.00–22.50]	23.10[20.50–25.86]	20.45[18.27–21.83]	22.20[20.00–25.61]	<0.01 *
SMI (kg/m²) §	6.25[5.78–7.10]	6.40[6.05–7.60]	6.00[5.40–6.70]	5.95[5.63–6.78]	0.01 *
ULMM (kg) §	3.81[3.19–4.71]	3.82[3.56–5.55]	3.28[2.86–4.04]	3.61[2.90–4.13]	0.03 *
LLMM (kg) §	12.44[10.21–14.43]	12.27[11.67–17.10]	11.04[9.92–13.63]	10.86[9.91–12.15]	<0.01 *
BFP (%)	22.54(7.31)	28.38(7.98)	23.76(7.08)	31.12(9.07)	<0.01 *
HGS/BW (kg/BW)	0.56(0.10)	0.49(0.11)	0.52(0.10)	0.44(0.13)	<0.01 *
KES/BW (kg/BW)	0.64(0.20)	0.62(0.16)	0.60(0.14)	0.53(0.16)	0.08
SLT (sec) §	60.00[60.00–60.00]	60.00[48.35–60.00]	60.00[25.12–60.00]	60.00[37.51–60.00]	0.23
MGS (m/sec) §	2.34[2.13–2.79]	2.25[2.05–2.73]	2.24[1.95–2.59]	2.13[1.81–2.33]	0.05
Flex (m)	0.39(0.10)	0.36(0.09)	0.38(0.11)	0.35(0.07)	0.44
30CS (time) §	24.00[19.75–29.00]	20.00[16.00–23.00]	21.00[18.00–29.00]	17.50[16.00–22.00]	<0.01 *
Renalase (mg/L) §	3.71[2.78–6.30]	4.85[2.71–6.28]	4.40[3.37–5.12]	4.13[3.45–4.95]	0.73
IL-6 (pg/mL) §	0.80[0.60–1.03]	0.90[0.75–1.45]	1.00[0.70–1.30]	1.70[1.10–2.08]	<0.01 *
UN (mg/dL)	13.23(2.87)	12.54(2.29)	14.72(2.62)	13.49(2.79)	0.02 *
CysC (mg/L) §	0.63[0.61–0.68]	0.66[0.61–0.69]	0.65[0.62–0.70]	0.68[0.61–0.70]	0.43
TG (mg/dL) §	65.50[46.50–81.75]	84.00[52.50–95.00]	58.00[43.00–78.00]	82.50[66.25–105.75]	0.01 *
Alb (g/dL)	4.50(0.29)	4.54(0.24)	4.55(0.32)	4.49(0.27)	0.74
Glu (mg/dL) §	93.00[87.50–99.25]	97.00[90.50–100.50]	99.00[94.00–108.00]	100.00[94.25–107.75]	0.02 *
insulin (μU/mL) §	4.05[2.98–5.95]	4.90[3.55–6.55]	3.70[2.70–6.80]	5.00[3.98–7.45]	0.10
HbA1c (%)	5.48(0.29)	5.55(0.31)	5.73(0.32)	5.79(0.39)	<0.01 *
AST (U/L)	21.19(4.50)	23.36(5.06)	24.39(4.87)	24.69(5.01)	0.04 *
ALT (U/L) §	16.00[12.00–17.25]	19.00[15.00–29.50]	18.00[15.00–21.00]	16.00[15.00–26.75]	0.05

These data are shown as mean (standard deviation) or median [interquartile range]. This is the result of one-way ANOVA or Kruskal-Wallis tests [§]. *: p < 0.05. sec: seconds, BW: body weight, SBP: systolic blood pressure, DBP: diastolic blood pressure, BMI: body mass index, SMI: skeletal mass index, ULMM: mass of muscle of upper limbs, LLMM: mass of muscle of lower limbs, BFP: body fat percentage, HGS/BW: handgrip strength/weight, KES: knee extensor muscle strength, SLT: single-leg stance time, MGS: maximum gait speed, Flex: long seat type body anteflexion, 30CS: chair rise test, IL-6: Interleukin-6, UN: urea nitrogen, CysC: cystatin C, TG: triglyceride, Alb: albumin, Glu: glucose, HbA1c: Glycosylated hemoglobin, AST: Aspartate transaminase, ALT: Alanine aminotransferase.

In the comparison between the four groups, one-way analysis of variance (ANOVA) for normality was performed while Kruskal-Wallis was performed for non-normality testing. Significant differences were found in SBP, DBP, Weight, BMI, SMI, ULMM, LLMM, BFP, HGS/BW, 30CS, IL-6, UN, TG, Glu, HbA1c, and AST. A post hoc test was calculated only on the parameters that were significantly different. Figure 1 shows the p-values of the parameters that were significantly different in the post hoc test. When Younger and Older are stratified, significant differences were found in SPB, DBP, BMI, HGS/BW, 30CS, IL-6, and TG only in the older group. BFP was significantly different in both younger and older groups. weight, SMI, ULMM, LLMM, UN, Glu, HbA1c, and AST were significantly different between the younger group and the older group.

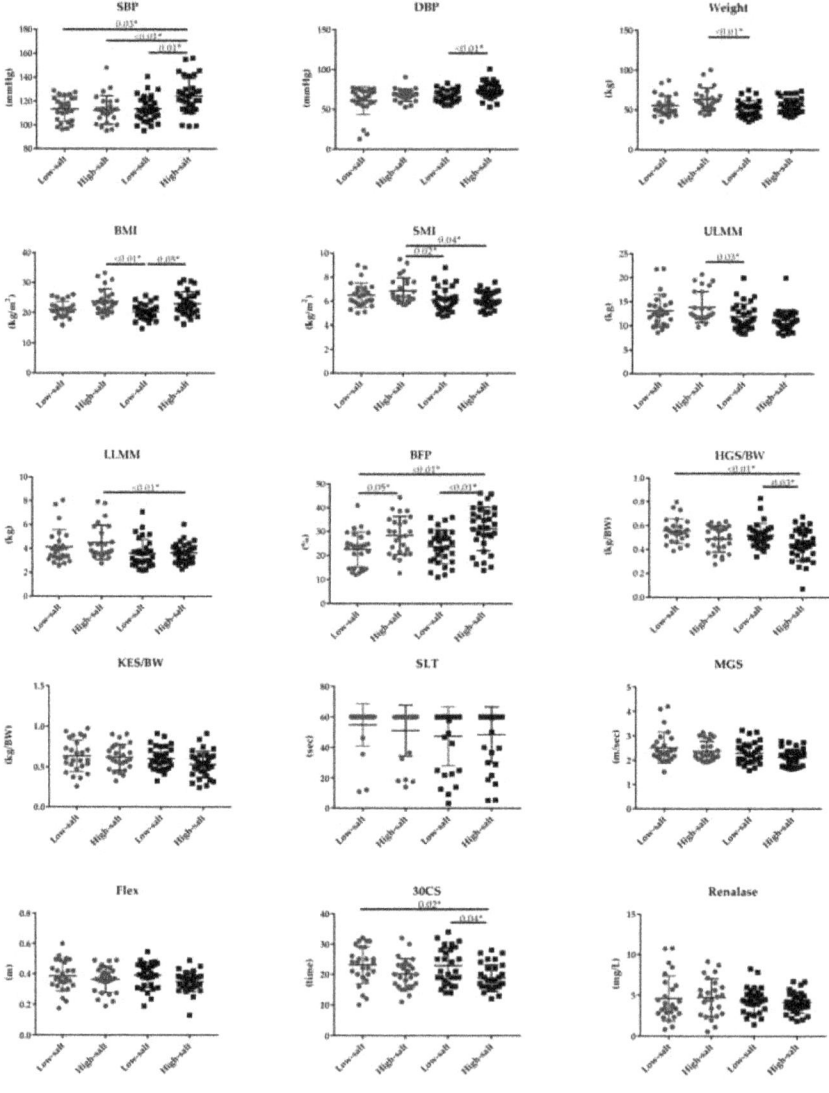

Figure 1. *Cont.*

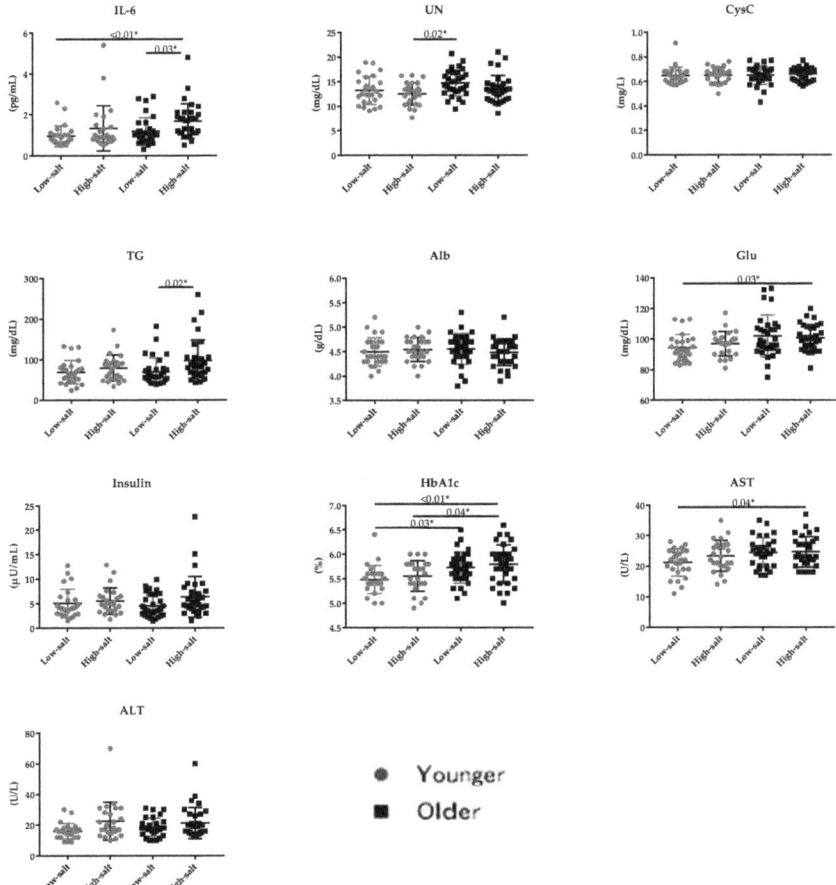

Figure 1. For comparison of the four groups, one-way ANOVA or Kruskal-Wallis test was performed, followed by a post hoc test. *: $p < 0.05$. sec: seconds, BW: body weight, SBP: systolic blood pressure, DBP: diastolic blood pressure, BMI: body mass index, SMI: skeletal muscle mass index, ULMM: mass of muscle of upper limbs, LLMM: mass of muscle of lower limbs, BFP: body fat percentage, HGS/BW: handgrip strength/weight, KES: knee extensor muscle strength, SLT: single-leg stance time, MGS: maximum gait speed, Flex: long seat type body anteflexion, 30CS: chair rise test, IL-6: interleukin-6, UN: urea nitrogen, CysC: cystatin C, TG: triglyceride, Alb: albumin, Glu: glucose, HbA1c: glycosylated hemoglobin, AST: aspartate transaminase, ALT: alanine aminotransferase.

3.4. Multivariate Analysis of Estimated Salt Intake and Sarcopenia Parameters

Multiple linear regression analysis used salt intake as the dependent variable. The independent variable populated all parameters related to sarcopenia risk. We then implemented the stepwise method. The adopted factors were BFP, ULMM, IL-6, SLT, LLMM, 30CS, ALT, and insulin, and the multiple regression equation for predicting salt intake (Y) was Y = 0.12 × (BFP) + 1.44 × (ULMM) + 0.46 × (IL-6) + 0.03 × (SLT) − 0.42 × (LLMM) − 0.08 × (30CS) + 0.05 × (ALT) − 0.14 × (insulin) + 5.09. The multiple correlation coefficient was 0.46, the adjusted coefficient of determination was 0.42, and the adjusted multiple correlation coefficient was 0.68. The value of the Burbin Watson test was 2.40. Residual analysis showed that the model was reliable.

4. Discussion

This study was conducted with a focus on salt intake, which pertains to nutritional intake. It is known that the salt intake of Japanese people is the highest in the world [52,53]. In this study, the estimated daily salt intake using the urine test values was high, with an average value of 9.32 g/day (2.14). This amount is close to the reported average Japanese salt intake and is almost twice the recommended amount given by the WHO [22,23].

All parameters that showed a significant difference are values indicating the degree of obesity and the amount of fat in the body. In addition, salt intake, BFP, and BMI showed positive correlations. These results suggest that excessive salt intake may contribute to fat accumulation and are consistent with previous studies reporting an association between excessive salt intake and obesity [18,54–56]. One factor that predicts sarcopenia is the increase of fat in muscle [57–60]. Excessive salt intake can lead to fat accumulation and sarcopenia risk, however, participants who consume excess salt may not have dietary controls other than salt, which may lead to fat accumulation and obesity. Since no dietary survey was conducted in this study, this cannot be clarified. In terms of assessment of physical performance, some parameters, such as muscle weakness, were significantly lower in the high-salt group than the low-salt group. Muscle weakness is one of the causes of sarcopenia [50,61]. However, according to the criteria of the AWGS [3], there were only five in the older group that had reduced grip strength. The high-salt: low-salt group ratio was 3:2. Furthermore, no decrease in the parameter (SIM) indicating muscle mass loss could be seen. Therefore, in this study, we can only say that there is a possibility of sarcopenia risk, and not sarcopenia. Regarding blood tests, the fact that IL-6 and insulin were significantly higher in the high-salt group may suggest insulin resistance. Insulin resistance contributes to obesity and aging, and skeletal muscle insulin secretion resistance is involved in the pathogenesis of sarcopenia. IL-6 has also been shown to induce insulin resistance. Therefore, when homeostasis model assessment as an index of insulin resistance (HOMA-IR) was calculated [62], the average value of low salt content and high salt content was 1.18 (0.69):1.49 (0.91), and HOMA-IR also increased significantly. Increased ALT in blood tests is associated with liver dysfunction. There are many reports of the risk of sarcopenia due to liver dysfunction, and there are also diagnostic criteria for liver disease in Japan [4]. Increases in all these parameters are associated with sarcopenia risk [4,12–19].

Next, we investigated the relationship between estimated salt intake, age, and a possibility of sarcopenia risk. There were 16 parameters with a significant difference. Parameters were stratified into the younger and older groups, the items that showed a significant difference only in older groups were the parameters related to fat and the parameters indicating the decrease in muscle strength or physical function. In addition, only BFP had significantly higher mean values in the high-salt group compared to the low-salt group in both the younger and older groups. In other words, the results of this study showed that excessive intake of salt was related with accumulated fat parameters in the bodies in both younger and older groups. The comparison of muscle strength in this study did not follow the sarcopenia definition of EWGSOP and AWGS, but HGS/BW, which indicates muscle strength, and 30CS, which indicates physical function, were significantly decreased in the high-salt group [2–4]. Therefore, in the older group, the high-salt group had fat accumulation and muscle weakness.

The expression of the renalase may also be related to salt intake and sarcopenia [30–32]. However, we observed no significant relation between blood renalase levels and sarcopenia in this study. A previous study reported that the daily intake of salt was 18 g, much higher than the 4.0–13.8 g/day of this experiment [30]. The results of this study did not reveal a link between renalase, salt intake, and sarcopenia.

Our study compared people with high and low salt intakes and found that those with high-salt intake had higher fat-related parameters. However, we could not investigate causal relationships and mechanisms. For example, fat accumulation is associated with a variety of factors. Salt intake can contribute to fat accumulation. It can also be inferred that fat accumulation changes depend on diet and physical activity. It cannot be ruled out that factors that have not been measured or considered may have confounded the observational results in this study. First, a detailed dietary and physical activity survey would be required to elucidate the association with salt intake. A second limitation of this study is water intake. "Inbody 770", which measures body composition, is affected by the amount of water in the body because it uses the bioelectrical impedance analysis method. Therefore, if the body composition is to be measured strictly, water restriction should be controlled from the previous day. The third, this study recruited adults over the age of 20, participants ranging from 22 to 81 years old, with an average age of 56 years. Further recruitment of participants over the age of 60 or 65 should have been recruited to investigate the association between salt intake and sarcopenia.

Our study does not directly show that excessive salt intake causes sarcopenia, but a diet with excessive salt is associated with fat accumulation and muscle weakness. Furthermore, aging without improving diet can lead to the development of sarcopenia. In addition, past papers have reported that skeletal muscle mass and skeletal muscle strength are maximized in the 20s and 30s [63], and there is a standard that the target age for sarcopenia is 60 or 65 years [3]. On the other hand, there are reports targeting people over 40 years old [64]. Controlling the diet from a young age can prevent various diseases, including the prevention of sarcopenia.

5. Conclusions

This study analyzed the relationship between salt intake and the risk of sarcopenia in the Japanese population. As a result, the parameters related to obesity were significantly increased and the parameters related to muscle strength were significantly decreased in the group of high-salt intake compared with the low-salt intake group. In addition, the results were more significant in the older group than the younger group. Excessive salt intake may be associated with risk of sarcopenia, although further analysis is needed.

Author Contributions: Y.Y. and K.K. conceived of and designed the research; Y.Y., K.K., M.M., M.Y., K.A. and T.K. performed the experiments; Y.Y., K.K., M.M. and M.Y. analyzed the data; Y.Y., K.K., T.S., R.M., M.K., K.Y., S.M. and K.T. interpreted the results of the experiments; Y.Y. and T.S. prepared the figures; Y.Y. drafted the manuscript; Y.Y., K.K., T.S., M.M., M.Y., K.A., T.K., R.M., M.K., K.Y., S.M. and K.T. edited and revised the manuscript. All authors have read and agreed to the published version of the manuscript.

Funding: This work was supported in part by a Grant-in-Aid for Scientific Research KAKENHI from the Ministry of Education, Culture, Sports, Science, and Technology, Japan (19H03995,18K17975); Y.Y. and K.K., K.K. and M.M. were recipients of a Grant-in-Aid for Research Fellowships of Japan Society for the Promotion of Science for Young Scientists (19J01099, 20J20892).

Acknowledgments: We wish to thank the members of S.M.'s laboratory (University of Tsukuba) for their technical assistance.

Conflicts of Interest: The authors declare no conflict of interest.

References

1. Aging Society White Paper. 2019. Available online: https://www8.cao.go.jp/kourei/whitepaper/index-w.html (accessed on 31 July 2020).
2. Cruz-Jentoft, A.J.; Baeyens, J.P.; Bauer, J.M.; Boirie, Y.; Cederholm, T.; Landi, F.; Martin, F.C.; Michel, J.P.; Rolland, Y.; Schneider, S.M.; et al. Sarcopenia: European consensus on definition and diagnosis: Report of the European Working Group on Sarcopenia in Older People. *Age Ageing* **2010**, *39*, 412–423. [CrossRef] [PubMed]
3. Chen, L.K.; Liu, L.K.; Woo, J.; Assantachai, P.; Auyeung, T.W.; Bahyah, K.S.; Chou, M.Y.; Chen, L.Y.; Hsu, P.S.; Krairit, O.; et al. Sarcopenia in Asia: Consensus report of the Asian Working Group for Sarcopenia. *J. Am. Med. Dir. Assoc.* **2014**, *15*, 95–101. [CrossRef] [PubMed]
4. Nishikawa, H.; Shiraki, M.; Hiramatsu, A.; Moriya, K.; Hino, K.; Nishiguchi, S. Japan Society of Hepatology guidelines for sarcopenia in liver disease (1st edition): Recommendation from the working group for creation of sarcopenia assessment criteria. *Hepatol. Res.* **2016**, *46*, 951–963. [CrossRef] [PubMed]
5. Arai, H. Clinical Management of Sarcopenia: Secondary Publication of Geriatrics & Gerontology International 2018;18 S1:1-44. *JMA J.* **2020**, *3*, 95–100.

6. Larsson, L.; Degens, H.; Li, M.; Salviati, L.; Lee, Y.I.; Thompson, W.; Kirkland, J.L.; Sandri, M. Sarcopenia: Aging-Related Loss of Muscle Mass and Function. *Physiol. Rev.* **2019**, *99*, 427–511. [CrossRef]
7. Marzetti, E.; Calvani, R.; Tosato, M.; Cesari, M.; Di Bari, M.; Cherubini, A.; Broccatelli, M.; Savera, G.; D'Elia, M.; Pahor, M.; et al. Physical activity and exercise as countermeasures to physical frailty and sarcopenia. *Aging Clin. Exp. Res.* **2017**, *29*, 35–42. [CrossRef]
8. Beaudart, C.; Dawson, A.; Shaw, S.C.; Harvey, N.C.; Kanis, J.A.; Binkley, N.; Reginster, J.Y.; Chapurlat, R.; Chan, D.C.; Bruyère, O.; et al. Nutrition and physical activity in the prevention and treatment of sarcopenia: Systematic review. *Osteoporos. Int.* **2017**, *28*, 1817–1833. [CrossRef]
9. Steffl, M.; Bohannon, R.W.; Sontakova, L.; Tufano, J.J.; Shiells, K.; Holmerova, I. Relationship between sarcopenia and physical activity in older people: A systematic review and meta-analysis. *Clin. Interv. Aging* **2017**, *12*, 835–845. [CrossRef]
10. Bosaeus, I.; Rothenberg, E. Nutrition and physical activity for the prevention and treatment of age-related sarcopenia. *Proc. Nutr. Soc.* **2016**, *75*, 174–180. [CrossRef]
11. Montero-Fernández, N.; Serra-Rexach, J.A. Role of exercise on sarcopenia in the elderly. *Eur. J. Phys. Rehabil. Med.* **2013**, *49*, 131–143.
12. Cruz-Jentoft, A.J.; Sayer, A.A. Sarcopenia. *Lancet* **2019**, *393*, 2636–2646. [CrossRef]
13. Sieber, C.C. Malnutrition and sarcopenia. *Aging Clin. Exp. Res.* **2019**, *31*, 793–798. [CrossRef] [PubMed]
14. Sinclair, A.J.; Abdelhafiz, A.H.; Rodríguez-Mañas, L. Frailty and sarcopenia newly emerging and high impact complications of diabetes. *J. Diabetes Complicat.* **2017**, *31*, 1465–1473. [CrossRef] [PubMed]
15. Moorthi, R.N.; Avin, K.G. Clinical relevance of sarcopenia in chronic kidney disease. *Curr. Opin. Nephrol. Hypertens.* **2017**, *26*, 219–228. [CrossRef]
16. Watanabe, H.; Enoki, Y.; Maruyama, T. Sarcopenia in Chronic Kidney Disease: Factors, Mechanisms, and Therapeutic Interventions. *Biol. Pharm. Bull.* **2019**, *42*, 1437–1445. [CrossRef]
17. Ponziani, F.R.; Gasbarrini, A. Sarcopenia in Patients with Advanced Liver Disease. *Curr. Protein Peptide Sci.* **2018**, *19*, 681–691. [CrossRef]
18. Kim, J.A.; Choi, K.M. Sarcopenia and fatty liver disease. *Hepatol. Int.* **2019**, *13*, 674–687. [CrossRef]
19. Dasarathy, S.; Merli, M. Sarcopenia from mechanism to diagnosis and treatment in liver disease. *J. Hepatol.* **2016**, *65*, 1232–1244. [CrossRef]
20. Garcia, M.; Seelaender, M.; Sotiropoulos, A.; Coletti, D.; Lancha, A.H., Jr. Vitamin D, muscle recovery, sarcopenia, cachexia, and muscle atrophy. *Nutrition* **2019**, *60*, 66–69. [CrossRef]
21. Naseeb, M.A.; Volpe, S.L. Protein and exercise in the prevention of sarcopenia and aging. *Nutr. Res.* **2017**, *40*, 1–20. [CrossRef]
22. Sodium Intake for Adults and Children Guideline WHO. 2012. Available online: http://apps.who.int/iris/bitstream/10665/77985/1/9789241504836_eng.pdf?ua=1&ua=1 (accessed on 31 July 2020).
23. National Health and Nutrition Survey. 2018. Available online: https://www.mhlw.go.jp/stf/newpage_08789.html (accessed on 31 July 2020).
24. Rust, P.; Ekmekcioglu, C. Impact of Salt Intake on the Pathogenesis and Treatment of Hypertension. *Adv. Exp. Med. Biol.* **2017**, *956*, 61–84.
25. Aaron, K.J.; Sanders, P.W. Role of dietary salt and potassium intake in cardiovascular health and disease: A review of the evidence. *Mayo Clin. Proc.* **2013**, *88*, 987–995. [CrossRef]
26. Kopp, C.; Linz, P.; Dahlmann, A.; Hammon, M.; Jantsch, J.; Müller, D.N.; Schmieder, R.E.; Cavallaro, A.; Eckardt, K.U.; Uder, M.; et al. 23Na magnetic resonance imaging-determined tissue sodium in healthy subjects and hypertensive patients. *Hypertension* **2013**, *61*, 635–640. [CrossRef]
27. Mandai, S.; Furukawa, S.; Kodaka, M.; Hata, Y.; Mori, T.; Nomura, N.; Ando, F.; Mori, Y.; Takahashi, D.; Yoshizaki, Y.; et al. Loop diuretics affect skeletal myoblast differentiation and exercise-induced muscle hypertrophy. *Sci. Rep.* **2017**, *7*, 46369. [CrossRef] [PubMed]
28. Tsuchiya, Y.; Nakashima, S.; Banno, Y.; Suzuki, Y.; Morita, H. Effect of high-NaCl or high-KCl diet on hepatic Na+- and K+-receptor sensitivity and NKCC1 expression in rats. *Am. J. Physiol. Regul. Integr. Comp. Physiol.* **2004**, *286*, R591–R596. [CrossRef] [PubMed]
29. Desir, G.V. Regulation of blood pressure and cardiovascular function by renalase. *Kidney Int.* **2009**, *76*, 366–370. [CrossRef] [PubMed]

30. Wang, Y.; Liu, F.Q.; Wang, D.; Mu, J.J.; Ren, K.Y.; Guo, T.S.; Chu, C.; Wang, L.; Geng, L.K.; Yuan, Z.Y. Effect of salt intake and potassium supplementation on serum renalase levels in Chinese adults: A randomized trial. *Medicine* **2014**, *93*, e44. [CrossRef] [PubMed]
31. Desir, G.V. Renalase deficiency in chronic kidney disease, and its contribution to hypertension and cardiovascular disease. *Curr. Opin. Nephrol. Hypertens.* **2008**, *17*, 181–185. [CrossRef] [PubMed]
32. Desir, G.V. Role of renalase in the regulation of blood pressure and the renal dopamine system. *Curr. Opin. Nephrol. Hypertens.* **2011**, *20*, 31–36. [CrossRef]
33. Tokinoya, K.; Yoshida, Y.; Sugasawa, T.; Takekoshi, K. Moderate-intensity exercise increases renalase levels in the blood and skeletal muscle of rats. *FEBS Open Bio* **2020**. [CrossRef]
34. Tokinoya, K.; Shiromoto, J.; Sugasawa, T.; Yoshida, Y.; Aoki, K.; Nakagawa, Y.; Ohmori, H.; Takekoshi, K. Influence of acute exercise on renalase and its regulatory mechanism. *Life Sci.* **2018**, *210*, 235–242. [CrossRef] [PubMed]
35. Yoshida, Y.; Sugasawa, T.; Hoshino, M.; Tokinoya, K.; Ishikura, K.; Ohmori, H.; Takekoshi, K. Transient changes in serum renalase concentration during long-distance running: The case of an amateur runner under continuous training. *J. Phys. Fit. Sports Med.* **2017**, *6*, 159–166. [CrossRef]
36. Tokinoya, K.; Shirai, T.; Ota, Y.; Takemasa, T.; Takekoshi, K. Denervation-induced muscle atrophy suppression in renalase-deficient mice via increased protein synthesis. *Physiol. Rep.* **2020**, *8*, e14475. [CrossRef] [PubMed]
37. Sato, S.; Shirato, K.; Tachiyashiki, K.; Imaizumi, K. Muscle plasticity and β_2-adrenergic receptors: Adaptive responses of β_2-adrenergic receptor expression to muscle hypertrophy and atrophy. *J. Biomed. Biotechnol.* **2011**, *2011*, 729598. [CrossRef]
38. Sugiura, T.; Takase, H.; Ohte, N.; Dohi, Y. Dietary Salt Intake is a Significant Determinant of Impaired Kidney Function in the General Population. *Kidney Blood Press. Res.* **2018**, *43*, 1245–1254. [CrossRef]
39. Wang, Y.; Xie, B.Q.; Gao, W.H.; Yan, D.Y.; Zheng, W.L.; Lv, Y.B.; Cao, Y.M.; Hu, J.W.; Yuan, Z.Y.; Mu, J.J. Effects of Renin-Angiotensin System Inhibitors on Renal Expression of Renalase in Sprague-Dawley Rats Fed With High Salt Diet. *Kidney Blood Press. Res.* **2015**, *40*, 605–613. [CrossRef]
40. Horio, M. [Development of evaluation of kidney function and classification of chronic kidney disease (CKD)–including CKD clinical practice guide 2012]. *Rinsho Byori. Jpn. J. Clin. Pathol.* **2013**, *61*, 616–621.
41. Koo, H.S.; Kim, Y.C.; Ahn, S.Y.; Oh, S.W.; Kim, S.; Chin, H.J.; Park, J.H. Estimating 24-hour urine sodium level with spot urine sodium and creatinine. *J. Korean Med. Sci.* **2014**, *29* (Suppl. S2), S97–S102. [CrossRef]
42. Tanaka, T.; Okamura, T.; Miura, K.; Kadowaki, T.; Ueshima, H.; Nakagawa, H.; Hashimoto, T. A simple method to estimate populational 24-h urinary sodium and potassium excretion using a casual urine specimen. *J. Hum. Hypertens.* **2002**, *16*, 97–103. [CrossRef]
43. Fang, W.H.; Yang, J.R.; Lin, C.Y.; Hsiao, P.J.; Tu, M.Y.; Chen, C.F.; Tsai, D.J.; Su, W.; Huang, G.S.; Chang, H.; et al. Accuracy augmentation of body composition measurement by bioelectrical impedance analyzer in elderly population. *Medicine* **2020**, *99*, e19103. [CrossRef]
44. Wang, H.; Hai, S.; Cao, L.; Zhou, J.; Liu, P.; Dong, B.R. Estimation of prevalence of sarcopenia by using a new bioelectrical impedance analysis in Chinese community-dwelling elderly people. *BMC Geriatr.* **2016**, *16*, 216. [CrossRef]
45. Hiraki, K.; Yasuda, T.; Hotta, C.; Izawa, K.P.; Morio, Y.; Watanabe, S.; Sakurada, T.; Shibagaki, Y.; Kimura, K. Decreased physical function in pre-dialysis patients with chronic kidney disease. *Clin. Exp. Nephrol.* **2013**, *17*, 225–231. [CrossRef]
46. Abro, A.; Delicata, L.A.; Vongsanim, S.; Davenport, A. Differences in the prevalence of sarcopenia in peritoneal dialysis patients using hand grip strength and appendicular lean mass: Depends upon guideline definitions. *Eur. J. Clin. Nutr.* **2018**, *72*, 993–999. [CrossRef] [PubMed]
47. Yeung, S.S.Y.; Reijnierse, E.M.; Trappenburg, M.C.; Blauw, G.J.; Meskers, C.G.M.; Maier, A.B. Knee extension strength measurements should be considered as part of the comprehensive geriatric assessment. *BMC Geriatr.* **2018**, *18*, 130. [CrossRef] [PubMed]
48. Ratkevicius, A.; Joyson, A.; Selmer, I.; Dhanani, T.; Grierson, C.; Tommasi, A.M.; DeVries, A.; Rauchhaus, P.; Crowther, D.; Alesci, S.; et al. Serum concentrations of myostatin and myostatin-interacting proteins do not differ between young and sarcopenic elderly men. *J. Gerontol. Ser. A* **2011**, *66*, 620–626. [CrossRef] [PubMed]
49. Hofmann, M.; Halper, B.; Oesen, S.; Franzke, B.; Stuparits, P.; Tschan, H.; Bachl, N.; Strasser, E.M.; Quittan, M.; Ploder, M.; et al. Serum concentrations of insulin-like growth factor-1, members of the TGF-beta superfamily and follistatin do not reflect different stages of dynapenia and sarcopenia in elderly women. *Exp. Gerontol.* **2015**, *64*, 35–45. [CrossRef] [PubMed]

50. Vieira, N.D.; Testa, D.; Ruas, P.C.; Salvini, T.F.; Catai, A.M.; De Melo, R.C. The effects of 12 weeks Pilates-inspired exercise training on functional performance in older women: A randomized clinical trial. *J. Bodyw. Mov. Ther.* **2017**, *21*, 251–258. [CrossRef] [PubMed]
51. Krupp, S.; Kasper, J.; Hermes, A.; Balck, F.; Ralf, C.; Schmidt, T.; Weisser, B.; Willkomm, M. The "Lübeck Worlds of Movement Model"-results of the effects evaluation. *Bundesgesundheitsblatt Gesundh. Gesundh* **2019**, *62*, 274–281. [CrossRef]
52. Mijnarends, D.M.; Meijers, J.M.; Halfens, R.J.; Ter Borg, S.; Luiking, Y.C.; Verlaan, S.; Schoberer, D.; Cruz Jentoft, A.J.; Van Loon, L.J.; Schols, J.M. Validity and reliability of tools to measure muscle mass, strength, and physical performance in community-dwelling older people: A systematic review. *J. Am. Med. Dir. Assoc.* **2013**, *14*, 170–178. [CrossRef]
53. Jones, C.J.; Rikli, R.E.; Beam, W.C. A 30-s chair-stand test as a measure of lower body strength in community-residing older adults. *Res. Q. Exerc. Sport* **1999**, *70*, 113–119. [CrossRef]
54. Asakura, K.; Uechi, K.; Sasaki, Y.; Masayasu, S.; Sasaki, S. Estimation of sodium and potassium intakes assessed by two 24 h urine collections in healthy Japanese adults: A nationwide study. *Br. J. Nutr.* **2014**, *112*, 1195–1205. [CrossRef] [PubMed]
55. Zhou, B.F.; Stamler, J.; Dennis, B.; Moag-Stahlberg, A.; Okuda, N.; Robertson, C.; Zhao, L.; Chan, Q.; Elliott, P. Nutrient intakes of middle-aged men and women in China, Japan, United Kingdom, and United States in the late 1990s: The INTERMAP study. *J. Hum. Hypertens.* **2003**, *17*, 623–630. [CrossRef] [PubMed]
56. Zhou, L.; Stamler, J.; Chan, Q.; Van Horn, L.; Daviglus, M.L.; Dyer, A.R.; Miura, K.; Okuda, N.; Wu, Y.; Ueshima, H.; et al. Salt intake and prevalence of overweight/obesity in Japan, China, the United Kingdom, and the United States: The INTERMAP Study. *Am. J. Clin. Nutr.* **2019**, *110*, 34–40. [CrossRef] [PubMed]
57. Lanaspa, M.A.; Kuwabara, M.; Andres-Hernando, A.; Li, N.; Cicerchi, C.; Jensen, T.; Orlicky, D.J.; Roncal-Jimenez, C.A.; Ishimoto, T.; Nakagawa, T.; et al. High salt intake causes leptin resistance and obesity in mice by stimulating endogenous fructose production and metabolism. *Proc. Natl. Acad. Sci. USA* **2018**, *115*, 3138–3143. [CrossRef] [PubMed]
58. Ma, Y.; He, F.J.; MacGregor, G.A. High salt intake: Independent risk factor for obesity? *Hypertension* **2015**, *66*, 843–849. [CrossRef]
59. Wannamethee, S.G.; Atkins, J.L. Muscle loss and obesity: The health implications of sarcopenia and sarcopenic obesity. *Proc. Nutr. Soc.* **2015**, *74*, 405–412. [CrossRef]
60. Oku, Y.; Tanabe, R.; Nakaoka, K.; Yamada, A.; Noda, S.; Hoshino, A.; Haraikawa, M.; Goseki-Sone, M. Influences of dietary vitamin D restriction on bone strength, body composition and muscle in rats fed a high-fat diet: Involvement of mRNA expression of MyoD in skeletal muscle. *J. Nutr. Biochem.* **2016**, *32*, 85–90. [CrossRef]
61. Conte, M.; Vasuri, F.; Trisolino, G.; Bellavista, E.; Santoro, A.; Degiovanni, A.; Martucci, E.; D'Errico-Grigioni, A.; Caporossi, D.; Capri, M.; et al. Increased Plin2 expression in human skeletal muscle is associated with sarcopenia and muscle weakness. *PLoS ONE* **2013**, *8*, e73709. [CrossRef]
62. Majid, H.; Masood, Q.; Khan, A.H. Homeostatic Model Assessment for Insulin Resistance (HOMA-IR): A Better Marker for Evaluating Insulin Resistance than Fasting Insulin in Women with Polycystic Ovarian Syndrome. *JCPSP* **2017**, *27*, 123–126.
63. Kim, H.K.; Lee, Y.J.; Lee, Y.K.; Kim, H.; Koo, K.H. Which Index for Muscle Mass Represents an Aging Process? *J. Bone Metab.* **2018**, *25*, 219–226. [CrossRef] [PubMed]
64. Dodds, R.M.; Granic, A.; Robinson, S.M.; Sayer, A.A. Sarcopenia, long-term conditions, and multimorbidity: Findings from UK Biobank participants. *J. Cachexia Sarcopenia Muscle* **2020**, *11*, 62–68. [CrossRef] [PubMed]

Publisher's Note: MDPI stays neutral with regard to jurisdictional claims in published maps and institutional affiliations.

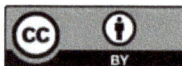

© 2020 by the authors. Licensee MDPI, Basel, Switzerland. This article is an open access article distributed under the terms and conditions of the Creative Commons Attribution (CC BY) license (http://creativecommons.org/licenses/by/4.0/).

MDPI
St. Alban-Anlage 66
4052 Basel
Switzerland
Tel. +41 61 683 77 34
Fax +41 61 302 89 18
www.mdpi.com

Nutrients Editorial Office
E-mail: nutrients@mdpi.com
www.mdpi.com/journal/nutrients

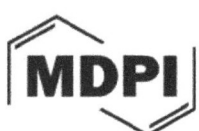

www.ingramcontent.com/pod-product-compliance
Lightning Source LLC
LaVergne TN
LVHW070418100526
838202LV00014B/1483